METHODS IN MOLECULAR BIOLOGY

Series Editor
John M. Walker
School of Life and Medical Sciences
University of Hertfordshire
Hatfield, Hertfordshire, AL10 9AB, UK

For further volumes:
http://www.springer.com/series/7651

Cancer Stem Cells

Methods and Protocols

Edited by

Gianpaolo Papaccio and Vincenzo Desiderio

Department of Experimental Medicine, University of Campania "Luigi Vanvitelli"
Naples, Italy

Humana Press

Editors
Gianpaolo Papaccio
Department of Experimental Medicine
University of Campania "Luigi Vanvitelli"
Naples, Italy

Vincenzo Desiderio
Department of Experimental Medicine
University of Campania "Luigi Vanvitelli"
Naples, Italy

ISSN 1064-3745 ISSN 1940-6029 (electronic)
Methods in Molecular Biology
ISBN 978-1-4939-7400-9 ISBN 978-1-4939-7401-6 (eBook)
DOI 10.1007/978-1-4939-7401-6

Library of Congress Control Number: 2017954499

Printed on acid-free paper

This Humana Press imprint is published by Springer Nature
The registered company is Springer Science+Business Media LLC
The registered company address is: 233 Spring Street, New York, NY 10013, U.S.A.

Preface

Back in 1997, Bonnet and Dick published, in *Nature Medicine*, a work describing, for the first time in acute myeloid leukemia, a subset of cells with the unique property of generating a new heterogenic tumor in immunocompromised mice. A few years later in 2003, Al-Hajj and Singh, almost at the same time, described a population of cells with tumor-initiating capacity in breast and brain tumors respectively, creating the base of the cancer stem cells (CSCs) theory. Since then, thousands of publications have been issued on this topic describing the presence and role of CSCs in almost all types of cancer with dramatic practical and clinical implications, although, looking at those publications, what immediately comes out at reader's eyes is the enormous variability in the approaches and techniques used for CSCs identification. Among these, there are surface marker expression, side population, spheres formation, ALDH activity, serial transplantation in immunocompromised mice, etc.; nevertheless, none of these techniques by themselves can be considered sufficient for the purpose of identifying and characterizing CSCs. Therefore, there is the need for the scientist who is interested in working with CSCs in any field and with any tumor type to have at least a basic knowledge of all the different procedures used and to be handy with few of them.

This is what this book is meant to be: a comprehensive collection of all the methods, protocols, and procedures used for the identification, characterization, and selection of cancer stem cells. Each chapter describes a single protocol authored by experts in that particular technique and, far from being merely a list of mechanical steps, it represents instead the summary of years of experience in that field, in which the protocol has been refined and tailored to fit the need of a specific purpose.

Being a professor of Human Embryology in the medical school, I have always seen the tumor as a development-related disease, in the sense that cancer cells are often activated by the same or similar pathways that are fundamental in embryo life, and that give to embryonic cells that plasticity that is so detrimental to the patient when possessed by cancer cells. For this reason, I'm firmly confident that CSCs represent the link between embryological pathways and disease and that targeting them will be of paramount importance for future cancer therapy.

Naples, Italy

Gianpaolo Papaccio
Vincenzo Desiderio

Contents

Contributors

ASHLEY A. ADILE • *McMaster Stem Cell and Cancer Research Institute, McMaster University, Hamilton, ON, Canada; Department of Biochemistry and Biomedical Science, Faculty of Health Sciences, McMaster University, Hamilton, ON, Canada*

MARIA LAURA DE ANGELIS • *Department of Oncology and Molecular Medicine, Istituto Superiore di Sanità, Rome, Italy*

MARTA BAIOCCHI • *Department of Oncology and Molecular Medicine, Istituto Superiore di Sanità, Rome, Italy*

DAVID BAKHSHINYAN • *McMaster Stem Cell and Cancer Research Institute, McMaster University, Hamilton, ON, Canada; Department of Biochemistry and Biomedical Science, Faculty of Health Sciences, McMaster University, Hamilton, ON, Canada*

ANNA DI BIASE • *The John van Geest Cancer Research Centre, Nottingham Trent University, Nottingham, UK*

MAGDALENA E. BUCZEK • *The John van Geest Cancer Research Centre, Nottingham Trent University, Nottingham, UK*

MICHELE CARAGLIA • *Department of Biochemistry, Biophysics and General Pathology, University of Campania "Luigi Vanvitelli", Naples, Italy*

CARLA CARUSO • *University of Tuscia, Viterbo, Italy*

ROGERIO MORAES CASTILHO • *Laboratory of Epithelial Biology, Department of Periodontics and Oral Medicine, University of Michigan School of Dentistry, Ann Arbor, MI, USA*

CHIRAYU CHOKSHI • *McMaster Stem Cell and Cancer Research Institute, McMaster University, Hamilton, ON, Canada; Department of Biochemistry and Biomedical Science, Faculty of Health Sciences, McMaster University, Hamilton, ON, Canada*

SUDIPTO DAS • *Department of Molecular and Cellular Therapeutics, Royal College of Surgeons in Ireland, Dublin, Ireland*

RENATO FRANCO • *Pathology Unit, University of Campania "Luigi Vanvitelli", Naples, Italy*

SEBASTIÁN A. GARCÍA • *Department of Gastrointestinal, Thoracic and Vascular Surgery, Medizinische Fakultät Carl Gustav Carus, Technische Universität Dresden, Dresden, Germany*

MONICA GARGIULO • *Pathology Unit, University of Campania "Luigi Vanvitelli", Naples, Italy*

VINOD GOPALAN • *Cancer Molecular Pathology, School of Medicine, Menzies Health Institute Queensland, Griffith University, Gold Coast, QLD, Australia*

MARTINA INTARTAGLIA • *Pathology Unit, University of Campania "Luigi Vanvitelli", Naples, Italy*

FARHADUL ISLAM • *Cancer Molecular Pathology, School of Medicine, Menzies Health Institute Queensland, Griffith University, Gold Coast, QLD, Australia*

MAYUR VILAS JAIN • *Division of Oto-Rhino-Laryngology, Head and Neck Surgery, Department of Clinical and Experimental Medicine, Faculty of Health Sciences, Linköping University, Linköping, Sweden; Department of Molecular Medicine and Gene Therapy, Lund Stem Cell Center, Lund University, Lund, Sweden*

MICHELLE M. KAMEDA-SMITH • *McMaster Stem Cell and Cancer Research Institute, McMaster University, Hamilton, ON, Canada; Department of Biochemistry and Biomedical Science, Faculty of Health Sciences, McMaster University, Hamilton, ON, Canada*

HIROMICHI KAWASAKI • *Department of Biochemistry, Biophysics and General Pathology, University of Campania "Luigi Vanvitelli", Naples, Italy; Drug Discovery Laboratory, Wakunaga Pharmaceutical Co., Ltd., Hiroshima, Japan*

MARTINA KONANTZ • *Departement of Biomedicine, University Hospital Basel and University of Basel, Basel, Switzerland*

ALFRED KING-YIN LAM • *Cancer Molecular Pathology, School of Medicine, Menzies Health Institute Queensland, Griffith University, Gold Coast, QLD, Australia*

CLAUDIA LENGERKE • *Departement of Biomedicine, University Hospital Basel and University of Basel, Basel, Switzerland; Division of Haematology, University Hospital Basel, Basel, Switzerland*

CARLO LEONETTI • *Experimental Chemotherapy Laboratory, UOSD SAFU, Regina Elena National Cancer Institute, Rome, Italy*

DAVIDE LICCARDO • *Department of Experimental Medicine, Medical School, University of Campania "Luigi Vanvitelli", Naples, Italy*

ANGELA LOMBARDI • *Department of Biochemistry, Biophysics and General Pathology, University of Campania "Luigi Vanvitelli", Naples, Italy*

RUGGERO DE MARIA • *Department of General Pathology, Università Cattolica del Sacro Cuore, Rome, Italy*

MANOELA DOMINGUES MARTINS • *Department of Oral Pathology, School of Dentistry, Federal University of Rio Grande do Sul, Porto Alegre, RS, Brazil*

GEETA MEHTA • *Department of Materials Science and Engineering, University of Michigan, Ann Arbor, MI, USA; Department of Biomedical Engineering, University of Michigan, Ann Arbor, MI, USA; Department of Macromolecular Science and Engineering, University of Michigan, Ann Arbor, MI, USA*

POOJA MEHTA • *Department of Materials Science and Engineering, University of Michigan, Ann Arbor, MI, USA*

LUIGI MELE • *Department of Experimental Medicine, Medical School, University of Campania "Luigi Vanvitelli", Naples, Italy*

AMANDA K. MILES • *The John van Geest Cancer Research Centre, Nottingham Trent University, Nottingham, UK*

BRUCE MORAN • *Cancer Biology and Therapeutics Laboratory, UCD Conway Institute of Biomedical and Biomolecular Research, University College Dublin, Dublin 4, Ireland*

CAYMEN NOVAK • *Department of Biomedical Engineering, University of Michigan, Ann Arbor, MI, USA*

YASUNORI OKADA • *Department of Pathology, Keio University School of Medicine, Tokyo, Japan; Department of Pathophysiology for Locomotive and Neoplastic Diseases, Juntendo University Graduate School of Medicine, Tokyo, Japan*

MASAHIDE OTA • *Department of Pathology, Keio University School of Medicine, Tokyo, Japan; Second Department of Internal Medicine and Respiratory Medicine, Nara Medical University, Nara, Japan*

ANNA M. PACZULLA • *Departement of Biomedicine, University Hospital Basel and University of Basel, Basel, Switzerland*

Antoinette S. Perry • *Cancer Biology and Therapeutics Laboratory, UCD Conway Institute of Biomedical and Biomolecular Research, University College Dublin, Dublin 4, Ireland*

Luca Pompili • *Experimental Chemotherapy Laboratory, UOSD SAFU, Regina Elena National Cancer Institute, Rome, Italy; University of Tuscia, Viterbo, Italy*

Manuela Porru • *Experimental Chemotherapy Laboratory, UOSD SAFU, Regina Elena National Cancer Institute, Rome, Italy*

Maleeha A. Qazi • *McMaster Stem Cell and Cancer Research Institute, McMaster University, Hamilton, ON, Canada; Department of Biochemistry and Biomedical Science, Faculty of Health Sciences, McMaster University, Hamilton, ON, Canada*

Shreya Raghavan • *Department of Materials Science and Engineering, University of Michigan, Ann Arbor, MI, USA*

Vijayalakshmi Rajendran • *Section of Immunity, Infection and Inflammation, School of Medicine, Medical Sciences and Nutrition, Institute of Medical Sciences, University of Aberdeen, Scotland, UK*

Stephen P. Reeder • *The John van Geest Cancer Research Centre, Nottingham Trent University, Nottingham, UK*

Tarik Regad • *The John van Geest Cancer Research Centre, Nottingham Trent University, Nottingham, UK*

Giovanna Roncador • *Monoclonal Antibody Unit, Spanish National Cancer Research Center, Madrid, Spain*

Rosalaura Sabetta • *Pathology Unit, University of Campania "Luigi Vanvitelli", Naples, Italy*

Sebastian Schölch • *Department of Gastrointestinal, Thoracic and Vascular Surgery, Medizinische Fakultät Carl Gustav Carus, Technische Universität Dresden, Dresden, Germany; German Cancer Consortium (DKTK), Dresden, Germany; German Cancer Research Center (DKFZ), Heidelberg, Germany*

Masayuki Shimoda • *Department of Pathology, Keio University School of Medicine, Tokyo, Japan*

Mohini Singh • *McMaster Stem Cell and Cancer Research Institute, McMaster University, Hamilton, ON, Canada; Department of Biochemistry and Biomedical Science, Faculty of Health Sciences, McMaster University, Hamilton, ON, Canada*

Sheila K. Singh • *McMaster Stem Cell and Cancer Research Institute, McMaster University, Hamilton, ON, Canada; Department of Biochemistry and Biomedical Science, Faculty of Health Sciences, McMaster University, Hamilton, ON, Canada; Department of Surgery, Faculty of Health Sciences, McMaster University, Hamilton, ON, Canada; Michael DeGroote Centre for Learning and Discovery, Stem Cell and Cancer Research Institute, McMaster University, Hamilton, ON, Canada*

Virginia Tirino • *Department of Experimental Medicine, Medical School, University of Campania "Luigi Vanvitelli", Naples, Italy*

Meenakshi Upreti • *Department of Pharmaceutical Sciences, College of Pharmacy, University of Kentucky, Lexington, KY, USA*

Chitra Venugopal • *McMaster Stem Cell and Cancer Research Institute, McMaster University, Hamilton, ON, Canada; Department of Surgery, Faculty of Health Sciences, McMaster University, Hamilton, ON, Canada*

VIVIAN PETERSEN WAGNER • *Department of Oral Pathology, School of Dentistry, Federal University of Rio Grande do Sul, Porto Alegre, RS, Brazil*
HUI WANG • *Departement of Biomedicine, University Hospital Basel and University of Basel, Basel, Switzerland*
LIANG WANG • *Department of Gastroenterology, Hepatology and Nutrition, The University of Texas MD Anderson Cancer Center, Houston, TX, USA*
MARIA WARD • *Department of Materials Science and Engineering, University of Michigan, Ann Arbor, MI, USA*
DAOYAN WEI • *Department of Gastroenterology, Hepatology and Nutrition, The University of Texas MD Anderson Cancer Center, Houston, TX, USA*
JÜRGEN WEITZ • *Department of Gastrointestinal, Thoracic and Vascular Surgery, Medizinische Fakultät Carl Gustav Carus, Technische Universität Dresden, Dresden, Germany; German Cancer Consortium (DKTK), Dresden, Germany; German Cancer Research Center (DKFZ), Heidelberg, Germany*
KEPING XIE • *Department of Gastroenterology, Hepatology and Nutrition, The University of Texas MD Anderson Cancer Center, Houston, TX, USA*
NICK YELLE • *McMaster Stem Cell and Cancer Research Institute, McMaster University, Hamilton, ON, Canada; Department of Biochemistry and Biomedical Science, Faculty of Health Sciences, McMaster University, Hamilton, ON, Canada*
FEDERICA ZITO MARINO • *Pathology Unit, University of Campania "Luigi Vanvitelli", Naples, Italy*
XIANGSHENG ZUO • *Department of Gastrointestinal Medical Oncology, The University of Texas MD Anderson Cancer Center, Houston, TX, USA*

Chapter 1

Introduction to Cancer Stem Cells: Past, Present, and Future

David Bakhshinyan, Ashley A. Adile, Maleeha A. Qazi, Mohini Singh, Michelle M. Kameda-Smith, Nick Yelle, Chirayu Chokshi, Chitra Venugopal, and Sheila K. Singh

Abstract

The Cancer Stem Cell (CSC) hypothesis postulates the existence of a small population of cancer cells with intrinsic properties allowing for resistance to conventional radiochemotherapy regiments and increased metastatic potential. Clinically, the aggressive nature of CSCs has been shown to correlate with increased tumor recurrence, metastatic spread, and overall poor patient outcome across multiple cancer subtypes. Traditionally, isolation of CSCs has been achieved through utilization of cell surface markers, while the functional differences between CSCs and remaining tumor cells have been described through proliferation, differentiation, and limiting dilution assays. The generated insights into CSC biology have further highlighted the importance of studying intratumoral heterogeneity through advanced functional assays, including CRISPR-Cas9 screens in the search of novel targeted therapies. In this chapter, we review the discovery and characterization of cancer stem cells populations within several major cancer subtypes, recent developments of novel assays used in studying therapy resistant tumor cells, as well as recent developments in therapies targeted at cancer stem cells.

Key words Cancer stem cells, Lung cancer, Colon cancer, Leukemia, Breast cancer, Brain cancer, CRISPR, Immunotherapy

1 History of Stem Cells

Although the term "stem cell" received its current definition in the late 1800s [1] it was not until the seminal work by Dr. James Till, Dr. Ernest McCulloch and colleagues in the 1960s that provided first definitive evidence of adult stem cells [2–4]. Through their adaptation of an in vivo spleen colony formation assay, where donor bone marrow cells (BMCs) were transplanted into a pre-irradiated recipient animal following the qualitative and quantitative analysis of colonies formed on the host's spleen, they were able to

The original version of this chapter was revised. An erratum to this chapter can be found at DOI 10.1007/978-1-4939-7401-6_19

Gianpaolo Papaccio and Vincenzo Desiderio (eds.), *Cancer Stem Cells: Methods and Protocols*, Methods in Molecular Biology, vol. 1692, DOI 10.1007/978-1-4939-7401-6_1, © Springer Science+Business Media LLC 2018

functionally describe and characterize adult stem cells. They first eluded to the fact that stem cell studies must be based on functional assays and defined the following properties of the cells capable of forming colonies in the recipient: (1) extensive proliferative capacity; (2) given rise to cells capable of differentiation; and (3) ability to self-renew. Following their work, adult stem cells have been shown to be present in blood, skin, and small intestines, all three associated with a high cell turnover and putative rare population of cells responsible for generating differentiated cells. In a review by Potten and Loeffler, an updated functional definition of stem cells was proposed as undifferentiated cells with (1) extensive proliferation capacity; (2) ability to self-renew; (3) potential to produce differentiated functional progenitors; (4) ability to regenerate tissue post injury; and (5) flexibility in the use of those abilities [5]. Interestingly, the existence of adult stem cells was thought to be limited to tissues with inherently high turnover rates up until early 1990s. However, with the development of increasingly enhanced culturing techniques, adult stem cells were discovered in more static tissues including breast [6], brain [7], and lungs [8].

2 Conceptualization of Cancer Stem Cells (CSCs)

Following an observation of phenotypic similarities between embryonic and cancer cells by Joseph Claude Anselme Recamier and Robert Remak in mid-1800s, the first putative notion of stem cells having the ability to give rise to cancers was postulated, termed embryonal rest theory of cancer. Formalized by Franco Durante and Julius Cohnheim the embryonal rest theory of cancer suggests that a small collection of persistent, undifferentiated embryonic tissue was the key to cancer initiation [9]. In the later half of the nineteenth century, the de-differentiation theory of cancer was brought into focus, acting as a substitute for the embryonal rest theory of cancer [10]. Unlike the embryonal rest theory, the dedifferentiation theory proposed that changes in the mature cells give rise to cancer due to the comparative properties of differentiated and cancer cells. A strong support for de-differentiation theory came from the observation made by Rudolf Virchow, who proposed that embryonic tissue in teratocarcinoma arose from chronic inflammation of connective tissue [11]. Other studies in the early 1900s suggesting that cancers could be caused by chemicals, infectious parasites, and loss of inhibitory influences of the body on tissues, were considered supporting of the de-differentiation hypothesis [10, 12]. It was not until the 1980s when the role of stem cells in cancer was brought back into the spot light through studies of teratocarcinoma and leukemia.

2.1 Teratocarcinoma

Teratocarcinomas are malignant cancers originating from germinal cells. During the analysis of cellular composition of teratocarcinomas, Barry Pierce and colleagues have demonstrated the similarities in the cellular composition between the malignant and normal tissue, as both contained differentiated cells, progenitor cells, and stem cells. Although over 90% of cells comprising teratocarcinomas were differentiated cells, the malignant cells were exclusively found in structures resembling early embryoid bodies [13]. More importantly, it was later demonstrated that it was the cells found in embryoid bodies that had the potential to be propagated in vitro and ability to initiate tumors upon transplantation [14, 15] Further experimentations by Leroy Stevens demonstrated that teratocarcinomas could arise from normal cells including early mouse embryo cells and testicular germ cells when transplanted from their natural site into abnormal tissues [16]. In the complementary experiments by Mintz and Illmensee, they found that when the stem cells isolated from teratocarcinomas were injected into the blastocyst of a normally developing embryo, they were able to give rise to normal tissue [17]. Together these studies have contributed to the understanding that not only malignant tissue had similar cellular hierarchy as normal tissue but that cancers were arising from maturation arrest of the stem cells found in normal tissues and not by dedifferentiation. Although originally thought to be limited to teratocarcinomas, conceptualization of stem cell driven tumorigenesis was further developed from studies done on leukemia.

3 Identification of Cancer Stem Cells

It has been largely accepted that cancer stem cells (CSCs) are endowed with conventional chemotherapy and radiation resistance, along with tumor-initiating and metastatic properties that are correlative with increased tumor recurrence and poor clinical outcome [18]. In stark contrast, non-CSCs are thought to be therapy-sensitive and lack any self-renewal capacity [19]. Studies involving human acute myeloid leukemia (AML) by Bonnet and Dick in 1997 provided the first compelling evidence of the existence of CSCs [20]. The existence of CSCs in solid tumors was reported in 2003 by Al Hajj who demonstrated the presence of CSCs in breast cancer [6]. Currently, CSCs have been proven to exist in various solid tumors including colon, lung, prostrate, pancreatic, brain, head and neck and liver, among others.

Current anti-cancer therapies have a tendency to kill bulk tumor, rather than specifically targeting the intrinsically resistant CSCs that proliferate following the completion of standard therapies. Interestingly, experiments with lung cancer cells have suggested that lung-CSCs rely on both symmetric and asymmetric cellular division, whereas non-CSCs undergo symmetric division [21]. With symmetric cell division, each CSC generates either two CSC progeny or two differentiated cells. Conversely, asymmetric division involves each CSC producing a differentiated progeny, along with a CSC. Despite their reliance on both types of cellular division, CSCs employ symmetric division particularly when subjected to cellular stress, such as chemotherapy [22], thus increasing the number of highly proliferative cells capable of repopulating the bulk tumor.

Whether tumors emerge from de-differentiation of a normal cell, or rather a transformation event of a normal stem cell or progenitor cell is largely elusive to researchers in the field. With significant tumor heterogeneity, a multipotent cell of origin is highly plausible, particularly due to the presence of several lineage phenotypes with distinct gene expression profiles and cell surface markers.

3.1 Leukemia

Leukemia, a malignant cancer of blood and immune system, is driven by a significant increase in immature white blood cells in circulation [20]. Through the course of the disease, normal white blood cells are rapidly replaced with the leukemic cells, resulting in diminished ability of patients to fight off any infection. Treatment of leukemia requires elimination of both leukemic stem cells (LSCs) and highly proliferative progenitor cells. In acute myeloid leukemia (AML), an excess of leukemic blasts with limited proliferation capacity is generated through an impairment in differentiation machinery. The human AML initiating cell, SCID leukemia initiating cell (SC-IC), was isolated and characterized through serial transplantation into immunocompromised mice [23]. A rare CD34+/CD38- fraction was shown to have the ability to recapitulate the entire diversity of leukemic hierarchy, analogous to the normal hematopoietic stem cells (HSCs) [20, 23]. Further similarities between normal HSCs and SC-ICs include their cell surface phenotype and presence in quiescent state, both suggesting that HSCs are the origin of malignant transformation [24, 25]. Although, chemo- and radiotherapies are effective in eliminating over 99% of the AML cells, only highly proliferative cells are affected. However, since the stem cell fraction of AML is normally in quiescent state, SC-ICs are spared and once therapy is discontinued, a rapid expansion of leukemia ensues.

3.2 Solid Tumors

3.2.1 Breast

Although therapeutic modalities for breast cancer have been evolving, disease relapse and metastasis, due to persistent subset of tumor cells, termed breast cancer stem cells (BCSCs) still constitute a major therapeutic concern [26]. The two prominent ideas of BCSCs' origins are deregulation of dormant normal stem cell [27] or de novo transformation a somatic cell [28], similarly to conclusion drawn by Mintz et al. from the studies of teratocarcinomas [29]. Since identification of BCSCs in 2003 based on the expression of two surface glycoproteins, $CD44^{+}/CD24^{-}$ phenotype has become a reliable isolation criterion [6, 30–33]. Increased levels of CD44 and low expression of CD24 contribute to increased capacity for proliferation, adhesion, migration, and invasion [34–36]. Some of the common sites for breast cancer metastasis are bone, lung, liver, and brain, all containing specific ligands for CD44, hyaluronan, and osteopontin [37]. Further in vivo and in vitro studies have also elucidated ALDH1 [38], CD133 [31], CD49f [39], and CD61 [40] as additional BCSC markers. Pathways relevant in embryogenesis, Notch, Hedgehog, and Wnt have also been implicated in contributing to the propagation of BCSCs and their inherit resistance to therapy [41, 42]. The ability of BCSCs to evade best available therapies is further associated with their ability to undergo epithelial-mesenchymal transition (EMT) and the reverse mesenchymal-epithelial transition (MET) [43], as cells persisting post therapy frequently exhibit both epithelial and mesenchymal markers, similar to the expression profiles of BCSCs, cytokeratin, and vimentin, respectively [44, 45]. More recent studies have highlighted the importance of investigating BCSCs in the context of tumor niche. An increased expression of TFGb and IL-8 in response to paclitaxel contributes to expansion of cancer stem cells in the triple-negative tumors [46]. Meanwhile, therapeutic targeting of IL-8 receptor, CXCR1, with an antibody has been shown to decrease tumor initiation in several preclinical models [47].

3.2.2 Brain

The discovery of brain tumor stem cells was made on the heels of work in breast cancer [6] and was among the first solid tumors where cells responsible for tumor initiation were identified [48]. Since the identification of normal neural stem cells (NSC) in mice and humans [7], several groups focused on whether NSC enrichment conditions could be used to identify a similar population in brain tumors. Hence, human brain tumors were grown in serum-free media with neural-specific growth factors, which led to the identification of small cell populations with clonogenic, self-renewing, and multi-lineage differentiation potential [48–51]. Utilizing prospective cell sorting through magnetic beads or fluorophore-conjugated antibodies, CD133 was the first protein that marked a cancer stem cell-like population in both pediatric and adult brain tumors [52] $CD133^+$ brain tumor cells gave rise to self-renewing colonies (termed neurospheres) in vitro and carried higher tumorigenic potential than $CD133^-$ cells when engrafted intracranially in immune-deficient mice. Tumors derived from $CD133^+$ cells were heterogeneous and a phenocopy of the patient's original tumor, suggesting the presence of cellular hierarchy originating from $CD133^+$ cell fraction [48]. In efforts to further characterize brain tumor stem cells, additional markers such as CD15 [53], integrin alpha 6 [54], L1CAM [55], ephrin family of receptors (EphA2, EphA3, EphB2) [56–58], as well as neural stem/precursor markers such as Nestin, Sox2 [59], Bmi [50], and Notch were subsequently identified. Although further characterization and purification of the brain tumor stem cell compartment is required, current knowledge already suggests that brain tumor stem cells play an important role in not only tumor initiation, but also tumor maintenance and therapy resistance. In adult malignant brain tumor, glioblastoma, the brain tumor stem cells seem to be localized to the perivascular niche, affording these cell populations to maintain tumor growth through access to the host vasculature. More significantly, brain tumor stem cells, marked especially by the expression of CD133, have been demonstrated to be resistant to radiation [60] and chemotherapy [61]. Hence, brain tumor stem cells can then also be seen as the source of therapy resistance and disease relapse observed in malignant brain tumors. The collective role that brain tumor stem cells have been shown to play in initiating and maintaining the tumor and allowing the tumor to escape therapy makes them a significant biological target for therapeutic development, making in vitro and in vivo brain tumor stem cell models pertinent platforms for future drug discovery.

3.2.3 Lung

Lung cancer is one of the most predominant causes of caner-related deaths worldwide [62]. Patient survival remains bleak despite recent advancements in treatment, with the 5-year survival at a mere 15% and dropping to 2% in patients with metastases [63]. As a disease, lung cancer is comprised of phenotypically different groups and subgroups. The first subdivision is into small cell lung carcinoma (SCLC, accounting for 20% of lung cancers) and non-small cell lung carcinoma (NSCLC, accounting for 80% of lung cancer). The latter is further distinguished into adenocarcinoma, squamous cell carcinoma, and neuroendocrine carcinoma. Within the heterogenous population of cell types that encompass the solid tumors, there exists a rare population of CSC that are able to resist typical chemotherapies and can re-populate the original tumor. Multiple studies investigating biological and functional markers of lung CSCs have identified an array of markers with a wide range of cellular functions. Through comparing functional differences between lung CSCs and non-CSC, two intriguing populations were identified. In 2007, Ho et al., using flow cytometry, have isolated a small population of cells capable of actively excluding Hoescht 33342 dye, termed side population (SP). These cells displayed an enhanced invasion, chemo-resistance, and tumorigenic properties [64]. Further characterization revealed association of high ABCG2 expression with SP cells and has been since used as a phenotypic marker of lung CSCs [64, 65]. In another study, chemo-resistant lung CSCs were identified based on their inherent trait to resist chemotherapeutic pressure, when treated with doxorubicin, cisplatin, and etoposide. The small number of surviving cells were found to display key CSC properties including expression of embryonic stem cell markers, self-renewal, and increased tumorigenic potential [66]. Analogous to other solid tumors, several markers have been used to identify lung CSC, including ALDH1,

CD44, CD133, CD166, and CD90. Increased ALDH1 activity in human lung cancer lines is associated with proliferation, self-renewal, and chemotherapy resistance [67]. Leung et al. (2010) showed $CD44^{+}$ populations in ten NSCLC lines to have increased stem properties, including sphere formation and enhanced tumor initiation potential [68]. Using both patient-derived and commercial cell lines, Chen et al. (2008) found $CD133^{+}$ cells exhibited stem-like properties like higher Oct4 expression, enhanced invasion and self-renewal, resistance to treatment, and increased CSC capabilities as compared with the $CD133^{-}$ populations [69]. Eramo et al. (2008) found $CD133^{+}$ cells isolated from lung cancer patient samples maintained spheroid growth in serum-free conditions and growth in vivo, properties that were lost when the cells were differentiated into $CD133^{-}$ cells [70]. Similar results were seen by Bertolini et al. (2009), where $CD133^{+}$ cells were also able to survive cisplatin treatment in vitro and in vivo [71]. Conversely, other studies have shown CD133 not to be a universal marker. Alternatively known as activated leukocyte adhesion molecule (ALCAM), CD166 has been a known CSC marker in several cancers, from colorectal [66] to prostate [72] to glioblastoma [73]. For NSCLC, CD166 was shown to be highly expressed in a small subset of patient tumor tissues, and in vivo $CD166^{+}$ cells displayed self-renewal and tumor initiation [74]. By screening the utility of CD44 and CD90 and markers of lung CSCs in several patient-derived lung cancer cell lines, Wang et al. identified a rare population to have high co-expression of both markers, which exhibited sphere formation, increased expression of mesenchymal markers as well as embryonic stem genes Oct4 and NANOG, and resistance to irradiation [75].

3.2.4 Colon

The remarkable renewal capacity of the intestinal epithelium, with nearly all of its cells in the epithelial lining replaced on a weekly basis, lends itself to the study of stem cell regulation. The colonic columnar cells originate from the stem cells situated within the colonic crypts. These cells have the capacity to differentiate into the complement of normal colonic crypt cells (i.e., enterocytes, endocrine cells, and goblet cells). It has been postulated that epigenetic and genetic aberrations to these cells result in the tumorigenesis of colorectal cancer (CRC) [76]. CRC has been identified as one of the most common human cancers worldwide with approximately 873,000 new cases each year [77]. CRCs are thought to contain as many as 80 mutations, which likely display significant cellular heterogeneity [78]. Two models currently exist to explain the process of CRC carcinogenesis. The first is the CRC somatic cell model suggesting that cancer cells originate from normal mature epithelial cells and undergo a series of epigenetic and genetic alterations such as MLH1 gene methylation and, KRAS and BRAF mutations, respectively. These initial mutations lead to the progression from low-grade to high-grade abnormal proliferation and subsequent accumulation of aberrant methylation and further mutations (e.g., *TP53, TGCBR2, BAX*) leads to malignant transformation of epithelial cells [79]. In contrast, the CRC stem cells are suggested to start at the precursor level with the capacity to differentiate into one cell type. Epigenetic changes such as aberrant methylation may result in silencing of genes (e.g., *p16, SFRPs, GATA4/5*, and *APC*) in these stem cells, committing them to a stem-like state that promotes abnormal clonal expansion, and ultimately transforming the colonic stem cell into a pre-invasive CRC stem cell [80]. Silencing key genes can direct cells to increase CRC-related pathways (i.e., Wnt Shh, and Notch pathways), resulting in genomic instability and mutations downstream genes (i.e., APC, β-catenin), which further activates these signaling pathways to promote tumorigenesis [76, 81–83]. Colorectal cancer (CRC) stem cells are a special subset of cells in CRC with the ability to initiate differentiation toward malignant cells and exhibit self-renewal and metastatic potential and are identified with genetic expression of *Lgr5* [84]. In humans, CRC CSCs have been defined using CD133, CD166, CD44, and CD24 markers [83, 85–90]. Current research is focused on experimentation on this rare fraction of cells to understand the mechanism by which they are associated with tumor burden, metastasis, and treatment evasion.

4 Future Technology

4.1 DNA Barcoding

Concept of cellular heterogeneity is displayed in both normal and cancer systems, with the presence of distinct cellular subpopulation. Intratumoral heterogeneity (ITH) at the cellular, genetic, and functional levels has been shown to occur to a startling degree in many cancers, and is increasingly appreciated as a key determinant of treatment failure and disease recurrence [91–93]. Pioneering work using lentivector-mediated clonal tracking of HSCs by John Dick demonstrated distinct clonal contribution of various cell populations to bone marrow engraftment in mice [94]. Resolution of clonal tracking was further improved by pairing cellular barcoding with sequence-based detection system, thus offering higher sensitivity for the identification of major and minor clones [95]. The application of cellular DNA barcoding technology has helped researchers to start appreciating the complexity tumoral heterogeneity and gain insights into temporal tumor evolution and how tumor cells respond to therapy. Through utilization of DNA barcoding technology in studies of acute lymphoblastic leukemia (ALL) [96], colorectal cancer [97, 98], and breast cancer [99], researchers were able to postulate that even when a presumably clonal population is transplanted in vivo the tumor growth is driven by a rare, pre-existing clonal cell subpopulation. However, in other studies by Connie Eaves group in breast cancer have demonstrated that multiple clonal population can be detected and a constant flux in clonal composition was observed [100]. Together these studies have highlighted polyclonality as an intrinsic property of tumor populations allowing for continuous adaptive potential under multiple environmental factors including chemo- and radiotherapies. Identification of clonal subpopulations responsible for driving tumor recurrence allows for development of novel therapeutic approaches that selectively targets treatment-refractory clones.

4.2 CRISPR-Cas Technology

The ability to target genomic locations in normal and cancer cells paves the way for evaluating the roles of specific genes in cancer involved in cancer development and resistance. Studies involving highly specific site-specific DNA manipulations in eukaryotic cells have been made easier after the development of Zinc Finger Nucleases (ZFNs) [101, 102], TALE domains in transcription activator-like effector nucleases (TALENs) [103], and CRISPR/Cas (clustered regularly interspaced palindromic repeats/CRISPR-associated) technology. Originally discovered as part of adaptive immunity in select bacteria and archaea, CRISPR allows these organisms to respond to and eliminate invading genetic materials than ZFNs and TALENs [104, 105], and has now been extensively adapted for eukaryotic genome engineering [106]. CRISPR allows for the precise manipulation of genetic locations in the mammalian genome, even if these regions are functionally silenced or structurally condensed [106]. Combined with the precise nature of CRISPR-Cas, the ease of generating large libraries of targeting constructs has poised this genomic editing system to discover novel therapeutic targets in cancer using loss-of-function (LoF) and gain-of-function screens (GoF).

CRISPR sgRNA genome-wide libraries have been developed for in vitro screening and, more recently, in vivo screening. First-generation CRISPR sgRNA LoF libraries were initially developed to target over 18,000 genes in the human genome, including over 1000 microRNAs (miRNA) [107, 108]. Recently, an improved CRISPR loss-of-function library targeting the human genome was developed by Hart et al., known as the Toronto KnockOut (TKO) library. The second-generation TKO CRISPR library contains ~2000 high-confidence fitness genes and demonstrates that knockout of context-dependent fitness genes is linked to pathway-specific genetic vulnerabilities [109]. Recently, Chen et al. have demonstrated the use of genome-wide CRISPR LoF screens in tumor growth and metastasis in vivo, by transplanting a mutant mouse cancer cell line using a genome scale library with ~68,000 sgRNAs into immunocompromised mice [110].

Using CRISPR sgRNA knockout-libraries, genome-wide LoF screens can be conducted on patient-derived or commercial cancer cell lines in vitro or in vivo. To begin with, patient-derived or commercial cancer cell lines are transduced with a pooled LoF CRISPR sgRNA library, containing either the whole or a subset of essential genes. Following selection and propagation of transduced Cas9-sgRNA clones, genetic vulnerabilities in the presence or absence of conventional chemoradiotherapy could be identified based on the in vitro and in vivo growth of cancer cells. Genomic samples of the transduced cells are collected at different time points and sequenced to identify an absence of particular sgRNA eluding to potential genetic vulnerability. Following validation, these genetic vulnerabilities can be targeted using small-molecule inhibitors or immunotherapeutic biologics.

4.3 Immunotherapy

Over the past decade, immunotherapy has become one of the most promising targeted therapeutic modalities in oncology. Although immunotherapy utilizes many aspects of the immune system, the more popular forms involve the creation or modification of antibodies for the treatment of cancers, due to their innate ability to target very specific, and sometimes unique, tumor-associated antigens (TAAs). Antibodies are central to the adaptive immune system as they can induce antibody-dependent cell-mediated cytotoxicity, activate the complement system, and prevent ligand-receptor interactions. Antibody-based cancer immunotherapies include the use of monoclonal antibodies (mAbs) [111, 112], bi-specific monoclonal antibodies (BsAbs) [113, 114], bi-specific T cell engagers (BiTEs) [115–117], and chimeric antigen receptors (CARs) [118–120]. While targeting binding between cell surface receptors and their respective ligands has been a major limitation of small-molecule-based therapies, Abs can block such interaction with high potency and specificity [121]. Furthermore, fully human monoclonal Abs have shown minimal "off-target" toxicity, in contrast to small-molecule inhibitors. Antibody-based immunotherapy can be used to bind to specific CSC antigens in order to neutralize them via cytotoxicity, or to inhibit T cell suppressing pathways (immune checkpoints) by blocking receptor-ligand interaction. Nevertheless, there is some limitation to Abs-based therapies including the inherit redundancy in cell signaling leading to cell proliferation, effects of microenvironment, activation of inhibitory receptors, and competition with circulation IgG [122]. In light of those limitations, an alternate strategy using BsAbs has been developed. BsAbs are very similar to mAbs; however, each of the two fragment antigen-binding (Fab) arms of the mAb recognizes and binds separate antigens [123]. Finally, a strategy involving chimeric antigen receptor (CAR)-T cells with genetically modified antigen-recognizing receptors unique to tumor cells has shown promising results in phase I and II clinical trials in patients with lymphoid leukemia [124–127].

References

1. Ramalho-Santos M, Willenbring H (2007) On the origin of the term "stem cell". Cell Stem Cell 1(1):35–38
2. Till JE, McCulloch EA (1961) A direct measurement of the radiation sensitivity of normal mouse bone marrow cells. Radiat Res 14:213–222
3. Siminovitch L, McCulloch EA, Till JE (1963) The distribution of colony-forming cells among spleen colonies. J Cell Physiol 62:327–336
4. McCulloch EA, Till JE, Siminovitch L (1965) The role of independent and dependent stem cells in the control of hemopoietic and immunologic responses. Wistar Inst Symp Monogr 4:61–68
5. Potten CS, Loeffler M (1990) Stem cells: attributes, cycles, spirals, pitfalls and uncertainties. Lessons for and from the crypt. Development 110(4):1001–1020
6. Al-Hajj M, Wicha MS, Benito-Hernandez A, Morrison SJ, Clarke MF (2003) Prospective identification of tumorigenic breast cancer cells. Proc Natl Acad Sci U S A 100 (7):3983–3988
7. Reynolds BA, Weiss S (1992) Generation of neurons and astrocytes from isolated cells of the adult mammalian central nervous system. Science 255(5052):1707–1710
8. Kajstura J, Rota M, Hall SR, Hosoda T, D'Amario D, Sanada F et al (2011) Evidence for human lung stem cells. N Engl J Med 364 (19):1795–1806
9. Cohnheim J (1875) Congenitales, quergestreiftes muskelsarkon der nireren. Virchows Arch:65–64
10. Rippert H. Geschwulstelehre fur Aerzte und Studierende. 1904
11. Virchow R. 1863. Dir Krankhoften Geschwulste. Vol II. Onkologie, Pt 1
12. Paget J (1853) Lectures on surgical pathology. Lindsay & Blakiston, Philadelphia
13. Pierce GB, Dixon FJ Jr (1959) Testicular teratomas. I. Demonstration of teratogenesis by metamorphosis of multipotential cells. Cancer 12(3):573–583
14. Mintz B, Illmensee K (1975) Normal genetically mosaic mice produced from malignant teratocarcinoma cells. Proc Natl Acad Sci U S A 72(9):3585–3589
15. Illmensee K (1978) Reversion of malignancy and normalized differentiation of teratocarcinoma cells in chimeric mice. Basic Life Sci 12:3–25
16. Stevens LC (1970) The development of transplantable teratocarcinomas from intratesticular grafts of pre- and postimplantation mouse embryos. Dev Biol 21(3):364–382
17. Stevens LC (1964) Experimental production of testicular teratomas in mice. Proc Natl Acad Sci U S A 52:654–661
18. Allen KE, Weiss GJ (2010) Resistance may not be futile: microRNA biomarkers for chemoresistance and potential therapeutics. Mol Cancer Ther 9(12):3126–3136
19. Nguyen LV, Vanner R, Dirks P, Eaves CJ (2012) Cancer stem cells: an evolving concept. Nat Rev Cancer 12(2):133–143
20. Bonnet D, Dick JE (1997) Human acute myeloid leukemia is organized as a hierarchy that originates from a primitive hematopoietic cell. Nat Med 3(7):730–737
21. Serrano D, Bleau AM, Fernandez-Garcia I, Fernandez-Marcelo T, Iniesta P, Ortiz-de-Solorzano C et al (2011) Inhibition of telomerase activity preferentially targets aldehyde dehydrogenase-positive cancer stem-like cells in lung cancer. Mol Cancer 10:96
22. Liu J, Xiao Z, Wong SK, Tin VP, Ho KY, Wang J et al (2013) Lung cancer tumorigenicity and drug resistance are maintained through ALDH(hi)CD44(hi) tumor initiating cells. Oncotarget 4(10):1698–1711
23. Lapidot T, Sirard C, Vormoor J, Murdoch B, Hoang T, Caceres-Cortes J et al (1994) A cell initiating human acute myeloid leukaemia after transplantation into SCID mice. Nature 367(6464):645–648
24. Wang JC, Dick JE (2005) Cancer stem cells: lessons from leukemia. Trends Cell Biol 15 (9):494–501
25. Warner JK, Wang JC, Hope KJ, Jin L, Dick JE (2004) Concepts of human leukemic development. Oncogene 23(43):7164–7177
26. Early Breast Cancer Trialists' Collaborative G (2005) Effects of chemotherapy and hormonal therapy for early breast cancer on recurrence and 15-year survival: an overview of the randomised trials. Lancet 365 (9472):1687–1717
27. Hartwig FP, Nedel F, Collares T, Tarquinio SB, Nor JE, Demarco FF (2014) Oncogenic somatic events in tissue-specific stem cells: a role in cancer recurrence? Ageing Res Rev 13:100–106
28. Wang RA, Li ZS, Zhang HZ, Zheng PJ, Li QL, Shi JG et al (2013) Invasive cancers are not necessarily from preformed in situ tumours - an alternative way of carcinogenesis

from misplaced stem cells. J Cell Mol Med 17 (7):921–926

29. Mintz B, Cronmiller C, Custer RP (1978) Somatic cell origin of teratocarcinomas. Proc Natl Acad Sci U S A 75(6):2834–2838
30. Ponti D, Costa A, Zaffaroni N, Pratesi G, Petrangolini G, Coradini D et al (2005) Isolation and in vitro propagation of tumorigenic breast cancer cells with stem/progenitor cell properties. Cancer Res 65(13):5506–5511
31. Wright MH, Calcagno AM, Salcido CD, Carlson MD, Ambudkar SV, Varticovski L (2008) Brca1 breast tumors contain distinct CD44+/CD24- and CD133+ cells with cancer stem cell characteristics. Breast Cancer Res 10(1): R10
32. Perrone G, Gaeta LM, Zagami M, Nasorri F, Coppola R, Borzomati D et al (2012) In situ identification of CD44+/CD24- cancer cells in primary human breast carcinomas. PLoS One 7(9):e43110
33. Wang LB, He YQ, Wu LG, Chen DM, Fan H, Jia W (2012) Isolation and characterization of human breast tumor stem cells. Xi Bao Yu Fen Zi Mian Yi Xue Za Zhi 28(12):1261–1264
34. Herrera-Gayol A, Jothy S (1999) Adhesion proteins in the biology of breast cancer: contribution of CD44. Exp Mol Pathol 66 (2):149–156
35. Gotte M, Yip GW (2006) Heparanase, hyaluronan, and CD44 in cancers: a breast carcinoma perspective. Cancer Res 66 (21):10233–10237
36. Schabath H, Runz S, Joumaa S, Altevogt P (2006) CD24 affects CXCR4 function in pre-B lymphocytes and breast carcinoma cells. J Cell Sci 119(Pt 2):314–325
37. Brown LF, Berse B, Van de Water L, Papadopoulos-Sergiou A, Perruzzi CA, Manseau EJ et al (1992) Expression and distribution of osteopontin in human tissues: widespread association with luminal epithelial surfaces. Mol Biol Cell 3(10):1169–1180
38. Ginestier C, Hur MH, Charafe-Jauffret E, Monville F, Dutcher J, Brown M et al (2007) ALDH1 is a marker of normal and malignant human mammary stem cells and a predictor of poor clinical outcome. Cell Stem Cell 1(5):555–567
39. Cariati M, Naderi A, Brown JP, Smalley MJ, Pinder SE, Caldas C et al (2008) Alpha-6 integrin is necessary for the tumourigenicity of a stem cell-like subpopulation within the MCF7 breast cancer cell line. Int J Cancer 122 (2):298–304
40. Vaillant F, Asselin-Labat ML, Shackleton M, Forrest NC, Lindeman GJ, Visvader JE (2008) The mammary progenitor marker CD61/beta3 integrin identifies cancer stem cells in mouse models of mammary tumorigenesis. Cancer Res 68(19):7711–7717
41. Peitzsch C, Kurth I, Kunz-Schughart L, Baumann M, Dubrovska A (2013) Discovery of the cancer stem cell related determinants of radioresistance. Radiother Oncol 108 (3):378–387
42. Karamboulas C, Ailles L (2013) Developmental signaling pathways in cancer stem cells of solid tumors. Biochim Biophys Acta 1830 (2):2481–2495
43. Singh A, Settleman J (2010) EMT, cancer stem cells and drug resistance: an emerging axis of evil in the war on cancer. Oncogene 29 (34):4741–4751
44. Creighton CJ, Li X, Landis M, Dixon JM, Neumeister VM, Sjolund A et al (2009) Residual breast cancers after conventional therapy display mesenchymal as well as tumor-initiating features. Proc Natl Acad Sci U S A 106(33):13820–13825
45. Creighton CJ, Chang JC, Rosen JM (2010) Epithelial-mesenchymal transition (EMT) in tumor-initiating cells and its clinical implications in breast cancer. J Mammary Gland Biol Neoplasia 15(2):253–260
46. Bhola NE, Balko JM, Dugger TC, Kuba MG, Sanchez V, Sanders M et al (2013) TGF-beta inhibition enhances chemotherapy action against triple-negative breast cancer. J Clin Invest 123(3):1348–1358
47. Ginestier C, Liu S, Diebel ME, Korkaya H, Luo M, Brown M et al (2010) CXCR1 blockade selectively targets human breast cancer stem cells in vitro and in xenografts. J Clin Invest 120(2):485–497
48. Singh SK, Hawkins C, Clarke ID, Squire JA, Bayani J, Hide T et al (2004) Identification of human brain tumour initiating cells. Nature 432(7015):396–401
49. Galli R, Binda E, Orfanelli U, Cipelletti B, Gritti A, De Vitis S et al (2004) Isolation and characterization of tumorigenic, stem-like neural precursors from human glioblastoma. Cancer Res 64(19):7011–7021
50. Hemmati HD, Nakano I, Lazareff JA, Masterman-Smith M, Geschwind DH, Bronner-Fraser M et al (2003) Cancerous stem cells can arise from pediatric brain tumors. Proc Natl Acad Sci U S A 100 (25):15178–15183
51. Ignatova TN, Kukekov VG, Laywell ED, Suslov ON, Vrionis FD, Steindler DA (2002) Human cortical glial tumors contain neural

stem-like cells expressing astroglial and neuronal markers in vitro. Glia 39(3):193–206
52. Singh SK, Clarke ID, Terasaki M, Bonn VE, Hawkins C, Squire J et al (2003) Identification of a cancer stem cell in human brain tumors. Cancer Res 63(18):5821–5828
53. Son MJ, Woolard K, Nam DH, Lee J, Fine HA (2009) SSEA-1 is an enrichment marker for tumor-initiating cells in human glioblastoma. Cell Stem Cell 4(5):440–452
54. Lathia JD, Gallagher J, Heddleston JM, Wang J, Eyler CE, Macswords J et al (2010) Integrin alpha 6 regulates glioblastoma stem cells. Cell Stem Cell 6(5):421–432
55. Bao S, Wu Q, Li Z, Sathornsumetee S, Wang H, McLendon RE et al (2008) Targeting cancer stem cells through L1CAM suppresses glioma growth. Cancer Res 68(15):6043–6048
56. Binda E, Visioli A, Giani F, Lamorte G, Copetti M, Pitter KL et al (2012) The EphA2 receptor drives self-renewal and tumorigenicity in stem-like tumor-propagating cells from human glioblastomas. Cancer Cell 22(6):765–780
57. Day BW, Stringer BW, Al-Ejeh F, Ting MJ, Wilson J, Ensbey KS et al (2013) EphA3 maintains tumorigenicity and is a therapeutic target in glioblastoma multiforme. Cancer Cell 23(2):238–248
58. Nakada M, Anderson EM, Demuth T, Nakada S, Reavie LB, Drake KL et al (2010) The phosphorylation of ephrin-B2 ligand promotes glioma cell migration and invasion. Int J Cancer 126(5):1155–1165
59. Alonso MM, Diez-Valle R, Manterola L, Rubio A, Liu D, Cortes-Santiago N et al (2011) Genetic and epigenetic modifications of Sox2 contribute to the invasive phenotype of malignant gliomas. PLoS One 6(11):e26740
60. Bao S, Wu Q, McLendon RE, Hao Y, Shi Q, Hjelmeland AB et al (2006) Glioma stem cells promote radioresistance by preferential activation of the DNA damage response. Nature 444(7120):756–760
61. Beier D, Schriefer B, Brawanski K, Hau P, Weis J, Schulz JB et al (2012) Efficacy of clinically relevant temozolomide dosing schemes in glioblastoma cancer stem cell lines. J Neuro-Oncol 109(1):45–52
62. Jemal A, Bray F, Center MM, Ferlay J, Ward E, Forman D (2011) Global cancer statistics. CA Cancer J Clin 61(2):69–90
63. Collins LG, Haines C, Perkel R, Enck RE (2007) Lung cancer: diagnosis and management. Am Fam Physician 75(1):56–63
64. Ho MM, Ng AV, Lam S, Hung JY (2007) Side population in human lung cancer cell lines and tumors is enriched with stem-like cancer cells. Cancer Res 67(10):4827–4833
65. Salcido CD, Larochelle A, Taylor BJ, Dunbar CE, Varticovski L (2010) Molecular characterisation of side population cells with cancer stem cell-like characteristics in small-cell lung cancer. Br J Cancer 102(11):1636–1644
66. Levina V, Marrangoni AM, DeMarco R, Gorelik E, Lokshin AE (2008) Drug-selected human lung cancer stem cells: cytokine network, tumorigenic and metastatic properties. PLoS One 3(8):e3077
67. Jiang F, Qiu Q, Khanna A, Todd NW, Deepak J, Xing L et al (2009) Aldehyde dehydrogenase 1 is a tumor stem cell-associated marker in lung cancer. Mol Cancer Res 7(3):330–338
68. Leung EL, Fiscus RR, Tung JW, Tin VP, Cheng LC, Sihoe AD et al (2010) Non-small cell lung cancer cells expressing CD44 are enriched for stem cell-like properties. PLoS One 5(11):e14062
69. Chen YC, Hsu HS, Chen YW, Tsai TH, How CK, Wang CY et al (2008) Oct-4 expression maintained cancer stem-like properties in lung cancer-derived CD133-positive cells. PLoS One 3(7):e2637
70. Eramo A, Lotti F, Sette G, Pilozzi E, Biffoni M, Di Virgilio A et al (2008) Identification and expansion of the tumorigenic lung cancer stem cell population. Cell Death Differ 15(3):504–514
71. Bertolini G, Roz L, Perego P, Tortoreto M, Fontanella E, Gatti L et al (2009) Highly tumorigenic lung cancer CD133+ cells display stem-like features and are spared by cisplatin treatment. Proc Natl Acad Sci U S A 106(38):16281–16286
72. Jiao J, Hindoyan A, Wang S, Tran LM, Goldstein AS, Lawson D et al (2012) Identification of CD166 as a surface marker for enriching prostate stem/progenitor and cancer initiating cells. PLoS One 7(8):e42564
73. Kijima N, Hosen N, Kagawa N, Hashimoto N, Nakano A, Fujimoto Y et al (2012) CD166/activated leukocyte cell adhesion molecule is expressed on glioblastoma progenitor cells and involved in the regulation of tumor cell invasion. Neuro-Oncology 14(10):1254–1264
74. Zhang WC, Shyh-Chang N, Yang H, Rai A, Umashankar S, Ma S et al (2012) Glycine decarboxylase activity drives non-small cell lung cancer tumor-initiating cells and tumorigenesis. Cell 148(1–2):259–272

75. Wang P, Gao Q, Suo Z, Munthe E, Solberg S, Ma L et al (2013) Identification and characterization of cells with cancer stem cell properties in human primary lung cancer cell lines. PLoS One 8(3):e57020
76. Medema JP, Vermeulen L (2011) Microenvironmental regulation of stem cells in intestinal homeostasis and cancer. Nature 474 (7351):318–326
77. Global Burden of Disease Cancer C, Fitzmaurice C, Dicker D, Pain A, Hamavid H, Moradi-Lakeh M et al (2015) The Global Burden of Cancer 2013. JAMA Oncol 1 (4):505–527
78. Wood LD, Parsons DW, Jones S, Lin J, Sjoblom T, Leary RJ et al (2007) The genomic landscapes of human breast and colorectal cancers. Science 318(5853):1108–1113
79. Markowitz SD, Bertagnolli MM (2009) Molecular origins of cancer: molecular basis of colorectal cancer. N Engl J Med 361 (25):2449–2460
80. Jones PA, Baylin SB (2007) The epigenomics of cancer. Cell 128(4):683–692
81. Baylin SB, Ohm JE (2006) Epigenetic gene silencing in cancer - a mechanism for early oncogenic pathway addiction? Nat Rev Cancer 6(2):107–116
82. Song L, Li Y, He B, Gong Y (2015) Development of small molecules targeting the Wnt signaling pathway in cancer stem cells for the treatment of colorectal cancer. Clin Colorectal Cancer 14(3):133–145
83. Vermeulen L, Todaro M, de Sousa MF, Sprick MR, Kemper K, Perez Alea M et al (2008) Single-cell cloning of colon cancer stem cells reveals a multi-lineage differentiation capacity. Proc Natl Acad Sci U S A 105 (36):13427–13432
84. Barker N, van Es JH, Kuipers J, Kujala P, van den Born M, Cozijnsen M et al (2007) Identification of stem cells in small intestine and colon by marker gene Lgr5. Nature 449 (7165):1003–1007
85. Todaro M, Alea MP, Di Stefano AB, Cammareri P, Vermeulen L, Iovino F et al (2007) Colon cancer stem cells dictate tumor growth and resist cell death by production of interleukin-4. Cell Stem Cell 1(4):389–402
86. Dalerba P, Dylla SJ, Park IK, Liu R, Wang X, Cho RW et al (2007) Phenotypic characterization of human colorectal cancer stem cells. Proc Natl Acad Sci U S A 104 (24):10158–10163
87. O'Brien CA, Pollett A, Gallinger S, Dick JE (2007) A human colon cancer cell capable of initiating tumour growth in immunodeficient mice. Nature 445(7123):106–110
88. Ricci-Vitiani L, Lombardi DG, Pilozzi E, Biffoni M, Todaro M, Peschle C et al (2007) Identification and expansion of human colon-cancer-initiating cells. Nature 445 (7123):111–115
89. Vermeulen L, De Sousa EMF, van der Heijden M, Cameron K, de Jong JH, Borovski T et al (2010) Wnt activity defines colon cancer stem cells and is regulated by the microenvironment. Nat Cell Biol 12(5):468–476
90. Kemper K, Sprick MR, de Bree M, Scopelliti A, Vermeulen L, Hoek M et al (2010) The AC133 epitope, but not the CD133 protein, is lost upon cancer stem cell differentiation. Cancer Res 70(2):719–729
91. Burrell RA, McGranahan N, Bartek J, Swanton C (2013) The causes and consequences of genetic heterogeneity in cancer evolution. Nature 501(7467):338–345
92. Swanton C (2015) Cancer evolution constrained by mutation order. N Engl J Med 372(7):661–663
93. Meacham CE, Morrison SJ (2013) Tumour heterogeneity and cancer cell plasticity. Nature 501(7467):328–337
94. Mazurier F, Gan OI, McKenzie JL, Doedens M, Dick JE (2004) Lentivector-mediated clonal tracking reveals intrinsic heterogeneity in the human hematopoietic stem cell compartment and culture-induced stem cell impairment. Blood 103(2):545–552
95. Gerrits A, Dykstra B, Kalmykowa OJ, Klauke K, Verovskaya E, Broekhuis MJ et al (2010) Cellular barcoding tool for clonal analysis in the hematopoietic system. Blood 115 (13):2610–2618
96. Turke AB, Zejnullahu K, Wu YL, Song Y, Dias-Santagata D, Lifshits E et al (2010) Preexistence and clonal selection of MET amplification in EGFR mutant NSCLC. Cancer Cell 17(1):77–88
97. Kreso A, O'Brien CA, van Galen P, Gan OI, Notta F, Brown AM et al (2013) Variable clonal repopulation dynamics influence chemotherapy response in colorectal cancer. Science 339(6119):543–548
98. Nolan-Stevaux O, Tedesco D, Ragan S, Makhanov M, Chenchik A, Ruefli-Brasse A et al (2013) Measurement of cancer cell growth heterogeneity through lentiviral barcoding identifies clonal dominance as a characteristic of in vivo tumor engraftment. PLoS One 8(6):e67316
99. Navin N, Kendall J, Troge J, Andrews P, Rodgers L, McIndoo J et al (2011) Tumour

evolution inferred by single-cell sequencing. Nature 472(7341):90–94
100. Nguyen LV, Cox CL, Eirew P, Knapp DJ, Pellacani D, Kannan N et al (2014) DNA barcoding reveals diverse growth kinetics of human breast tumour subclones in serially passaged xenografts. Nat Commun 5:5871
101. Bibikova M, Beumer K, Trautman JK, Carroll D (2003) Enhancing gene targeting with designed zinc finger nucleases. Science 300 (5620):764
102. Porteus MH, Baltimore D (2003) Chimeric nucleases stimulate gene targeting in human cells. Science 300(5620):763
103. Boch J, Scholze H, Schornack S, Landgraf A, Hahn S, Kay S et al (2009) Breaking the code of DNA binding specificity of TAL-type III effectors. Science 326(5959):1509–1512
104. Mojica FJ, Diez-Villasenor C, Garcia-Martinez J, Soria E (2005) Intervening sequences of regularly spaced prokaryotic repeats derive from foreign genetic elements. J Mol Evol 60(2):174–182
105. Bolotin A, Quinquis B, Sorokin A, Ehrlich SD (2005) Clustered regularly interspaced short palindrome repeats (CRISPRs) have spacers of extrachromosomal origin. Microbiology 151(Pt 8):2551–2561
106. Knight SC, Xie L, Deng W, Guglielmi B, Witkowsky LB, Bosanac L et al (2015) Dynamics of CRISPR-Cas9 genome interrogation in living cells. Science 350 (6262):823–826
107. Shalem O, Sanjana NE, Hartenian E, Shi X, Scott DA, Mikkelsen TS et al (2014) Genome-scale CRISPR-Cas9 knockout screening in human cells. Science 343 (6166):84–87
108. Wang T, Wei JJ, Sabatini DM, Lander ES (2014) Genetic screens in human cells using the CRISPR-Cas9 system. Science 343 (6166):80–84
109. Hart T, Chandrashekhar M, Aregger M, Steinhart Z, Brown KR, MacLeod G et al (2015) High-resolution CRISPR screens reveal fitness genes and genotype-specific cancer liabilities. Cell 163(6):1515–1526
110. Chen S, Sanjana NE, Zheng K, Shalem O, Lee K, Shi X et al (2015) Genome-wide CRISPR screen in a mouse model of tumor growth and metastasis. Cell 160 (6):1246–1260
111. Stern M, Herrmann R (2005) Overview of monoclonal antibodies in cancer therapy: present and promise. Crit Rev Oncol Hematol 54(1):11–29
112. Vennepureddy A, Singh P, Rastogi R, Atallah JP, Terjanian T (2016) Evolution of ramucirumab in the treatment of cancer - A review of literature. J Oncol Pharm Pract
113. Chames P, Baty D (2009) Bispecific antibodies for cancer therapy: the light at the end of the tunnel? MAbs 1(6):539–547
114. Muller D, Kontermann RE (2010) Bispecific antibodies for cancer immunotherapy: current perspectives. BioDrugs 24(2):89–98
115. Wolf E, Hofmeister R, Kufer P, Schlereth B, Baeuerle PA (2005) BiTEs: bispecific antibody constructs with unique anti-tumor activity. Drug Discov Today 10 (18):1237–1244
116. Wong R, Pepper C, Brennan P, Nagorsen D, Man S, Fegan C (2013) Blinatumomab induces autologous T-cell killing of chronic lymphocytic leukemia cells. Haematologica 98(12):1930–1938
117. Suryadevara CM, Gedeon PC, Sanchez-Perez L, Verla T, Alvarez-Breckenridge C, Choi BD et al (2015) Are BiTEs the "missing link" in cancer therapy? Oncoimmunology 4(6): e1008339
118. Porter DL, Levine BL, Kalos M, Bagg A, June CH (2011) Chimeric antigen receptor-modified T cells in chronic lymphoid leukemia. N Engl J Med 365(8):725–733
119. Till BG, Jensen MC, Wang J, Qian X, Gopal AK, Maloney DG et al (2012) CD20-specific adoptive immunotherapy for lymphoma using a chimeric antigen receptor with both CD28 and 4-1BB domains: pilot clinical trial results. Blood 119(17):3940–3950
120. Sampson JH, Choi BD, Sanchez-Perez L, Suryadevara CM, Snyder DJ, Flores CT et al (2014) EGFRvIII mCAR-modified T-cell therapy cures mice with established intracerebral glioma and generates host immunity against tumor-antigen loss. Clin Cancer Res 20(4):972–984
121. Reichert JM (2010) Antibodies to watch in 2010. MAbs 2(1):84–100
122. Chames P, Van Regenmortel M, Weiss E, Baty D (2009) Therapeutic antibodies: successes, limitations and hopes for the future. Br J Pharmacol 157(2):220–233
123. Baeuerle PA, Kufer P, Bargou R (2009) BiTE: teaching antibodies to engage T-cells for cancer therapy. Curr Opin Mol Ther 11 (1):22–30
124. Gross G, Waks T, Eshhar Z (1989) Expression of immunoglobulin-T-cell receptor chimeric molecules as functional receptors with antibody-type specificity. Proc Natl Acad Sci U S A 86(24):10024–10028

125. Maude SL, Frey N, Shaw PA, Aplenc R, Barrett DM, Bunin NJ et al (2014) Chimeric antigen receptor T cells for sustained remissions in leukemia. N Engl J Med 371 (16):1507–1517

126. Cruz CR, Micklethwaite KP, Savoldo B, Ramos CA, Lam S, Ku S et al (2013) Infusion of donor-derived CD19-redirected virus-specific T cells for B-cell malignancies relapsed after allogeneic stem cell transplant: a phase 1 study. Blood 122(17):2965–2973

127. Brentjens RJ, Davila ML, Riviere I, Park J, Wang X, Cowell LG et al (2013) CD19-targeted T cells rapidly induce molecular remissions in adults with chemotherapy-refractory acute lymphoblastic leukemia. Sci Transl Med 5(177):177ra38

Chapter 2

Surface Markers for the Identification of Cancer Stem Cells

Vinod Gopalan, Farhadul Islam, and Alfred King-yin Lam

Abstract

Cancer stem cells have genetic and functional characteristics that can turn them resistant to standard cancer therapeutic targets. Identification of these cells is challenging and is mostly done by detecting the expression of their antigens in a group of stem cells. Currently, there are a significant number of surface markers available which can detect the cancer stem cells by directly targeting their specific antigens present in cells. These markers possess differential expression patterns and sub-localizations in cancer stem cells when compared to non-neoplastic stem cells and somatic cells. In addition to molecular markers, multiple analytical methods and techniques including functional assays, cell sorting, filtration approaches, and xenotransplantation methods are used to identify cancer stem cells. This chapter will overview the functional significance of cancer stem cells, its biological correlations, specific markers, and detection methods.

Key words Stem cell, Cancer, Detection, Markers, Methods, Isolation

1 Introduction

Cancer stem cells (CSCs) or tumor initiating cells can be defined as a group of undifferentiated cells within a tumor that can self-renew and drive carcinogenesis [1]. These cells possess distinct genetic, epigenetic, and functional heterogeneity which in turn can resist therapy and may later initiate metastatic process [2–4]. Previous studies have proven that increased genetic instabilities in normal stem cells may lead to the formation of CSCs suggesting that stemness are attained from the additional genetic modifications [5, 6]. CSCs represent approximately 0.1–10% of all tumor cells and they express characteristically low levels of their antigens compared to established tumor-associated antigens [7]. Identification of CSC antigens was done not based on their overexpression but on their expression in a group of cells with stem-cell-like properties [8–11].

Origin and development of CSCs are highly regulated by a key cellular process called epithelial-mesenchymal transition (EMT) which is a key determinant of cancer growth and metastasis

Gianpaolo Papaccio and Vincenzo Desiderio (eds.), *Cancer Stem Cells: Methods and Protocols*, Methods in Molecular Biology, vol. 1692, DOI 10.1007/978-1-4939-7401-6_2, © Springer Science+Business Media LLC 2018

[1, 4]. EMT makes the epithelial cells polarize and develop stem-like properties by losing their epithelial characteristics and gaining mesenchymal properties which lead to increased invasion and motility. Thus, the detection of EMT changes during or prior to cancer development provides a valuable prognostic tool and therapeutic target [3]. Also, the increased expressions of some of these markers in cancer tissues may be used to predict the response of targeted therapy developed against these groups of cancer cells. Thus, the quality of life and survival rates of patients could be improved by developing exclusive therapies that target CSCs, particularly for patients that suffer from metastatic disease.

The existence of CSCs in vivo was first confirmed in 1997 in acute myeloid leukaemia by Bonnet and Dick [8]. The authors have identified $CD34^{+}$ $CD38^{-}$ subpopulation cells in the leukaemia, similar to normal hematopoietic stem cells, and were found proficient of initiating acute myeloid leukaemia once transplanted into non-obese diabetic/severe combined immuno deficient mice [8]. Since then, CSCs have been identified in several cancers using specific molecular markers. It was demonstrated that collective markers for detecting CSCs in general are unlikely as CSCs are generally tissue specific [1]. Also, varied expression levels and co-expression of antigens from normal stem cells have made the detection of antigens specific for identifying or targeting CSCs difficult [7].

Every cell surface in the body is coated with specialized proteins, namely receptors, which have the ability to selectively bind or adhere to other signaling molecules [12]. The identification of receptors is generally based on the increased expression of specific markers in different cell types [13]. These receptors are noted in specific cell types including cancer stem cells [12]. Expressions of specific cell-surface antigens that enrich for cells with CSC properties remain the most common approach of identifying CSCs [13]. Primarily, many of these antigens are targeted due to their identified expressions on endogenous stem cells. Currently, there is no universal marker that can identify CSCs in every cancer. Therefore, multiple genetic markers are used in combination to achieve high specificity in CSC detections. A brief overview of common markers used in multiple cancers is listed in Table 1.

1.1 CSC Surface Markers

In recent years, there is a significant increase in the number of surface marker molecules to detect and characterize CSCs. Till now, CSCs and their specific markers have been identified from various cancers including those from the breast, brain, blood (leukaemia), prostate, skin, thyroid, lung, gastrointestinal tract, reproductive tract, and head a/neck. Stemness activity or presence is generally defined by either increased expression or absence of certain markers [14]. Also, many markers that are expressed in non-neoplastic stem cells are also expressed in cancer stem cells (Table 2). The detection and specificity of these markers depends

Table 1
Cell surface markers for the identification cancer stem cells in common cancers

Cancer	Markers	References
Haematological	CD34, CD38, CD19, CD26	[30–32]
Breast	CD44, CD24, CD29, CD133	[33–36]
Colon	CD44, CD24, CD26, CD29, CD133, CD166, Ep-CAM	[37–40]
Brain	CD90, CD133, CD15	[41–43]
Head and neck	CD44, CD271	[44, 45]
Skin	CD20, CD271	[45, 46]
Liver	CD44, CD90, CD133, CD13, Ep-CAP	[47]
Lung	CD44, CD133, CD166	[48]
Pancreas	CD44, CD24, CD133	[49]
Prostate	CD44, CD24, CD133, CD166, CD151	[50]
Oesophagus	CD271, CD44, CD24, CD90	[51]
Cervix	CD13, CD29, CD44, CD105	[52]
Stomach	CD44, CD133	[53]

Table 2
Cell surface markers expresses on normal stem cells and cancer stem cells

Marker	Normal expression	Cancer stem cell expression
CD19	B lymphocytes	B cell malignancies
CD20	B lymphocytes	Melanoma
CD24	B lymphocytes; neuroblasts	Pancreatic carcinoma, lung carcinoma
CD34	Haemopoietic cells; endothelial cells	Haemopoietic malignancies
CD38	B and T lymphocytes	Negative on acute myeloid leukaemia
CD44	Multiple tissues	Breast, liver, head and neck, pancreas carcinomas
CD90	T lymphocytes, neurons	Liver carcinoma
CD133	Multiple tissues	Brain, colorectal, lung, liver carcinomas
EpCAM/ESA	Epithelial cells	Colorectal and pancreas carcinomas
ABCB5	Keratinocytes	Melanoma

ABCB5: ATP-binding cassette subfamily B member 5

upon the type of stem cells they target. For example, some markers can specifically differentiate embryonic stem cells from adult stem cells or pluripotent from progenitor cells [14]. At present, there is no clear distinction between the expression patterns and detection of stem cell markers across non-neoplastic and cancer stem cells. Onco-fetal stem cell markers, defined as markers that are undetectable in adult tissues but expressed in embryos or foetuses and with re-expression in cancers, are currently surfaced as a best option for the identification of cancer cells [14, 15].

Majority of stem cell markers identified so far are proteins and a small group of markers are noted to be glycans (e.g., glycoprotein) which in turn bound to proteins or lipids. For example, CD15 is a stage-specific embryonic antigen that is carried on lipids or proteins in CSCs from glioblastoma [16]. These markers, through their various genetic modifications, have the ability to be physically isolated as distinct subpopulations of CSCs with differing biological features. Overall, these markers are either upregulated (e.g., ATP-binding cassette (ABC) transporter G subfamily [ABCG]) [17], absent, mutated (e.g., Notch homolog 1, translocation-associated (Drosophila) [NOTCH1]) [18] or show differential expression patterns with their isotypes (e.g., CD44v) [19].

Another interesting feature of stem cell markers includes their difference in physical localizations such as cell surface or intra-cytoplasmic (either in nucleus/cytoplasmic). CSC markers such as CD133 represent cell-surface antigens that are expressed by their corresponding adult stem cells. In the meantime, aldehyde dehydrogenase 1 (ALDH1) is located in the cytoplasm. It is a soluble protein that is used to detect CSCs in various cancers, including leukaemia [20], breast cancer [21], and colon cancer [22]. Hoechst 33342 is a nuclear dye. It is used for the detection of non-neoplastic stem cells as well as CSCs in side population cells [23]. The differential expression patterns and sub-localizations of these markers imply that CSCs possesses complex epigenetic and genetic alterations.

1.2 Isolation and Detection

Isolation and detection of CSCs depends on its specific biological and molecular features such as ability of spheres formation, generation of new tumors in mice, and positivity/differential expression patterns of stemness markers. The current analytical techniques for the CSC detection focus on functional, image-based, molecular, cytological sorting, filtration approaches, and xenotransplantation [24–26]. A graphical illustration of CSC isolation and characterization is illustrated in Fig. 1. Functional differences between CSCs and non-CSCs are identified by colony formation, sphere formation, side population (SP) analysis, aldehyde dehydrogenase (ALDH) activity, and therapy resistance assays [27]. In addition, CSCs can be specifically isolated from non-CSCs by sorting these cells by cell sorting methods like flow-cytometry and MACS (magnetic-activated cell sorting) using CSC-specific cell surface marker/s [28]. Furthermore, molecular methods to identify the expression (mRNA and protein) profiling of CSC markers using quantitative PCR, immunofluorescence, and immunohistochemistry are also widely used

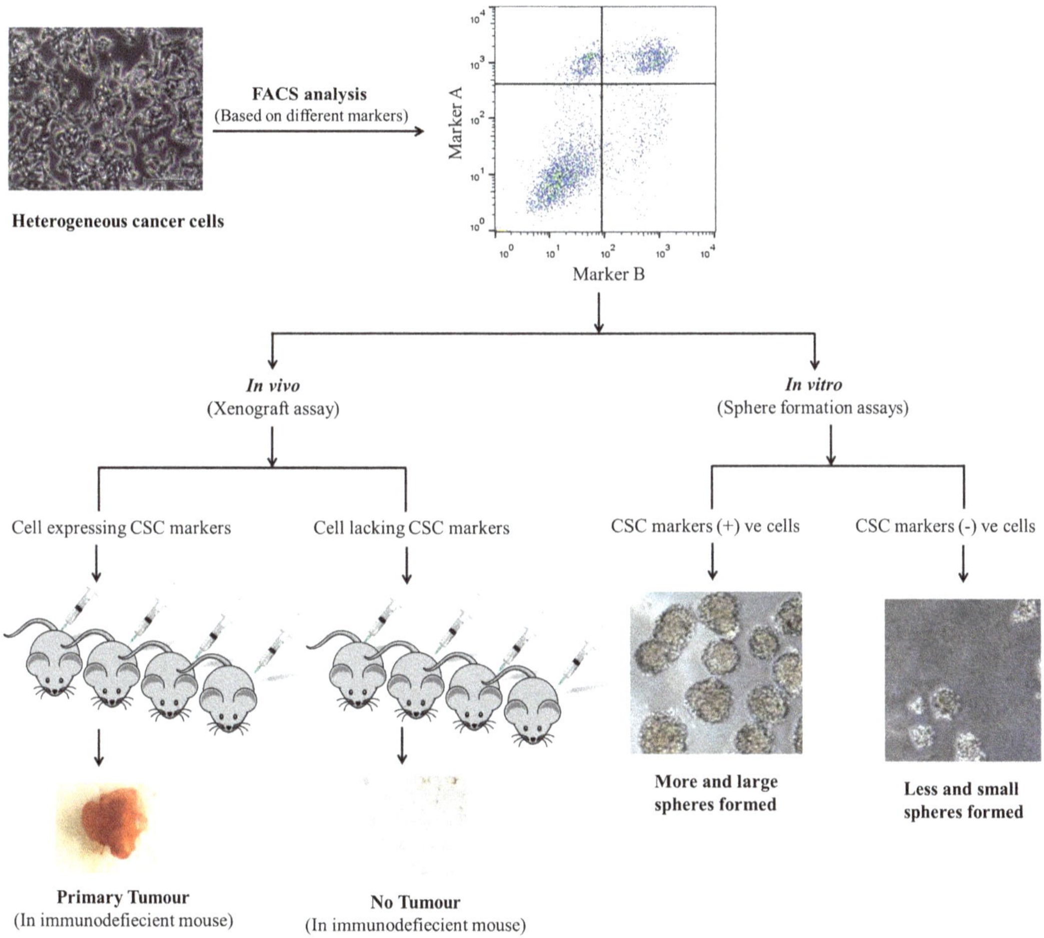

Fig. 1 Isolation and characterization of CSCs using FACS, in-vitro and in-vivo techniques. Surface markers play a key role in the further characterization or confirmation of CSCs. These cells can later undergo various in-vitro and in-vivo xenograft models to validate their biological characteristics

by researchers to confirm localization of the surface markers [24]. Recent studies have confirmed that the gold standard for the confirmation of CSCs is xenotransplantation into immune-deficient animals [29]. These methods are practiced in combination to achieve a sensitive/specific detection CSC isolation and detection in various tumors. Detailed methodology and steps are described below.

2 Materials

2.1 Cell Culture

1. Cancer cell lines.
2. Culture media: Rosewell Park Memorial Institute (RPMI) or Dulbecco's Modified Eagle Medium (DMEM).

3. Supplementary materials: 10% foetal bovine serum (FBS), 1% of 100 g/mL streptomycin, or/and 100 U/mL penicillin.
4. Cell dissociation solution: 0.25% Trypsin-ethylenediaminetetraacetic acid (EDTA).
5. Extra supplements: L-ascorbic acid, L-glutamine, bovine serum antigen, transferrin, insulin, 2-mercaptoethanol, etc. are required based on the tissue/cell type.
6. Cell counting device and microscope.

2.2 Cell Sorting and CSC Surface Markers

1. Aldefluor assay kit: specific for identification, evaluation, and isolation of stem and progenitor cells expressing high levels of ALDH.
2. Inhibitor of ALDH enzyme.
3. Dimethyl sulfoxide (DMSO).
4. 2 N Hydrochloric acid (HCl).
5. Diethylaminobenzaldehyde (DEAB).
6. A fluorescence-activated cell sorting (FACS) machine: e.g., MoFlow XDP Beckman Coulter Modular Flow Sorter or BD FACS Aria (*see* **Note 1**).
7. Antibodies for labeling: Antibodies include CD24, CD29, CD44, CD45, CD90, CD133, CD326, and cytokeratin (*see* **Note 2**).

2.3 Materials for Detecting CSC Functions

2.3.1 Sphere-Forming Assay

1. *Isolated CSCs cell population.*
2. *Culture plates*: 6-well ultra-low attachment plates.
3. Serum-free media: RPMI or DMEM medium supplemented with 20 ng/mL epidermal growth factor (EGF), 20 ng/mL basic fibroblast growth factor (bFGF), and B27 supplement (1: 50 ratio).
4. Phase-contrast microscope.

2.3.2 Western Blotting

The essential materials required for this step include

1. 200–600 μL protein buffer comprised of 10% cell lysis buffer.
2. 10% protease inhibitor cocktail.
3. 80% distilled water.
4. Bicinchoninic acid (BCA) protein assay kit.
5. 10% 2D polyacrylamide gel electrophoresis (PAGE) gel.
6. Gel electrophoresis.
7. 1× Laemmli running buffer (100 mL of 10× Laemmli stock in 1 L of distilled water).
8. 40 μg of extracted protein from CSCs.

9. Coomassie brilliant blue dye mixture.
10. Protein standard ladder.
11. Polyvinylidene fluoride (PVDF) membrane.
12. 1× blotting buffer (Tris/Lysate/10% methanol).
13. 5% Milk power solution.
14. Tris-Buffered Saline and Tween 20 (TBST) buffer.
15. Image development and detection system.

2.3.3 Immunostaining

1. Cell culture plates: 12-well or any other desired plates.
2. Sterile cover slips.
3. 70% ethanol.
4. 5% BSA (bovine serum albumin) in PBS.
5. Immunofluorescence compatible antibodies.
6. 4′,6-diamidino-2-phenylindole (DAPI).
7. Mounting media.
8. Confocal microscope.

2.3.4 Polymerase Chain Reaction (PCR)

1. Commercial mRNA/total RNA extraction kits (*see* **Note 3**).
2. cDNA conversion kit.
3. Cell lysis buffer.
4. RNase-free water.
5. DNase enzyme.
6. Nano-drop or other spectrometers to measure RNA concentration and quality.
7. Primers for PCR amplification of target genes.
8. Sybr-PCR master mix.
9. Real-time PCR machine.

3 Methods

3.1 Isolation and Sorting

The primary objective of this method is to identify and isolate the Aldefluor bright cells and CD44 or other desired stem cell markers in high population from the selected cancer cell groups. The key steps involved in this method are listed below in a sequential order.

1. Aldefluor reagent should be resuspended in 25 μL Dimethyl sulfoxide (DMSO) and allowed to stand for 1 min at room temperature. Then add 25 μL of 2 N hydrochloric acid (HCl) and incubate at room temperature for 15 min after mixing. Add 360 μL of Aldefluor assay buffer to this mixture and store in 2–8 °C.

2. Cells (~1 × 10^6 cells) should be detached using trypsin and then washed thrice with PBS. Resuspend this cell suspension with 1 mL of the Aldefluor assay buffer and select ~1 × 10^5 cells per milliliter using a haemocytometer or an automatic cell counter (*see* **Note 4**).
3. Antibody labeling: Dive each cell lineLineage into two tubes labeled as "test" and "control." The test tube cells will be treated with CD44-FITC-conjugated antibody, while the control test tube cells should be treated with RAE Control (S)-FITC mouse isotype control. Incubate the cells on ice for 30 min and kept in the dark with proper wrapping in aluminum foil for better efficiency. Afterward, centrifuge the cells at 800 rpm for 10 min at 4 °C. Remove the supernatant and resuspend the cells in 1% bovine serum albumin in phosphate-buffered saline (PBS) (100 mL).
4. Cell sorting: Elute the Aldefluor tested cells into 50 mL falcon tubes with their recommended culture media as well as FBS and 1% of penicillin- streptomycin antibiotic. During sorting, the cells expressing high levels of aldehyde dehydrogenase (ALDH) should be isolated and cultured to a healthy confluence of ~85% before the CD44 antibody sorting. After CD44 sorting, cells will be eluted into 1.5 mL Eppendorf tubes based on their CD44 expression. Cells expressing high levels of CD44 can be labeled as CSCs while the cells expressing lower levels of CD44 can be used as control cells (*see* **Note 5**).

3.2 In-Vitro Growth Properties of CSCs

Tumor sphere formation assay is the most commonly performed method to confirm the enrichment of cancer stemness and the self-renewal capacity. After sorting (as detailed above), plate the isolated CD44+ and ALDH+ cells in ultra-low attachment plates at a density of ~1000 viable cells per well. Growth of these cells should be maintained in a serum-free medium, at 37 °C in 5% carbon dioxide. Tumor spheres can be collected carefully after 7–10 days of growth and centrifuged gently (800 rpm/min) for 5 min (Fig. 2) (*see* **Note 6**).

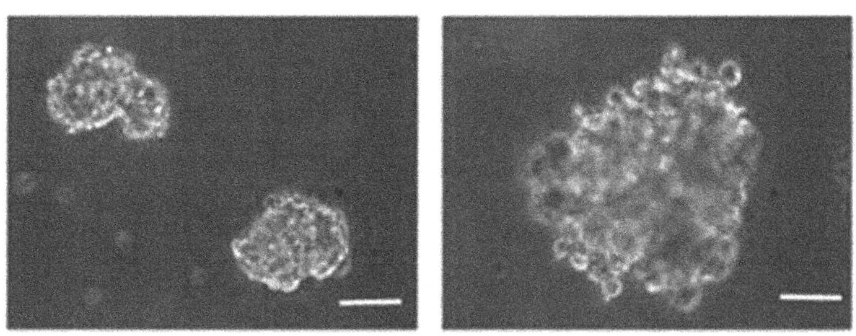

Fig. 2 Tumor sphere formation of CSC after isolation from FACS

3.3 Molecular Expression of CSC Markers

PCR and immunological methods are the commonly used methods to detect the expression and localization of surface markers in CSC after isolation. The key steps involved in each method are detailed below.

3.3.1 PCR

Following a commercial protocol, the total RNA was extracted following cell lysis. Then, filter with specific spin columns and follow with membrane-washing steps. Elute the RNA with an elution buffer and measure quality and purity by quantifying absorbance at 260 nm (A260) and 280 nm (A280) with a spectrophotometer (NanoDrop). The extracted RNA should undergo cDNA conversion following the manufacturer's guidelines (Eg- miSript reverse transcription kit, Qiagen). Once converted to cDNA, store them at −20 °C until used for PCR. A quantitative real-time PCR using specific primers of the cell surface markers (e.g., CD44, CD133, etc.) can be performed to detect the mRNA expression changes. PCR results of the CSC markers should be normalized to control gene/s such as alpha tubulin, beta actin, or glyceraldehyde 3-phosphate dehydrogenase (GAPDH). Detection of annealing and melting temperature can be obtained commercially or through running a graded PCR.

3.3.2 Western Blot

This method requires extraction of total proteins from tumor spheres and also from control cells. Approximately 40ug of the total protein should be used for this analysis. The key steps involved in this method are detailed below.

1. The total proteins were separated using 4–16% polyacrylamide gel and transferred onto the polyvinylidene difluoride (PVDF) membrane.
2. Block the PVDF membrane using 5% of nonfat milk for 90-min at room temperature, before incubating overnight with the CSC-specific antibodies at 4 °C.
3. Wash the membrane thrice with PBS-T and incubate with secondary antibody at room temperature for 30–90 min.
4. Detect the protein bands by enhanced chemiluminescence (ECL) and visualize them using a VersaDoc-MP Imaging system (BioRad) (*see* **Note** 7).

3.3.3 Immunological Analysis

Cellular distribution and qualitative expression of the stem cell markers can be confirmed with immunofluorescence analysis. First, seed the CSC spheres or cells directly on the sterile cover slips at a density of ~1×10^4 cm^2 and incubate them at 37 °C for 16 h. Succeeding incubation, wash cells with ice-cold PBS. For 30 min after incubation, fix the cells with 70% cold ethanol, subsequently wash again with PBS and block with 5% of BSA for 1 h at room temperature. After washing, incubate the cells with desired

CSC marker/s' antibodies at 4 °C overnight. With PBS, cells should be rinsed again and incubated with secondary antibody for 90 min at room temperature and light protected. After a final rinse with PBS-T three times for 10 min on a shaker, remove the cover slips with sterilized forceps and affix on a glass slide, with a drop of DAPI (and mounting media). Slides should be left to dry for 48 h and then observed by a confocal microscope.

4 Notes

1. The cells could be cultured in serum-free RPMI medium, supplemented with 20 ng/mL epidermal growth factor (EGF), 20 ng/mL basic fibroblast growth factor (bFGF), and B27 supplement (1: 50 ratio) at 37 °C in 5% carbon dioxide.
2. Based on the sensitivity of the assays, one to three or more antibodies can be used for labeling the stem cells from somatic cancer cell lines. A FITC-conjugated RAE (retinoid acid early inducible gene) control (S) antibody clone REA293 (a universal isotype control) is required for recognizing the cell surface antigens.
3. RNA extraction followed by cDNA conversion is required to confirm the CSC properties in the isolated cells using RT-qPCR. This semi-quantitative test will help in confirming the Western blot and immunological studies.
4. Prepare two separate tubes of selected cell populations the "test" and "control" tubes. Add 1 mL of the cell suspension into each of the tubes. Add 5 μL of the Aldefluor DEAB reagent into the "control" tube and add a same volume of the earlier activated Aldefluor reagent to each of the "test" samples, mix and transfer 0.5 mL of the mixture to the DEAB "control" tube. Incubate the samples for 30–45 min at 37 °C. Then, centrifuge for 5 min at 250 × g and remove the supernatant. After washing, the cell pellets should be resuspended again in 0.5 mL of Aldefluor assay buffer and stored on ice for flow cytometry.
5. To avoid the cells clumping during the cell sorting they will be resuspended in a buffer comprising of PBS, 10% FBS, and 2 mM EDTA.
6. Cells obtained from dissociation can be sieved through a 40 μm sieve and analyzed microscopically for single cellularity. If groups of cells were present at a frequency >150 for 10,000 single cells, mechanical dissociation and sieving can be repeated.
7. High protein expression is correlated with a strong/thick band and lower expression of proteins is represented as a thin/weak band.

References

1. Islam F, Gopalan V, Smith RA, Lam AK (2015) Translational potential of cancer stem cells: a review of the detection of cancer stem cells and their roles in cancer recurrence and cancer treatment. Exp Cell Res 335:135–147
2. Frank NY, Schatton T, Frank MH (2010) The therapeutic promise of the cancer stem cell concept. J Clin Invest 120:41–50
3. Zhou BB, Zhang H, Damelin M, Geles KG, Grindley JC, Dirks PB (2009) Tumour-initiating cells: challenges and opportunities for anticancer drug discovery. Nat Rev Drug Discov 8:806–823
4. Islam F, Qiao B, Smith RA, Gopalan V, Lam AK (2015) Cancer stem cell: fundamental experimental pathological concepts and updates. Exp Mol Pathol 98:184–191
5. Major AG, Pitty LP, Farah CS (2013) Cancer stem cell markers in head and neck squamous cell carcinoma. Stem Cells Int 2013:319489
6. Sayed SI, Dwivedi RC, Katna R, Garg A, Pathak KA, Nutting CM, Rhys-Evans P, Harrington KJ, Kazi R (2011) Implications of understanding cancer stem cell (CSC) biology in head and neck squamous cell cancer. Oral Oncol 47:237–243
7. Deonarain MP, Kousparou CA, Epenetos AA (2009) Antibodies targeting cancer stem cells: a new paradigm in immunotherapy? MAbs 1:12–25
8. Bonnet D, Dick JE (1997) Human acute myeloid leukemia is organized as a hierarchy that originates from a primitive hematopoietic cell. Nat Med 3:730–737
9. Collins AT, Berry PA, Hyde C, Stower MJ, Maitland NJ (2005) Prospective identification of tumourigenic prostate cancer stem cells. Cancer Res 65:10946–10951
10. O'Brien CA, Pollett A, Gallinger S, Dick JE (2007) A human colon cancer cell capable of initiating tumour growth in immunodeficient mice. Nature 445:106–110
11. Dirks PB (2008) Brain tumour stem cells: bringing order to the chaos of brain cancer. J Clin Oncol 26:2916–2924
12. Zhao W, Ji X, Zhang F, Li L, Ma L (2012) Embryonic stem cell markers. Molecules 17:6196–6236
13. Shah A, Patel S, Pathak J, Swain N, Kumar S (2014) The evolving concepts of cancer stem cells in head and neck squamous cell carcinoma. Sci World J 2014:842491
14. Karsten U, Goletz S (2013) What makes cancer stem cell markers different? Springerplus 2:301
15. Hsu CC, Chiang CW, Cheng HC, Chang WT, Chou CY, Tsai HW, Lee CT, Wu ZH, Lee TY, Chao A, Chow NH, Ho CL (2011) Identifying LRRC16B as an oncofetal gene with transforming enhancing capability using a combined bioinformatics and experimental approach. Oncogene 30:654–667
16. Hennen E, Faissner A (2012) Lewis X: A neural stem cell specific glycan? Int J Biochem Cell Biol 44:830–833
17. Monzani E, Facchetti F, Galmozzi E, Corsini E, Benetti A, Cavazzin C, Gritti A, Piccini A, Porro D, Santinami M, Invernici G, Parati E, Alessandri G, LaPorta CA (2007) Melanoma contains CD133 and ABCG2 positive cells with enhanced tumourigenic potential. Eur J Cancer 43:935–946
18. Guo W, Lasky JL, Chang C-J, Mosessian S, Lewis X, Xiao Y, Yeh JE, Chen JY, Iruela-Arispe ML, Varella-Garcia M, Wu H (2008) Multi-genetic events collaboratively contribute to Pten-null leukemia stem-cell formation. Nature 453:529–533
19. Günthert U, Hofmann M, Rudy W, Reber S, Zöller M, Haussmann I, Matzku S, Wenzel A, Ponta H, Herrlich P (1991) A new variant of glycoprotein CD44 confers metastatic potential to rat carcinoma cells. Cell 65:13–24
20. Cheung AM, Wan TS, Leung JC, Chan LY, Huang H, Kwong YL, Liang R, Leung AY (2007) Aldehyde dehydrogenase activity in leukemic blasts defines a subgroup of acute myeloid leukemia with adverse prognosis and superior NOD/ SCID engrafting potential. Leukemia 21:1423–1430
21. Ginestier C, Hur MH, Charafe-Jauffret E, Monville F, Dutcher J, Brown M, Jacquemier J, Viens P, Kleer CG, Liu S, Schott A, Hayes D, Birnbaum D, Wicha MS, Dontu G (2007) ALDH1 is a marker of normal and malignant human mammary stem cells and a predictor of poor clinical outcome. Cell Stem Cell 1:555–567
22. Carpentino JE, Hynes MJ, Appelman HD, Zheng T, Steindler DA, Scott EW, Huang EH (2009) Aldehyde dehydrogenase-expressing colon stem cells contribute to tumorigenesis in the transition from colitis to cancer. Cancer Res 69:8208–8215
23. Li R, Wu X, Wei H, Tian S (2013) Characterization of side population cells isolated from the gastric cancer cell line SGC7901. Oncol Lett 5:877–883
24. Lianidou ES, Markou A (2011) Circulating tumor cells in breast cancer: detection systems,

molecular characterization, and future challenges. Clin Chem 57:1242–1255
25. Tirino V, Desiderio V, Paino F, De Rosa A, Papaccio F, La Noce M, Laino L, De Francesco F, Papaccio G (2013) Cancer stem cells in solid tumors: an overview and new approaches for their isolation and characterization. FASEB J 27:13–24
26. Milne AN, Carneiro F, O'Morain C, Offerhaus GJ (2009) Nature meets nurture: molecular genetics of gastric cancer. Hum Genet 126:615–628
27. Podberezin M, Wen J, Chang CC (2013) Cancer stem cells: a review of potential clinical applications. Arch Pathol Lab Med 137:1111–1116
28. Greve B, Beller C, Cassens U, Sibrowski W, Göhde W (2006) The impact of erythrocyte lysing procedures on the recovery of hematopoietic progenitor cells in flow cytometric analysis. Stem Cells 24:793–799
29. Fulawka L, Donizy P, Halon A (2014) Cancer stem cells - the current status of an old concept: literature review and clinical approaches. Biol Res 47:66
30. Wang K, Wei G, Liu D (2012) CD19: a biomarker for B cell development, lymphoma diagnosis and therapy. Exp Hematol Oncol 1:36
31. Ferrero E, Malavasi F (1999) The metamorphosis of a molecule: from soluble enzyme to the leukocyte receptor CD38. J Leukoc Biol 65:151–161
32. Andrews RG, Singer JW, Bernstein ID (1989) Precursors of colony-forming cells in humans can be distinguished from colony-forming cells by expression of the CD33 and CD34 antigens and light scatter properties. J Exp Med 169:1721–1731
33. Ponta H, Sherman L, Herrlich PA (2003) CD44: from adhesion molecules to signaling regulators. Nat Rev Mol Cell Biol 4:33–45
34. Snyder EL, Bailey D, Shipitsin M, Polyak K, Loda M (2009) Identification of CD44v6(+)/CD24- breast carcinoma cells in primary human tumors by quantum dot-conjugated antibodies. Lab Investig 89:857–866
35. Vassilopoulos A, Chisholm C, Lahusen T, Zheng H, Deng CX (2014) A critical role of CD29 and CD49f in mediating metastasis for cancer-initiating cells isolated from a Brca1-associated mouse model of breast cancer. Oncogene 33:5477–5482
36. Lv X, Wang Y, Song Y, Pang X, Li H (2016) Association between ALDH1+/CD133+ stem-like cells and tumor angiogenesis in invasive ductal breast carcinoma. Oncol Lett 11:1750–1756
37. Farhana L, Antaki F, Anees MR, Nangia-Makker P, Judd S, Hadden T, Levi E, Murshed F, Yu Y, Van Buren E, Ahmed K, Dyson G, Majumdar AP (2016) Role of cancer stem cells in racial disparity in colorectal cancer. Cancer Med 5:1268–1278
38. Grunt TW, Hebar A, Laffer S, Wagner R, Peter B, Herrmann H, Graf A, Bilban M, Posch M, Hoermann G, Mayerhofer M, Eisenwort G, Zielinski CC, Selzer E, Valent P (2015) Prominin-1 (CD133, AC133) and dipeptidyl-peptidase IV (CD26) are indicators of infinitive growth in colon cancer cells. Am J Cancer Res 5:560–574
39. Mărgaritescu C, Pirici D, Cherciu I, Bărbălan A, Cârtână T, Săftoiu A (2014) CD133/CD166/Ki-67 triple immunofluorescence assessment for putative cancer stem cells in colon carcinoma. J Gastrointestin Liver Dis 23:161–170
40. Vaiopoulos AG, Kostakis ID, Koutsilieris M, Papavassiliou AG (2012) Colorectal cancer stem cells. Stem Cells 30:363–371
41. He J, Liu Y, Zhu T, Zhu J, Dimeco F, Vescovi AL, Heth JA, Muraszko KM, Fan X, Lubman DM (2012) CD90 is identified as a candidate marker for cancer stem cells in primary high-grade gliomas using tissue microarrays. Mol Cell Proteomics 11:M111.010744
42. Singh SK, Hawkins C, Clarke ID, Squire JA, Bayani J, Hide T, Henkelman RM, Cusimano MD, Dirks PB (2004) Identification of human brain tumour initiating cells. Nature 432:396–401
43. Dahlrot RH, Hermansen SK, Hansen S, Kristensen BW (2013) What is the clinical value of cancer stem cell markers in gliomas? Int J Clin Exp Pathol 6:334–348
44. Prince ME, Sivanandan R, Kaczorowski A, Wolf GT, Kaplan MJ, Dalerba P, Weissman IL, Clarke MF, Ailles LE (2007) Identification of a subpopulation of cells with cancer stem cell properties in head and neck squamous cell carcinoma. Proc Natl Acad Sci U S A 104:973–978
45. Murillo-Sauca O, Chung MK, Shin JH, Karamboulas C, Kwok S, Jung YH, Oakley R, Tysome JR, Farnebo LO, Kaplan MJ, Sirjani D, Divi V, Holsinger FC, Tomeh C, Nichols A, Le QT, Colevas AD, Kong CS, Uppaluri R, Lewis JS Jr, Ailles LE, Sunwoo JB (2014) CD271 is a functional and targetable marker of tumor-initiating cells in head and neck squamous cell carcinoma. Oncotarget 5:6854–6866

46. Fang D, Nguyen TK, Leishear K, Finko R, Kulp AN, Hotz S, Van Belle PA, Xu X, Elder DE, Herlyn M (2005) A tumorigenic subpopulation with stem cell properties in melanomas. Cancer Res 65:9328–9337
47. Sun JH, Luo Q, Liu LL, Song GB (2016) Liver cancer stem cell markers: progression and therapeutic implications. World J Gastroenterol 22:3547–3557
48. Miyata T, Yoshimatsu T, So T, Oyama T, Uramoto H, Osaki T, Nakanishi R, Tanaka F, Nagaya H, Gotoh A (2015) Cancer stem cell markers in lung cancer. Personalized Medicine Universe 4:40–45
49. Zhu YY, Yuan Z (2015) Pancreatic cancer stem cells. Am J Cancer Res 5:894–906
50. Moltzahn F, Thalmann GN (2013) Cancer stem cells in prostate cancer. Transl Androl Urol 2:242–253
51. Qian X, Tan C, Wang F, Yang B, Ge Y, Guan Z, Cai J (2016) Esophageal cancer stem cells and implications for future therapeutics. Onco Targets Ther 9:2247–2254
52. Yao T, Lu R, Zhang Y, Zhang Y, Zhao C, Lin R, Lin Z (2015) Cervical cancer stem cells. Cell Prolif 48:611–625
53. Brungs D, Aghmesheh M, Vine KL, Becker TM, Carolan MG, Ranson M (2016) Gastric cancer stem cells: evidence, potential markers, and clinical implications. J Gastroenterol 51:313–326

Chapter 3

The Role of CD44 and Cancer Stem Cells

Liang Wang, Xiangsheng Zuo, Keping Xie, and Daoyan Wei

Abstract

Solid tumors are composed of mutually interacting cancer cells and tumor microenvironment. Many environmental components, such as extracellular matrix (ECM), mesenchymal stem cells, endothelial and immune cells, and various growth factors and cytokines, provide signals, either stimulatory or inhibitory, to cancer cells and determine their fates. Meanwhile, cancer cells can also educate surrounding cells or tissues to undergo changes that are in favorable of tumor progression. CD44, as a transmembrane receptor for hyaluronic acid (HA) and many other ECM components and a coreceptor for growth factors and cytokines, is a critical cell surface molecule that can sense, integrate, and transduce cellular microenvironmental signals to membrane-associated cytoskeletal proteins or to cell nucleus to regulate a variety of gene expressions that govern cell behaviors. Mounting evidence suggests that CD44, particularly CD44v isoforms, are cancer stem cell (CSC) markers and critical regulators of cancer stemness, including self-renewal, tumor initiation, and metastasis. Thus, CD44 is widely used alone or in combination with other cell surface markers to isolate or enrich CSCs through fluorescence-activated cell sorting of dissociated single cells that originate from the patient, xenograft tumor tissues, or tumor cell cultures. Sorted cells are cultured in a specialized culture medium for spheroid formation or inoculated into immunodeficient mice for the analysis of tumorigenic or metastatic potential. In this chapter, detailed experimental methods regarding $CD44^+$ tumor cell isolation, spheroid culture, and characterization will be described.

Key words CD44, Cancer stem cell, Methods, Cell sorting, Biomarker, Splicing variants, Tumor spheroid, Therapeutic target, Tumor microenvironment

1 Introduction

Heterogeneity is a common feature of tumors. Within a tumor mass, the genetic and phenotypic characteristics of cancer cells, including cellular morphology, gene expression, metabolism, proliferation, and metastatic potential, can vary [1]. The heterogeneity of cancer cells brings significant challenges both clinically, in designing effective treatment strategies, and experimentally, in understanding the causes and pathogenesis of disease. Accumulating evidence suggests that only a small population of cells within a tumor mass is responsible for the tumor heterogeneity. These cells are termed cancer stem cells (CSCs) and characterized by their

Gianpaolo Papaccio and Vincenzo Desiderio (eds.), *Cancer Stem Cells: Methods and Protocols*, Methods in Molecular Biology, vol. 1692, DOI 10.1007/978-1-4939-7401-6_3, © Springer Science+Business Media LLC 2018

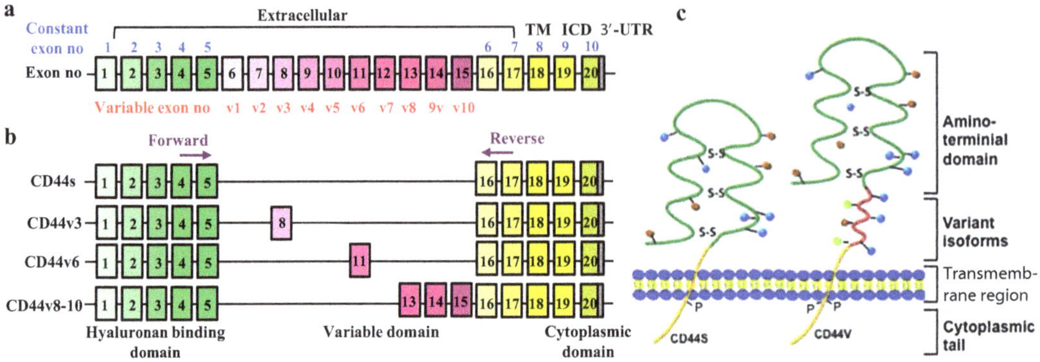

Fig. 1 Diagrammatic structure of the CD44 gene and protein. (**a**) Schematic structure of the CD44 gene. This gene consists of several exons, some of which are constant exons that are used in every CD44 mRNA and protein (*green* and *yellow boxes*). Others are variant exons (*pink boxes*) that are used in the CD44 splicing variant (CD44v) mRNAs and proteins. (**b**) Schematic structure of CD44 pre-mRNAs. The standard CD44 (CD44s) does not contain any variant exons, whereas CD44 splicing variants contain distinct variable exons. Examples shown here are CD44v3, CD44v6, and CD44v8-10. A reverse transcriptase PCR-based DNA sequence analysis using a pair of PCR primers that cover the constant exon 5 and exon 16 regions (*purple arrows*) is often used to identify specific CD44 variants in different cells or tissues. (**c**) CD44 protein structural domains. The CD44 protein is composed of an extracellular link domain, a stalk-like region in the extracellular domain close to the transmembrane region, where the variant exon products (*red*) are inserted, the transmembrane region, and the intracellular cytoplasmic domain. Abbreviation: *TM* transmembrane region, *ICD* intracellular cytoplasmic domain, *UTR* untranslated region. (Adapted from Yongmin Yan, Xiangsheng Zuo, and Daoyan Wei, Stem Cells Translational Medicine, 2015; 4:1033–1043. ©AlphaMed Press 2015 (*9*).)

abilities to self-renew and differentiate into multiple cell types. CSCs are thus responsible for tumor initiation, progression, recurrence, and metastasis [2]. Therapies specifically targeting CSCs hold great promise for improving survival outcomes in patients with cancer. Over the past few decades, tremendous efforts have been made to identify and characterize CSCs in various tumors. Identifying CSC-specific markers to isolate or target CSCs remains the fundamental technical challenge and primary research focus in the field of CSCs.

CD44, a multistructural and multifunctional transmembrane glycoprotein, is encoded by the highly conserved CD44 gene on chromosome 11 in humans [3]. The full-length CD44 gene has 20 exons and 19 introns (Fig. 1), of which 10 exons are expressed in all isoforms (known as “constant” exons), while the 10 central exons (known as “variable” exons) undergo extensive alternative splicing via inclusion or excision in various combinations in the membrane-proximal stem region to generate splicing variants (CD44v isoforms). The so-called standard isoform (CD44s) is the smallest one, which lacks all variant exons in the extracellular domains and is expressed on most vertebrate cells; whereas CD44v isoforms, often acquiring a new function as a coreceptor for many growth factors and nonreceptor protein-tyrosine kinases, or as a cofactor interacting with other proteins when inclusion of different combinations of exons v1-v10, are expressed only on some cells under specific conditions. For instance, the sequence encoded by exon v3 has a heparin-sulfate site, which allows CD44v3 to bind several heparan sulfate-binding growth factors such as fibroblast growth factors (FGFs) and epidermal growth factor (EGF) [4], whereas CD44 v8-10 is able to interact with and stabilizes xCT, a subunit of the cystine-glutamate transporter xc(−), and thereby promotes cystine uptake to enhance GSH synthesis, which is the primary intracellular antioxidant [5]. The enhanced resistance to reactive oxidative species (ROS) endows CSCs with survival advantage and thus, drives tumor growth, metastasis, and chemoresistance. The inclusion of variant exons has been found to be regulated, at least in part, by mitogenic or oncogenic signals [6, 7]. Therefore, cancer cells often express a large variety of CD44 variants, particularly when the cancer is in an advanced stage [8].

Importantly, CD44 has been identified as a typical CSC surface marker, individually or in combination with other marker(s) such as CD24, CD133, CD34, and c-Met, for isolating or enriching CSCs in various types of cancer [9]. Initially, breast tumor cells with $CD44^{+}CD24^{-/low}Lineage^{-}$ markers were isolated from breast cancer tissues and demonstrated to have tumor initiating potential. As few as 100 cells carrying this phenotype were able to form tumors in immunocompromised mice, whereas tens of thousands of cells bearing alternate phenotypes failed to do so. The tumorigenic subpopulation could be serially passaged, and the new tumors generated in each round of passage contain phenotypically diverse mixed $CD44^{+}CD24^{-/low}Lineage^{-}$ tumorigenic cells and other populations of nontumorigenic cells [10]. This was the first demonstration that a subpopulation of $CD44^{+}CD24^{-/low}Lineage^{-}$ cells is putative breast CSCs. Later, $CD44^{+}$ cells were identified as gastric cancer initiating cells from a panel of human gastric cancer cell lines [11]. $CD44^{+}$ cells showed spheroid colony formation in serum-free medium in vitro, as well as tumorigenic ability when injected into stomach or skin of severe combined immunodeficient (SCID) mice in vivo. Also, the $CD44^{+}$ gastric cancer cells displayed the stem cell properties of self-renewal and the ability to form differentiated progeny and gave rise to $CD44^{-}$ cells. Additionally, the $CD44^{+}$ gastric cancer cells exhibited increased resistance to radiation- or chemotherapy-induced cell death. On the contrary, CD44 knockdown led to much reduced spheroid colony formation and smaller tumor production in SCID mice, and the $CD44^{-}$ populations had significantly decreased tumorigenic ability in vitro and in vivo, whereas other potential CSC markers, such as CD24, CD133, stage-specific embryonic antigen-1 (SSEA-1), or sorting for side population, did not show any association with tumorigenicity in vitro or in vivo. These results indicate the existence of gastric CSCs and identified CD44 as a reliable cell surface marker for gastric CSCs. More significantly, the functional role of CD44 as a biomarker as well as a regulator of CSC was further demonstrated by CD44 direct reprogramming of $CD44^-$ colon cancer cells into $CD44^+$ stem-like cancer cells [12], whereas down-regulation of CD44 expression revealed the opposite effect in head and neck cancer cells [13].

The unique expression pattern and function of CD44v makes it more attractive and clinically significant to investigate as a potential CSC marker. Indeed, recent studies showed that CD44v6 functions as a CSC marker in colon cancer [14], whereas CD44v8-10 is a CSC marker specific to gastric cancer and CD44v3 is a CSC marker specific to head and neck cancer [15, 16]. Mechanistically, CD44, and particularly the CD44v isoform, can serve as a CSC marker not only because of its specific expression on the cell surface but also, more importantly, because of its profound effects on regulating CSC properties. These regulatory effects range from integrating and transmitting tumor environmental and cellular signaling to the nucleus for self-renewal to protecting the cell from stress-induced damage or apoptosis by ROS or other adverse stimuli [9]. This basic knowledge may help in the design of rational experiments to further identify and characterize CSCs in various cancers. This chapter presents detailed experimental methods for $CD44^+$ cell isolation, spheroid culture, and characterization, and pancreatic cancer will be used as an example.

2 Materials

2.1 Single-Cell Suspension Preparation

1. Complete medium. Dulbecco's modified Eagle medium supplemented with 10% fetal bovine serum (FBS) and 100 units/mL penicillin/streptomycin. Store at 4 °C.
2. Cell dissociation buffer. Dulbecco's modified Eagle medium supplemented with 200 U/mL collagenase type IV and 0.6 U/mL Dispase. This is freshly made before every use.
3. 40 μm Steriflip filter units.
4. Red blood cell lysing buffer.
5. CSC medium. Serum-free Dulbecco's modified Eagle medium/nutrient mixture F-12 HAM medium supplemented with 2 mM glutamine, 20 ng/mL human recombinant epidermal growth factor, 10 ng/mL human recombinant basic fibroblast growth factor, 2% N2, and 1% B27 supplements (Life Technologies, Carlsbad, CA) (*see* **Note 1**).
6. Gelatin solution (Sigma-Aldrich).
7. Trypan blue.
8. Phosphate-buffered saline.
9. Trypsin-EDTA solution.

2.2 Cell Staining for Flow Cytometry

1. Sterile 5 mL polystyrene round-bottom tubes (12 × 75 mm style).
2. Bovine serum albumin (BSA).
3. 4′,6-diamidino-2-phenylindole, dihydrochloride (DAPI).
4. Antibodies: FITC-conjugated rat anti-human c-Met antibody, PE-conjugated mouse anti-human CD44 antibody (*see* **Note 2**), and Biotin-labeled anti-mouse H2K antibody and APC Streptavidin dye (secondary for anti-mouse H2K antibody).
5. Fluorescence-activated cell sorting (FACS) machine for flow cytometry.

2.3 Tumor Spheroid Culture

1. CSC medium is the same as that in Subheading 2.1.
2. Ultra-low attachment plate (Corning, Corning, NY).
3. StemProAccutase (Life Technologies).
4. siPORT NeoFx transfection agent (Ambion/Invitrogen, Carlsbad, CA) or equivalent.
5. Opti-MEM I reduced serum media.
6. Control and human CD44 siRNA.

3 Methods

3.1 Preparation of Single-Cell Suspension of Tumor Cells

3.1.1 Generation of Cell Suspensions from Tumor Tissues

1. Tumor tissue can be obtained from surgically removed patient specimens or patient-derived xenografts from mice. Tumor tissues can be temporarily stored in complete medium at 4 °C but should be processed within 24 h of surgical resection for maximal cell viability.
2. In a sterile biosafety cabinet, transfer the tumor tissue to a 60 × 15 mm cell culture dish containing 1 mL of sterile cell dissociation buffer (*see* **Note 3**). Mechanically mince tumors into 1 to 5 mm pieces using a sterile scalpel and forceps (Fig. 2a, b).
3. Add 1 mL of cell dissociation buffer to the cell culture dish. Repeat the trituration step until the tissue is completely dissociated—usually three to four repetitions are required.
4. Transfer the total tumor cell suspension to a 50 mL conical tube using a 5 mL serologic pipet. The tumor pieces should be small enough that they do not clog the pipet.
5. Add cell dissociation buffer to a final volume of 20 mL and vortex at maximum speed (approximately 3200 rotations per minute) for 1 min.
6. Incubate the tumor cell suspension at 37 °C for 30 min, with intermittent shaking every 10 min.

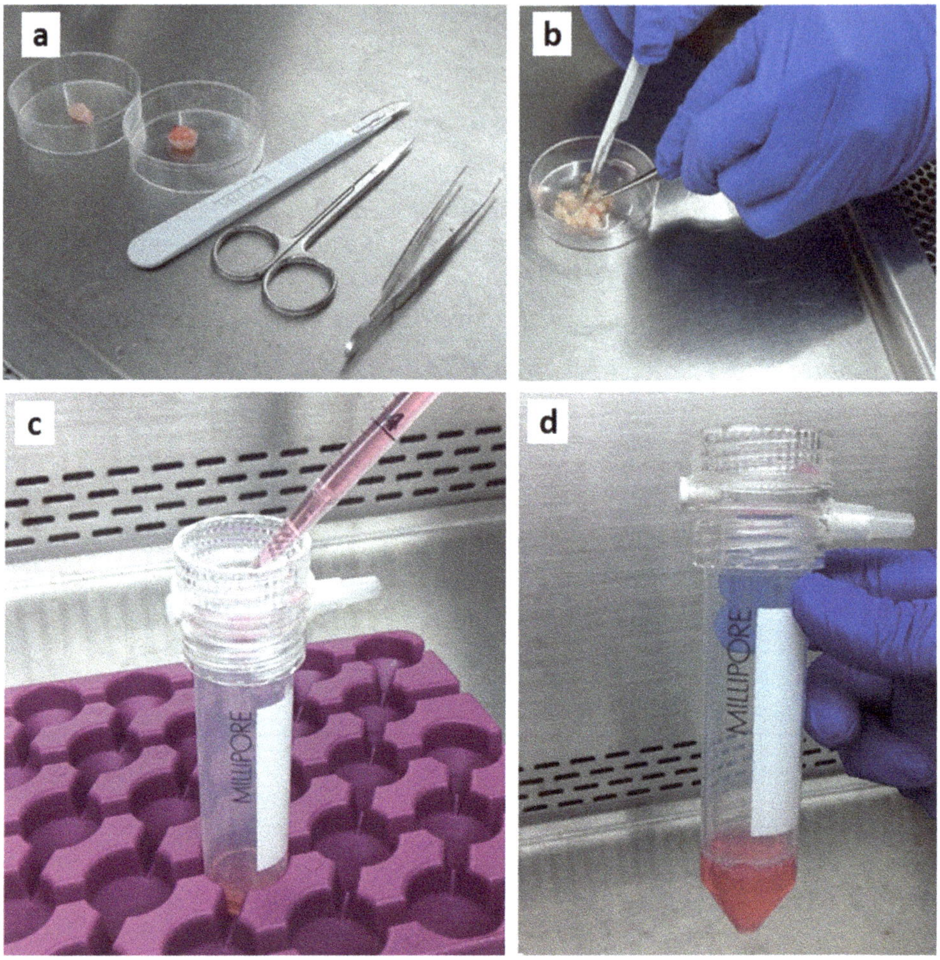

Fig. 2 Preparation of single-cell suspension from tumor tissues. (**a**) Mouse xenograft tumor tissues and tools used for cell dissociation. (**b**) Mechanical dissociation using a scalpel and forceps. (**c**) Cell suspension filtered through a cell strainer. (**d**) Collected follow-through cell suspension

7. After 30 min of incubation, filter the resulting suspension through a 40 μm cell strainer and collect follow-through cells into a second sterile 50 mL conical tube (Fig. 2c, d).
8. Centrifuge the tube at 1000 rotations per minute for 5 min to get cell pellet.
9. Gently decant the supernatant and add 5 mL of red blood cell lysing buffer to resuspend the cell pellet. Incubate the solution for 5 min at room temperature. Remove the red blood cell lysis buffer using centrifugation at 1000 rotations per minute for 5 min at room temperature.
10. Optional (*see* **Note 4**): Resuspend the cell pellet in the CSC medium. Plate the pellet on a gelatin-coated dish and incubate

it at 37 °C for 1 h. After incubation, carefully recover the cell suspension in the dish.

11. Quantify the number of viable (trypan blue-negative) cells using a hemocytometer or automated cell counter. Generate a suspension of 1×10^6 cells/mL. This can be kept on ice for antibody staining.

3.1.2 Generation of Cell Suspensions from Tumor Cell Lines

1. When cells reach 80–90% confluence in a 100 mm culture dish (5–10 million cells per dish), wash cells once with sterile PBS.
2. Detach the cells from dishes using Trypsin-EDTA and centrifuge at 1000 rotations per minute for 5 min to get cell pellet.
3. Resuspend the cell pellet in 1× PBS and adjust the cell concentration to 1×10^6 cells/mL. The cell suspension can be kept on ice for antibody staining.

3.2 Cell Staining with Antibody for FACS

1. Prepare single-cell suspensions in Dulbecco's PBS (DPBS)/1% BSA solution (*see* **Note 5**) at a concentration of 1 to 5×10^6 cells/mL. All the solutions should be on ice during the whole process and centrifugation should be done at 4 °C.
2. Prepare the single-color-staining controls by aliquoting 200 μL cell suspensions into four individual tubes. Label the tubes DAPI, H2K, CD44-PE, and c-Met-FITC. For primary cancer cells from patient specimens and human cell lines, three single-color-staining controls (DAPI, CD44-PE, and c-Met-FITC) are needed because H2K (mouse histocompatibility class I) is an antibody used to remove mouse-specific cells and is needed only for patient-derived xenograft samples collected from mice. Label another tube as the experimental tube and aliquot a 1 mL cell suspension into it for FACS of CSCs.
3. Avoid exposure to light from this step forward. Add each antibody (except DAPI) to the appropriate control tube and add all antibodies to the experimental tube at a 1:40 dilution. Incubate all tubes for 30 min on ice (*see* **Note 6**).
4. After incubation, wash all the samples twice with DPBS/1% BSA solution.
5. If the H2K antibody was used, resuspend cells in a H2K tube and an experimental tube to the original volume with DPBS/1% BSA solution. Then add APC Streptavidin dye to the H2K tube and experimental tube at a dilution of 1:200. Incubate both the tubes for 20 min on ice.
6. Spin down all tubes, carefully aspirate the supernatant, and resuspend cells in DPBS/1% BSA solution containing 1 μg/mL DAPI.
7. Run all single-color-staining controls individually, to adjust the voltage and gates.

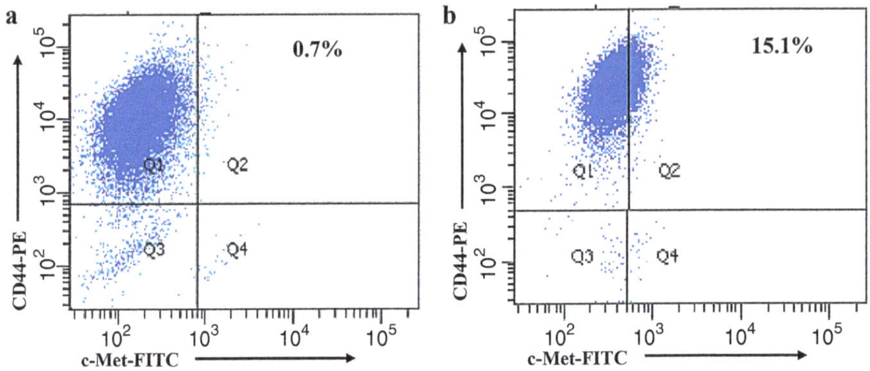

Fig. 3 Isolation of pancreatic cancer stem cells by fluorescence-activated cell sorting. The plots depicted are representative examples of patterns of CD44 and c-Met staining of two pancreatic cancer cell lines, the parental Colo357 (**a**) and its metastatic deviant L3.7 (**b**). The subpopulation of Q2 are CD44 and c-Met double-positive cells, which have been demonstrated to be pancreatic cancer stem cells [17]

8. Prerun the sample and set the gates for sorting, and then sort the sample. In all experiments using human xenograft tissue, eliminate any infiltrating mouse cells by discarding $H2K^+$ cells during flow cytometry. Eliminate dead cells by using the viability dye DAPI. Eliminate cell doublets using side-scatter and forward-scatter profiles. Examples of FACS results for CD44-PE and c-Met-FITC sorting from two pancreatic cancer cell lines are shown in Fig. 3.
9. Reanalyze the cells for purity to confirm complete separation of different subpopulations (*see* **Note 7**).

3.3 Tumor Spheroid Formation Assay

3.3.1 Primary Spheroid Formation Assay

1. Adjust the sorted cells from the last step to a concentration of 2000 cells/mL with CSC medium (*see* **Note 8**).
2. Seed 2 mL of the cells to each well of the 6-well ultra-low attachment plate with three replicates for each sample. Gently rock the plate first back and forth and then left and right to distribute cells evenly in the wells before placing the plate into the incubator.
3. Incubate the cells at 37 °C in a 5% CO_2 incubator for 2–4 weeks. During this period of culture, fresh CSC medium can be added every other day to maintain a proper concentration of growth factors. A significant fraction of cells grown in these conditions will die in the first few days. If there are too many dead cells, they may interfere with the growth of living cells, and the medium needs to be changed. To change the medium, transfer the cell culture from each well to a 15 mL conical tube, centrifuge the tube at low speed (<800 rotations per minute) for 5 min, and aspirate the supernatant carefully to remove dead cells and cell debris. Be cautious not to disturb the spheroid-forming cells at the bottom. Next, add fresh CSC

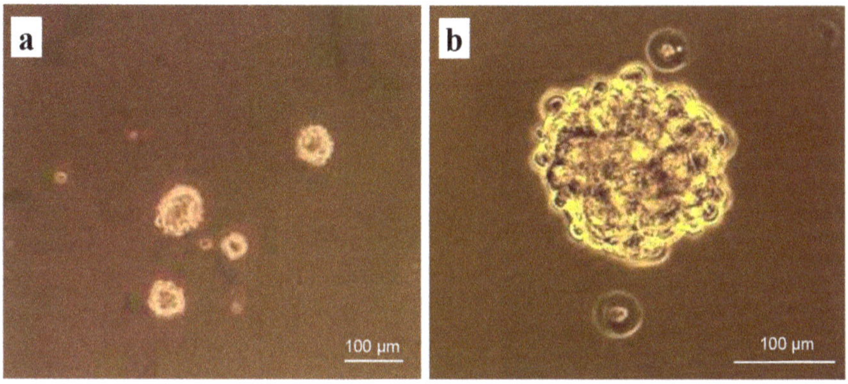

Fig. 4 Primary tumor spheroid formation from sorted CD44^{+}/c-Met^{+} PANC-1 pancreatic cancer cells. (**a**) Small spheroids appear at day 7 of incubation. (**b**) A large spheroid is formed at day 14 of incubation

medium into individual 15 mL conical tubes to make cell (or cell cluster) suspensions, then transfer cell suspensions to a new set of wells in the 6-well ultra-low attachment plate for continuing culture. Non-adherent spherical clusters of cells (spheroids) will form in about 7–10 days, and larger spheroids can be observed in about 2–3 weeks (Fig. 4).

4. The typical primary spheres with >50 cells isolated from the culture spheres can be digested with StemProAccutase to prepare a single-cell suspension for secondary spheroid formation assay, or other functional assays to identify features of cancer cell stemness, such as drug or radiation resistance or in vivo tumorigenic and metastatic potential (detailed protocols and troubleshooting of such assays can be found in related chapters of this book), or to define the function of a specific gene in the regulation of cancer stemness (*see* below).

3.3.2 CD44 Knockdown on Secondary Spheroid Formation

1. Collect primary spheres by centrifugation at 800 rotations per minute for 5 min. Wash the pellet once with sterile PBS and perform centrifugation again for 5 min. Digest primary spheres with StemProAccutase for 15–20 min in a 37 °C incubator.
2. During digestion, prepare the siRNA transfection complexes using control or CD44 siRNA and siPORT NeoFx Tranfection Agent according to the manufacturer's instructions (*see* **Note 9**). In brief, individually dilute siPORT NeoFX Transfection Agent and siRNA oligos (siCtrl or siCD44) in Opti-MEM I medium and incubate for 10 min at room temperature. Mix diluted siRNA and diluted siPORT NeoFX Transfection Agent together and incubate for 10 min at room temperature to allow transfection complexes to form. Then, dispense the transfection complexes into the wells of a 24-well ultra-low attachment plate.

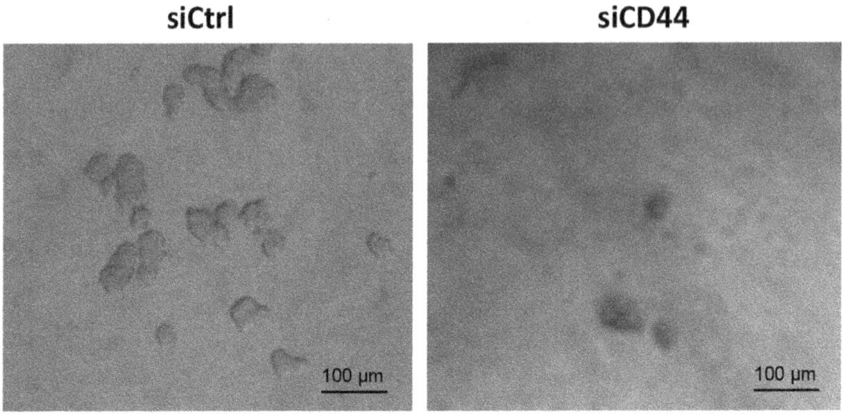

Fig. 5 CD44 knockdown inhibits secondary spheroid formation. In this representative image, primary spheroids were digested into single-cell suspension and transfected with control small interfering RNA (siCtrl) or CD44-siRNA (siCD44). Secondary spheroid formation was evaluated on day 10 after transfection

3. After 15 min of digestion, check the cell viability and dispersal status by mixing 10 μL of cell suspension with 10 μL of trypan blue, and count the percentage of viable (trypan blue-negative) cells using a hemocytometer. If multiple-cell clusters still exist, extend the digestion time until single-cell suspension is reached.
4. Stop digestion by centrifugation at 1000 rotations per minute for 5 min and carefully aspirate the supernatant. Resuspend cell pellet with the CSC medium to prepare a cell concentration of 1000 viable cells/mL. Overlay 0.5 mL cell suspensions onto the transfection complexes in each well and gently tilt the 24-well plate to mix cells with transfection complexes.
5. Place the cells in a 37 °C incubator supplied with 5% CO_2 for 10–14 days. To allow undisturbed formation of tumor spheres, do not change the medium. However, a fresh CSC medium can be added to the cell culture every other day to maintain a favorable concentration of growth factors because they are not stable in culture medium.
6. On day 10 after transfection, assess the number of tumor spheres formed in each well. Only tumor spheres with a diameter of at least 40 μm should be considered. A representative result is shown in Fig. 5.

4 Notes

1. Epidermal growth factor and basic fibroblast growth factor should be aliquoted and stored at −80 °C, and N2 and B27 supplements should be stored at −20 °C as stock. We recommend preparing a complete CSC medium for a relatively small

amount, i.e., 100 mL, every time and using it up within 2 weeks because these growth factors are not stable in culture medium.

2. CD44 antibody used in this chapter is generated to recognize all splicing variants of CD44 molecules, but isoform-specific CD44 antibodies have been generated by some research groups [5] and some are commercially available (such as CD44v6). These antibodies have been reported to isolate or enrich CSCs from specific tumor types, such as CD44v8-10 for gastric cancer [15] and CD44v6 for colon cancer [14].
3. Cellular aggregation can be reduced by adding 100 U/mL DNase I to cell dissociation buffer when necessary.
4. Performing this step will remove most of the fibroblast cells that quickly attach to the plate. For tumor tissues that contain many stromal cells, such as pancreatic tumors, this step is highly recommended.
5. Single-cell suspensions for FACS can be prepared in DPBS supplemented with 1% FBS. However, some growth factors in FBS, even at very low concentrations, can induce stem cell differentiation, which is unfavorable for following functional assays. Therefore, we recommend using BSA instead of FBS. The BSA solution should be filtered through a 0.22 μm filter to guarantee sterility.
6. Before FACS is conducted, the reactivity and specificity of each antibody should be determined, and the best antibody dilution should be empirically adjusted for different antibodies and cells.
7. If the purity of sorted cells is not desired, a secondary sorting can be processed to improve the purity. However, it should be noted that up to 30% of the cells obtained from the first sorting may be lost with secondary sorting.
8. The initial number of cells plated for tumor spheroid formation may vary and depend on factors such as cell and tissue type, duration of growth, and the desired size of the spheroid at the time of assessment. In general, more cells are needed for seeding if stem cells isolated from patient tumor specimens are used because the proportion of CSCs is very low in such samples.
9. The reagent amounts suggested in the manufacturer's instructions can be used in the first experiments, and optimization should be performed as needed on the basis of the results. Because transfection reagent is not removed from the cell culture in this assay, we recommend using a relatively low amount of reagent to reduce cytotoxicity.

Acknowledgment

The authors would like to thank Eric A Goodoff for helpful comments. The work was supported in part by grants 1R01CA195651 and 1R01CA198090; and grant R03CA124523 from the National Cancer Institute, NIH, and grants from the American Institute for Cancer Research (#10A073), Texas Medical Center Digestive Disease Center, and M.D. Anderson Cancer Center Institutional Research program.

References

1. Egeblad M, Nakasone ES, Werb Z (2010) Tumors as organs: complex tissues that interface with the entire organism. Dev Cell 18 (6):884–901
2. Shackleton M, Quintana E, Fearon ER, Morrison SJ (2009) Heterogeneity in cancer: cancer stem cells versus clonal evolution. Cell 138 (5):822–829
3. Goldstein LA, Zhou DF, Picker LJ, Minty CN, Bargatze RF, Ding JF et al (1989) A human lymphocyte homing receptor, the hermes antigen, is related to cartilage proteoglycan core and link proteins. Cell 56(6):1063–1072
4. Grimme HU, Termeer CC, Bennett KL, Weiss JM, Schopf E, Aruffo A et al (1999) Colocalization of basic fibroblast growth factor and CD44 isoforms containing the variably spliced exon v3 (CD44v3) in normal skin and in epidermal skin cancers. Br J Dermatol 141 (5):824–832
5. Ishimoto T, Nagano O, Yae T, Tamada M, Motohara T, Oshima H et al (2011) CD44 variant regulates redox status in cancer cells by stabilizing the xCT subunit of system xc(−) and thereby promotes tumor growth. Cancer Cell 19(3):387–400
6. Cheng C, Yaffe MB, Sharp PA (2006) A positive feedback loop couples Ras activation and CD44 alternative splicing. Genes Dev 20 (13):1715–1720
7. Weg-Remers S, Ponta H, Herrlich P, Konig H (2001) Regulation of alternative pre-mRNA splicing by the ERK MAP-kinase pathway. EMBO J 20(15):4194–4203
8. Matsumura Y, Tarin D (1992) Significance of CD44 gene products for cancer diagnosis and disease evaluation. Lancet (London, England) 340(8827):1053–1058
9. Yan Y, Zuo X, Wei D (2015) Concise review: emerging role of CD44 in cancer stem cells: a promising biomarker and therapeutic target. Stem Cells Transl Med 4(9):1033–1043
10. Al-Hajj M, Wicha MS, Benito-Hernandez A, Morrison SJ, Clarke MF (2003) Prospective identification of tumorigenic breast cancer cells. Proc Natl Acad Sci U S A 100 (7):3983–3988
11. Takaishi S, Okumura T, Tu S, Wang SS, Shibata W, Vigneshwaran R et al (2009) Identification of gastric cancer stem cells using the cell surface marker CD44. Stem cells (Dayton, Ohio) 27 (5):1006–1020
12. Su YJ, Lai HM, Chang YW, Chen GY, Lee JL (2011) Direct reprogramming of stem cell properties in colon cancer cells by CD44. EMBO J 30(15):3186–3199
13. Kidwai F, Costea DE, Hutchison I, Mackenzie I (2013) The effects of CD44 down-regulation on stem cell properties of head and neck cancer cell lines. J Oral Pathol Med 42(9):682–690
14. Todaro M, Gaggianesi M, Catalano V, Benfante A, Iovino F, Biffoni M et al (2014) CD44v6 is a marker of constitutive and reprogrammed cancer stem cells driving colon cancer metastasis. Cell Stem Cell 14(3):342–356
15. Lau WM, Teng E, Chong HS, Lopez KA, Tay AY, Salto-Tellez M et al (2014) CD44v8-10 is a cancer-specific marker for gastric cancer stem cells. Cancer Res 74(9):2630–2641
16. Bourguignon LY, Wong G, Earle C, Chen L (2012) Hyaluronan-CD44v3 interaction with Oct4-Sox2-Nanog promotes miR-302 expression leading to self-renewal, clonal formation, and cisplatin resistance in cancer stem cells from head and neck squamous cell carcinoma. J Biol Chem 287(39):32800–32824
17. Li C, Wu JJ, Hynes M, Dosch J, Sarkar B, Welling TH et al (2011) c-Met is a marker of pancreatic cancer stem cells and therapeutic target. Gastroenterology 141(6):2218–27.e5

Chapter 4

Evaluation and Isolation of Cancer Stem Cells Using ALDH Activity Assay

Luigi Mele, Davide Liccardo, and Virginia Tirino

Abstract

The aldehyde dehydrogenase (ALDH) is a polymorphic enzyme responsible for the oxidation of aldehydes to carboxylic acids. In this chapter, it is described the role of ALDH in the identification of cancer stem cells (CSCs), having been shown that stem cells express high levels of ALDH. Here, we present a method called ALDEFLUOR assay used for the identification, evaluation, and isolation of normal, cancer stem and progenitor cells.

Key words Aldehyde dehydrogenase (ALDH), CSCs, Aldefluor, Cancer, Progenitor cells

1 Introduction

Aldehyde dehydrogenases (ALDHs) are a family of enzymes that catalyze the oxidation of endogenous aldehyde substrates to their corresponding carboxylic acids and conversion of retinol to retinoic acid. The human genome contains 19 ALDH genes that code for enzymes involved in detoxification from aldehydes produced by physiological metabolic processes or environmental agents and cytotoxic drugs [1]. For this reason, an increase in ALDH activity may confer cells more resistance to chemotherapeutic treatments [2]. ALDH1 has three isoforms (A1, A2, A3) and is considered a marker for normal and cancer stem cells (CSCs). Indeed, this subpopulation of stem-like tumor cells is responsible for tumor initiation, invasive growth, and metastasis formation, and has high levels and high activity of this enzyme. *Hilton J* [3] first showed the role of high ALDH activity in chemotherapeutic resistance to cyclophosphamide, an alkylating agent, in leukemia stem cells. In addition to drug resistance, ALDH maintains low levels of reactive oxygen species (ROS) by preventing apoptosis of CSCs [4]. High ALDH activity has been demonstrated in CSCs of liver, lung, breast, colon and head and neck cancers [5–9]. Generally,

Gianpaolo Papaccio and Vincenzo Desiderio (eds.), *Cancer Stem Cells: Methods and Protocols*, Methods in Molecular Biology, vol. 1692, DOI 10.1007/978-1-4939-7401-6_4, © Springer Science+Business Media LLC 2018

ALDH1A1 isoform is commonly considered to be responsible for increasing ALDH activity in CSCs, although recent studies have shown that other isoforms contribute to increased activity, in particular the ALDH1A3 isoform [10]. However, the expression and activity of this enzyme can be considered a reliable marker in tissues that normally do not express or express low levels of ALDH1A1 (breast, lung), but cannot be considered a tissue marker that already expresses high levels of ALDH1A1 (liver, pancreas) [1]. The method used to identify and select high ALDH activity cells is Aldefluor assay kit (StemCell Technologies, Durham, NC, USA). The viable cells with high expression of ALDH become brightly fluorescent and can be detected using the green fluorescence channel of a standard flow cytometer or isolated by cell sorting. High ALDH activity in the Aldefluor assay has been attributed to the expression of ALDH1, but it is not possible to understand which of the three isoforms of this enzyme (A1, A2, A3) is due. Aldefluor assay is based on conversion of substrate BODIPY-aminoacetaldehyde (BAAA) to the fluorescence product BODIPY-aminoacetate (BAA). In conclusion, we provide here a staining protocol based on the evaluation of ALDH activity using flow cytometry.

2 Materials

2.1 Reagents

1. ALDEFLUOR™ Kit by STEMCELL Technologies.
2. 12 × 75 mm tubes compatible with the cytometer used low-speed centrifuge (capable of 250 × *g*).
3. 37 °C heating device (water bath or heat block).
4. Flow cytometer equipped with a 488 nm blue argon ion laser for excitation and an optical filter set to defected 515–545 nm (green) fluorescence.
5. Refrigerator (2–8 °C) or ice.
6. Erythrocyte lysing agent (without detergent or fixatives).

2.2 Sample Preparation

1. Prepare fresh or frozen test samples according to standard procedures for the sample type.
2. If using samples containing blood and the erythrocyte to leukocyte ratio (RBC:WBC) of the specimen is >2:1, lyse the erythrocytes with an ammonium chloride-based buffered solution that does not contain detergents or fixatives.
3. If using sphere-forming cells to separate them and obtain single-cell solution, centrifuge the sample for 5 min at 250 × *g*, remove the supernatant, and suspend cells in 1× trypsin-EDTA and incubate at 37 °C for 10 min, then neutralize the trypsin with medium supplemented with serum.

4. Centrifuge the sample for 5 min at 250 × *g*, remove the supernatant, and suspend the cells in 1 ml of ALDEFLUOR Assay Buffer.
5. Perform a cell count.
6. Adjust sample to a concentration of 1 × 10^6 cells/ml with ALDEFLUOR Assay Buffer.

3 Methods

3.1 ALDEFLUOR Assay

1. Obtain a single viable cells suspension.
2. Count cells using Coulter counter.
3. Spin cells at 250 × *g* for 5 min.
4. Decant media and resuspend cells at 1 × 10^6 cells/ml in Aldefluor assay buffer (*see* **Note 1**).
5. Label one 11 × 75 flow tube (Falcon) for each of the following: with 1 μg/ml propidium iodide (PI) or 7-actinoaminomycin-D (7-AAD) only, DEAB, ALDH. If a cell sort is required, label an additional ALDH tube for every 500,000 cells(500 μl) of sample to be sorted (*see* **Note 2**).
6. Transfer 500 μl (500,000 cells) into each flow tube. Due to the nature of the bioassay, no tube may contain more than 500 μl of volume or 500,000 cells, as it is a very concentration-specific assay.
7. Add 5 μl of DEAB into the tube labeled DEAB and mix well.
8. Add 2.5 μl of Aldefluor substrate into each tube, except the tube labeled with PI or 7-AAD only. Add the substrate to the tube labeled DEAB last. Mix all the tubes well.
9. Place all the tubes (including PI or 7-ADD only tube) into a water bath preset to 37 °C, making sure that there is a lid as the reaction is light-sensitive.
10. Incubate the tube at 37 °C for 30–60 min (*see* **Note 3**). Do not exceed 60 min (*see* **Note 4**).
11. After a 30–60-min incubation, the tubes can be removed from the water bath and brought back to the flow hood. If there is no sorting required, and there are only three tubes (PI or 7-AAD only, DEAB,ALDH) proceed to **step 13**.
12. If the cells are going to be sorted, pipette all the volume in the tubes labeled ALDH into a single tube labeled ALDH and centrifuge for 5 min at 250 × *g*. Resuspend the sample in Aldefluor assay buffer to a concentration of 2,000,000 cells/ml (this is half the volume used during the incubation) and proceed to **step 13**.

13. Add 2 µl of 1 µg/ml dye probe to PI or 7-AAD tube, DEAB tube and the ALDH tube if for analysis only. If the ALDH tube is to be sorted and has more than 500,000 cells in it, add 20 µl for ml of volume in the ALDH tube (*see* **Note 5**).

3.2 Flow Cytometer Set Up and Data Acquisition

3.2.1 Prepare an Acquisition Template

1. Create a Forward Scatter (FCS) vs. Side Scatter (SSC) dot plot, to select in a gate (P1) nucleated cells population based on scatter excluding RBCs and debris.
2. Create a Fluorescence Channel 1 (FL1) vs. SSC dot plot, gated on P1 (*see* **Note 6**).

3.2.2 To Set Up Analyzer and Acquire Data

1. Place DEAB negative control sample on the cytometer.
2. Adjust the FL1 photo-multiplier voltage so that the stained population is placed at second log decade and gated on P1.
3. Remove the tube.
4. Place the ALDH test sample on the cytometer. Create a gate (P2) to encompass the $ALDH^{bright}$ population using the same instrument settings (*see* **Note 7**).
5. $ALDH^{bright}$ cells derived from fresh biopsies or heterogeneous cell populations can have different SCC characteristics and the gate must be set correctly. For example, if epithelia cells are used, it is a good practice to stain the cells with an epithelial marker and gated on epithelial cells.
6. To exclude dead cells, create an FSC vs. viability stain dot plot gated on P1, and gate on cells within the first log decade on the viability stain axis.
7. Sometimes, depending on DNA probe used, it is necessary to perform a compensation setting. PI dye emits in PE fluorescence and ALDH in FITC fluorescence. PE emission is largely detected in the detector specific for PE but the emission tail lies within the range of the bandpass filter used for the detection of FITC. This will be seen as "false positive" signals in the FITC channel and fluorescence compensation is needed to correct for this overlap.
8. To perform a compensation, run a sample stained only with a PE-labeled dye such as PI. Observe the signal in both PE and FITC channels.
9. Adjust the compensation settings until no PE signal is seen in the FITC channel: ***(FITC+ PE overlap) – (PE overlap) = accurate FITC results***
10. Collect almost 100,000 events in P1 for each sample.

3.2.3 Cell Sorting

1. The sorting gates are established using as negative controls the cells stained with PI or 7-ADD only.
2. First to perform cell sorting, it is important to exclude doublets. Doublet exclusion is to ensure count single cells and

exclude doublets from the analysis. If a doublet containing a fluorescence positive and negative cell passes through the laser, it will produce a positive pulse leading to false positives in both analysis and sorting experiments.

3. Doublet exclusion is performed by plotting the height or width against the area for forward scatter or side scatter. Doublets will have double the area and width values of single cells while the height is roughly the same. Therefore, disproportions between height, width, and area can be used to identify doublets.
4. $ALDH^{bright}$ and $ALDH^{-}$ fractions are sorted.
5. Aliquots of $ALDH^{bright}$ and $ALDH^{-}$ sorted cells are evaluated for purity by flow cytometry. The purity must be almost 80%.
6. $ALDH^{bright}$ and $ALDH^{-}$ sorted cell populations are cultured in a standard medium, used for in vivo and in vitro experiments, analyzed for stemness markers and spheres formation assay (*see* **Note 8**).

4 Notes

1. Optimal cell concentration may vary among different cell types. Therefore, it is necessary to individuate the cell concentration that gives the strongest fluorescence intensity of $ALDH^{bright}$ cells and the highest signal-to-background ratio and, for heterogeneous cell samples, the best distinction between $ALDH^{bright}$ and $ALDH^{low}$ cells. Suggested concentrations of cells per ml of ALDEFLUORTM samples can be: 1×10^5, 2×10^5, 5×10^5, 1×10^6, 2×10^6. Moreover, it is good practice to use cells that have a high ALDH activity as positive control. Usually, A549 cell line can be used as positive control cell line for ALDH activity.
2. If the samples contain fewer than 90% viable cells, it is recommended to stain the cells with a DNA dye, such as propidium or 7-actinoaminomycin-D, to stain dead cells.
3. The cells will settle to the bottom of the tube and each tube must be mixed every 15 min for the assay to work.
4. Optimal incubation times may vary among different cell types. Therefore, it is necessary to test different times. Suggested incubation times can be 15 min, 30 min, 45 min, and 60 min.
5. To perform double staining with a cell surface marker (example $ALDH^{bright}$/CD44), after **step 13**, incubate for 15–30 min at 2°C to 8 °C samples with antibody. Centrifuge test control tube with antibody, DEAB and ALDH at $250 \times g$ for 5 min, then remove the supernatant for each tube. Resuspend each cell pellet in 0.5 ml Aldefluor Assay Buffer.
6. FL1 is assumed to correspond to green fluorescence signal.

7. Cells with high ALDH activity are identified in comparison with DEAB negative control sample.
8. Sorted cells are cultured in media supplemented with an excess of gentamicin to avoid contamination being the sorting semi-sterile.

References

1. Tomita H, Tanaka K, Tanaka T, Hara A (2016) Aldehyde dehydrogenase 1A1 in stem cells and cancer. *Oncotarget* 7(10):11018–11032
2. Tirino V, Desiderio V, Paino F, De Rosa A, Papaccio F, La Noce M, Laino L, De Francesco F, Papaccio G (2013) Cancer stem cells in solid tumors: an overview and new approaches for their isolation and characterization. FASEB J 27:13–24
3. Hilton J (1984) Role of aldehyde dehydrogenase in cyclophosphamide-resistant L1210 leukemia. Cancer Res 44(11):5156–5160
4. Xu X, Chai S, Wang P, Zhang C, Yang Y, Yang Y, Wang K (2015) Aldehyde dehydrogenases and cancer stem cells. Cancer Lett 369 (1):50–57
5. Ma S, Chan KW, Lee TK-W, Tang KH, Wo JY-H, Zheng B-J, Guan X-Y (2008) Aldehyde dehydrogenase discriminates the CD133 liver cancer stem cell populations. Mol Cancer Res 6 (7):1146–1153
6. Jiang F, Qiu Q, Khanna A, Todd NW, Deepak J, Xing L, Wang H, Liu Z, Su Y, Stass SA, Katz RL (2009) Aldehyde dehydrogenase 1 is a tumor stem cell-associated marker in lung cancer. Mol Cancer Res 7(3):330–338
7. Marcato P, Dean CA, Pan D, Araslanova R, Gillis M, Joshi M, Helyer L, Pan L, Leidal A, Gujar S, Giacomantonio CA, Lee PW (2011) Aldehyde dehydrogenase activity of breast cancer stem cells is primarily due to isoform ALDH1A3 and its expression is predictive of metastasis. Stem Cells 29(1):32–45
8. Giraud J, Failla LM, Pascussi J-M, Lagerqvist EL, Ollier J, Finetti P, Bertucci F, Ya C, Gasmi I, Bourgaux J-F, Prudhomme M, Mazard T, Ait-Arsa I, Houhou L, Birnbaum D, Pélegrin A, Vincent C, Ryall JG, Joubert D, Pannequin J, Hollande F (2016) Autocrine secretion of Progastrin promotes the survival and self-renewal of colon cancer stem–like cells. Cancer Res 76(12):3618–3628
9. Desiderio V, Papagerakis P, Tirino V et al (2015) Increased fucosylation has a pivotal role in invasive and metastatic properties of head and neck cancer stem cells. Oncotarget 6 (1):71–84
10. Marcato P, Dean CA, Giacomantonio CA, Lee PW (2011) Aldehyde dehydrogenase: its role as a cancer stem cell marker comes down to the specific isoform. Cell Cycle 10(9):1378–1384

Chapter 5

Isolation of Cancer Stem Cells by Side Population Method

Masayuki Shimoda, Masahide Ota, and Yasunori Okada

Abstract

The Hoechst side population (SP) method is a flow cytometry technique used to obtain stem cells based on the dye efflux properties of the ATP-binding cassette (ABC) transporters. The SP cells are characterized by their capability to efflux the fluorescent DNA-binding dye Hoechst 33342 through their ABC transporters and are enriched in stem cells, which are endowed with a self-renewal capacity and multilineage differentiation potential and express the stemness genes including ABC multidrug transporters. The protocols outlined in this book chapter describe the isolation method of the SP cells from human lung carcinoma cell lines by using Hoechst 33342. In addition, we refer to the propagation method of SP cells by successive rounds of fluorescence-activated cell sorting analysis for SP cells. These approaches will be helpful for the establishment of novel in vitro and in vivo models using cancer stem cells, which may play a key role during carcinogenesis and/or tumor progression.

Key words Side population, Main population, Cancer stem cell, Hoechst 33342, Flow cytometry, Propagation of side population cells, Lung carcinoma cell lines

1 Introduction

The Hoechst side population (SP) method is based on the differential potential of cells to efflux the fluorescent DNA-binding Hoechst dye via the verapamil-sensitive ATP-binding cassette (ABC) transporters expressed within the cell membrane [1, 2]. ABC transporters belong to the superfamily of membrane pumps that perform ATP-dependent transport of various endogenous materials and xenobiotics from the cells. The SP cells expressing a sufficient number of ABC transporters are able to actively efflux the dye out of the cells. The protocol for the isolation of SP cells was originally established for murine bone marrow hematopoietic stem cells (HSCs) [1]. The bone marrow SP cells have been shown to be highly enriched for functional HSCs and also overlap with the phenotypically defined $CD117^{+}Sca\text{-}1^{+}Lin^{-}Thy1^{lo}$ HSC population [3, 4]. This method has been adapted for stem cell isolation in

Gianpaolo Papaccio and Vincenzo Desiderio (eds.), *Cancer Stem Cells: Methods and Protocols*, Methods in Molecular Biology, vol. 1692, DOI 10.1007/978-1-4939-7401-6_5,

other tissues including the umbilical cord blood [5], skeletal muscle [6], kidney [7], liver [8], mammary glands [9], lung [10], and forebrain [11]. Importantly, stem cells that exhibit SP properties are rare in most tissues and often constitute a heterogeneous population, depending on organ type and stage of development.

Accumulated lines of evidence have indicated that malignant neoplastic cells contain a small subpopulation of cells with properties of tumor initiation, self-renewal, resistance to chemotherapy, and metastatic potential, which are called cancer stem cells (CSCs) or tumor initiating cells [12]. CSCs were initially identified in the hematopoietic malignancies [13] and then observed in various solid tumors such as the prostate [14], ovarian [15], gastric [16], breast [17], and lung [18] carcinomas. In most cases, current therapies targeting the bulk of cancers do not eradicate CSCs completely, and thus the development of therapeutic strategies targeting CSCs is necessary. Techniques focusing on the CSC-specific cell surface markers, the aldehyde dehydrogenase activity, or the ability of floating sphere formation in serum-free medium have been applied to isolate CSCs from malignant tissues and established cell lines [19]. Besides these methodologies, the Hoechst SP technique is a useful method that enables us to isolate CSCs from various cancer tissues and/or cell lines by using fluorescence-activated cell sorting (FACS) [20–28]. The SP cells are present in a number of cancer tissues and shown to display increased capability of self-renewal and tumorigenicity when transplanted into immunocompromised mice. Moreover, the SP cells from the colon, breast, and lung carcinomas display high expression of stem cell-related genes [23, 29, 30]. Therefore, the SP cells are thought to represent one of the putative cancer stem cell populations.

The Hoechst SP technique is commonly used for stem cell isolation. However, as compared to the isolation method utilizing cell surface markers, this method requires an additional dye incubation step for the appropriate equilibration of the Hoechst dye between the extracellular and intracellular compartments prior to dye efflux by the action of the ABC transporters. The ABC transporter-mediated dye efflux is a dynamic biological process that is highly sensitive to modifications in the staining conditions such as Hoechst concentration, temperature, duration, and light conditions. In addition, the percentage of SP cells depends on the cell culture conditions including cell density, nutrient composition, serum and oxygen levels. Thus, experimental results may occasionally have a problem in reproducibility. In this chapter, we describe the protocol for the Hoechst SP method to obtain the reproducible results and mention the propagation of the SP fraction by successive rounds of the FACS analysis of the SP cells.

2 Materials

1. Cell Lines: Lung carcinoma cell lines including A549, PC-9, and H1650 are available from American Type Culture Collection (Manassas, VA, USA) or Immuno-Biological Laboratories (Gunma, Japan) or other sources.
2. Culture medium: RPMI 1640 medium supplemented with 10% fetal bovine serum (FBS), 100 UI/mL penicillin, and 100 μg/mL streptomycin.
3. Dissociation solution: Trypsin-EDTA solution consisting of 0.05% Trypsin and 0.53 mM EDTA or Cell Dissociation Buffer (Invitrogen, Carlsbad, CA, USA).
4. Incubation solution: RPMI 1640 medium, 5% FBS, and 10 mM HEPES.
5. Running solution: ice-cold PBS solution containing 2% FBS and 10 mM HEPES.
6. Hoechst 33342 solution (10 mg/mL in distilled water). The solution is diluted at a concentration of 1 mg/mL with distilled water, filter-sterilized and then stored at −20 °C in 1 mL aliquots in the dark. The "working" stock solution is covered with aluminum foil and kept at 4 °C.
7. Verapamil, an ABC transporter inhibitor, is dissolved at a concentration of 100 mM in 95% ethanol and stored at −80 °C in 2.5 μL aliquots in the dark. The aliquot of 100 mM verapamil is diluted to 5 mM with phosphate-buffered saline (PBS), and added to cell suspension at a final concentration of 100 μM. The remains of the diluted solution should be discarded without re-use.
8. Propidium iodide (PI) solution (1 mg/mL solution in distilled water) is stored at 4 °C in 100 μL aliquots in the dark. The "working" stock solution should be covered with aluminum foil and kept at 4 °C.
9. FACS analyses of the SP fractions can be carried out by using a flow cytometer such as Moflo (Beckman, Brea, CA, USA) or equivalent and a FlowJo software (Tree Star, Ashland, OR, USA) or equivalent.
10. Freezing solution: CELLBANKER® (Nippon Zenyaku Kogyo Co., Ltd. Koriyama, Fukushima, Japan) or FBS with 10% dimethyl sulfoxide (DMSO).

3 Methods

3.1 Cell Preparation Protocol

1. All the cell lines are grown in culture dishes within a chamber with a humidified atmosphere in a 37 °C incubator supplied with 5% CO_2.

2. When they reach at 50–75% confluence, the culture medium is discarded from the dishes (*see* **Note 1**).
3. The cells are washed once with Ca^{2+}/Mg^{2+}-free PBS solution.
4. They are dissociated by incubation with dissociation solution (1–2 mL per 10-cm dish) in a CO_2 incubator at 37 °C. The cell layer is detached usually within 3–5 min in 0.05% Trypsin/0.53 mM EDTA solution or within 10–15 min in Cell Dissociation Buffer (*see* **Note 2**).
5. Culture medium, which inactivates proteinase activity of trypsin and stops the action of Cell Dissociation Buffer, is added to the culture dishes (3–6 mL per 10 cm dish), and cells are dissociated into single cells by gently pipetting.
6. The cell suspension is transferred to a centrifuge tube, and spun down at 1000 rpm ($190 \times g$) for 5 min at room temperature.

3.2 Hoechst SP Method Protocol

1. The cell pellet is suspended at 1.0×10^6 cells per mL in the incubation solution (*see* **Note 3**). The cell suspension is supplemented with a certain concentration of Hoechst 33342 (*see* **Note 4**) in the absence or presence of 100 μM verapamil, an ABC transporter inhibitor (*see* **Note 5**).
2. The cells in suspension in the incubation solution supplemented with Hoechst 33342 in the absence or presence of verapamil are incubated in a water bath at 37 °C for 90 min by gently agitating every 30 min.
3. After the incubation, the cells are spun down at 190 g for 5 min at room temperature.
4. The cell pellet is resuspended at 1.0×10^6 cells per mL in the running solution.
5. The suspended cells are supplemented with 2 μg/mL of PI and left on ice about 5 min before FACS analysis. This step allows us to exclude dead cells and cell debris as PI permeates cells that do not have an intact membrane.
6. The SP and non-SP, i.e., main population (MP), cell fractions in the viable cells are analyzed by flow cytometer. When two or more cell samples are analyzed, the cell suspensions are maintained at 4 °C before flow cytometry analysis.
7. During flow cytometry analysis, the Hoechst dye is excited with a UV laser at 355 nm and its fluorescence emission is measured with both 505 long-pass 670/40 filter (Hoechst Red) and 450/50 filter (Hoechst Blue). The representative Hoechst dye efflux profiles showing the SP and MP cell fractions of A549 or PC-9 cells in the absence or presence of verapamil are shown as Fig. 1 (*see* **Note 6**).
8. The SP and MP cell fractions are collected by FACS in 1 mL of the culture medium.

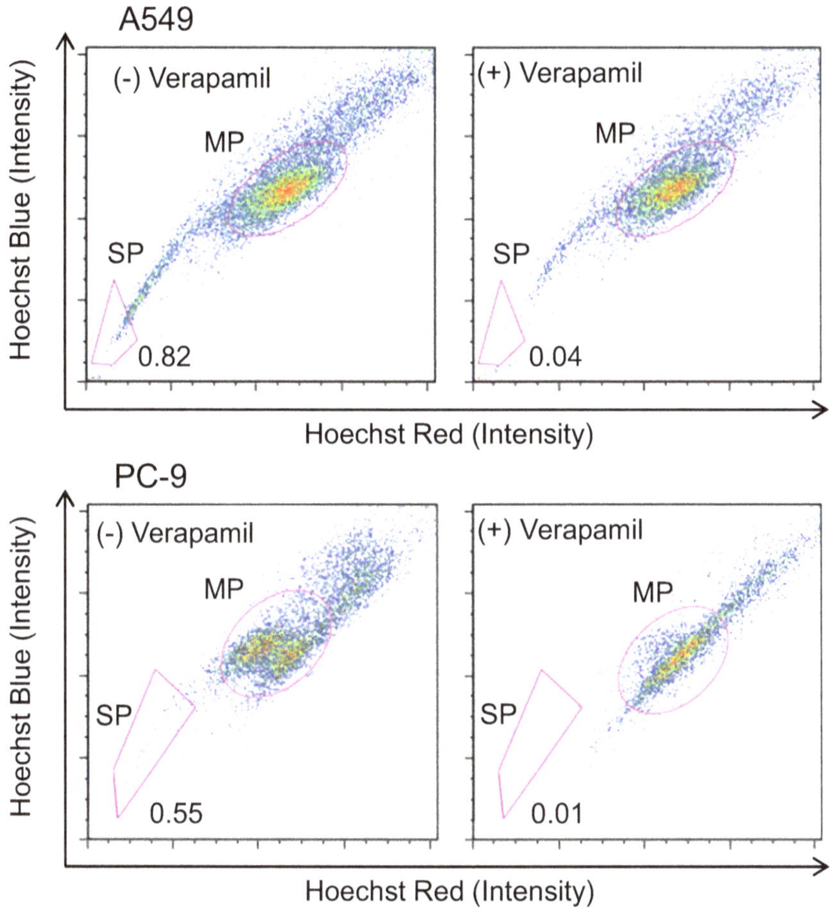

Fig. 1 Representative flow cytometric profiles obtained after staining A549 and PC-9 lung carcinoma cell lines with 5 μg/mL Hoechst 33342 in the absence (*left panel*) or presence of verapamil (*right panel*). The SP and MP factions are outlined, showing their percentages

9. Both the collected SP and MP cells are centrifuged at 190 × *g* for 5 min at room temperature.
10. The cell pellets are washed more than twice with the culture medium (*see* **Note 7**), and the cells are resuspended in the same medium.
11. They are either used directly for further experiments of characterizations of the SP and MP cells or cultured in a CO_2 incubator at 37 °C to increase number of the cells sufficient for further studies.

3.3 Propagation of SP Fraction Protocol

1. The SP cells collected by FACS analysis are centrifuged at 190 × *g* for 5 min at room temperature.
2. The cell pellets are washed more than twice with the culture medium (*see* **Note 7**), and the cells were suspended in the same medium.

3. They are then cultured in the medium in a CO_2 incubator at 37 °C by changing the medium every three days.
4. When the cells reach at 50–75% confluence after culturing for 4–7 days, they are subjected to the Hoechst SP method by following the steps as described in Subheading 3.2, and this step is repeated several times (*see* **Note 8**). The Hoechst dye efflux profiles showing the SP and MP cell fractions of A549 cells sequentially sorted up to nine times are presented in Fig. 2. Note that percentage of the SP cells ~10-fold increases after the propagation.

3.4 Freezing and Thawing of SP Cells

1. The SP cells or the propagated SP cells in culture are washed once with Ca^{2+}/Mg^{2+}-free PBS solution.
2. They are dissociated by incubation with the dissociation solution in a CO_2 incubator at 37 °C. The cell layer is detached usually within 3–5 min in 0.05% Trypsin/0.53 mM EDTA solution or within 10–15 min in Cell Dissociation Buffer (*see* **Note 2**).
3. Culture medium is added to the culture dishes, and the cells are dissociated into single cells by gently pipetting.
4. After centrifugation at 190 × *g* for 5 min, the cell pellets are washed once with the culture medium, and suspended in the freezing solution at 1.0×10^6 cells/mL.
5. The suspension is transferred into 2 mL cryogenic vials, gradually cooled down at a rate of 1 °C/min, and stored in liquid nitrogen.
6. When thawing the frozen cells, they were quickly thawed by immersion of the vials in a 37 °C water bath.
7. They are suspended in 10 mL of the culture medium and rinsed once with the same medium prior to culture on dishes.
8. The cells are cultured and dissociated when they reach 50–75% confluency. The cell suspension is used for the Hoechst SP method as mentioned above in Subheading 3.3.

4 Notes

1. Percentage of SP cells to total cells is influenced by culture conditions such as cell density. To obtain the reproducible data on the SP analysis, the conditions for cell preparation and culture, especially confluency of the cells, should be similar each time.
2. Agents used for cell dissociation depend on the purpose of the following experiments. The 0.05% Trypsin/0.53 mM EDTA solution is commonly used, but Cell Dissociation Buffer is

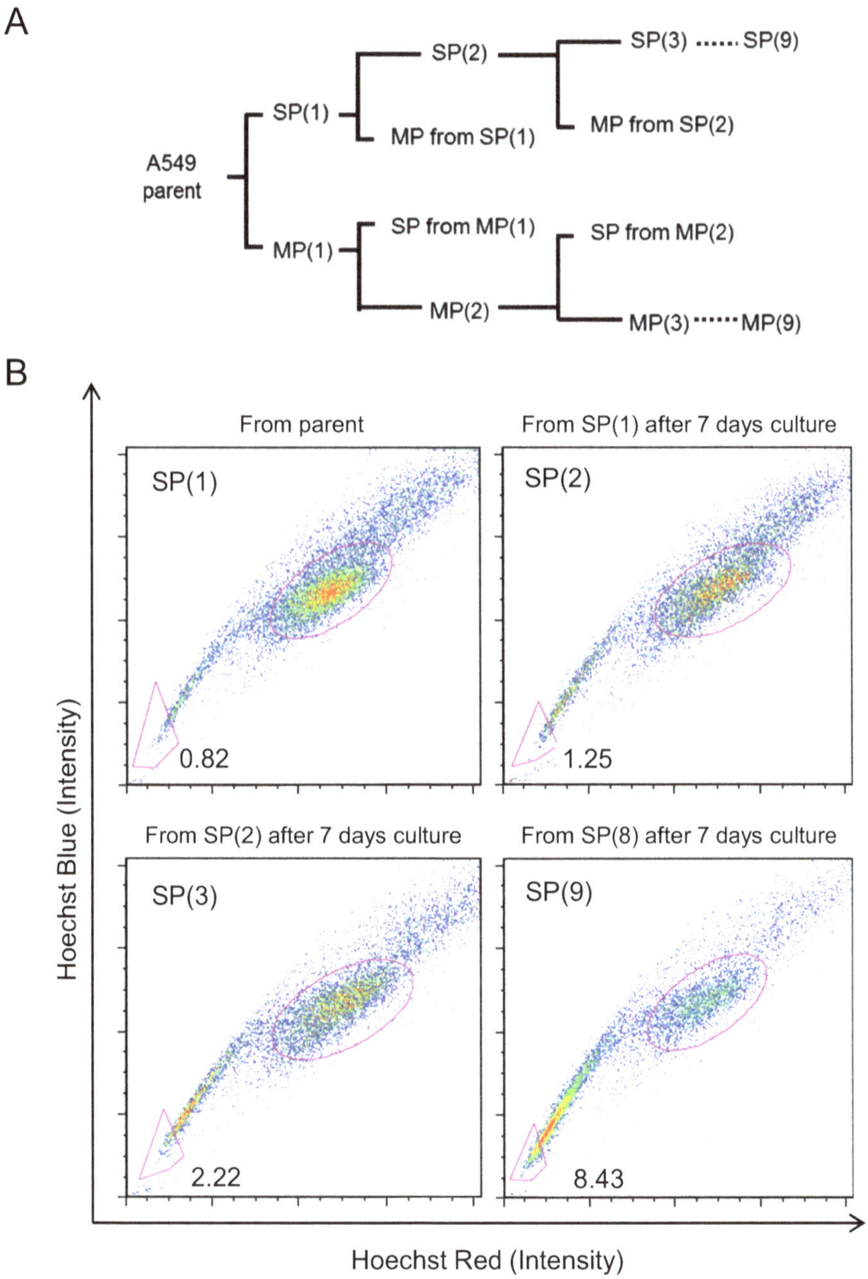

Fig. 2 Propagation of A549-derived SP cells by successive rounds of FACS. (**A**) Schematic presentation of propagation of A549-derived SP and MP cells. Both SP and MP cell fractions were sequentially sorted up to nine times by applying the each fraction. Numbers in brackets indicate times of FACS analysis. (**B**) Representative Hoechst-stained profiles of A549-derived SP(1), SP(2), SP(3), or SP(9) cells. The SP fractions are outlined, showing their percentages

suitable for the experiments such as cell adhesion assay immediately after the isolation of the SP cells by FACS.

3. A concentration of 5% FBS is recommended, because the use of a serum free-medium may result in low viability or low tumorigenicity of the cells.

4. Appropriate concentrations of Hoechst 33342, usually ranging from 1 to 10 μg/mL depending on cell types, should be determined by titration curves for SP cell fractions (Fig. 3).

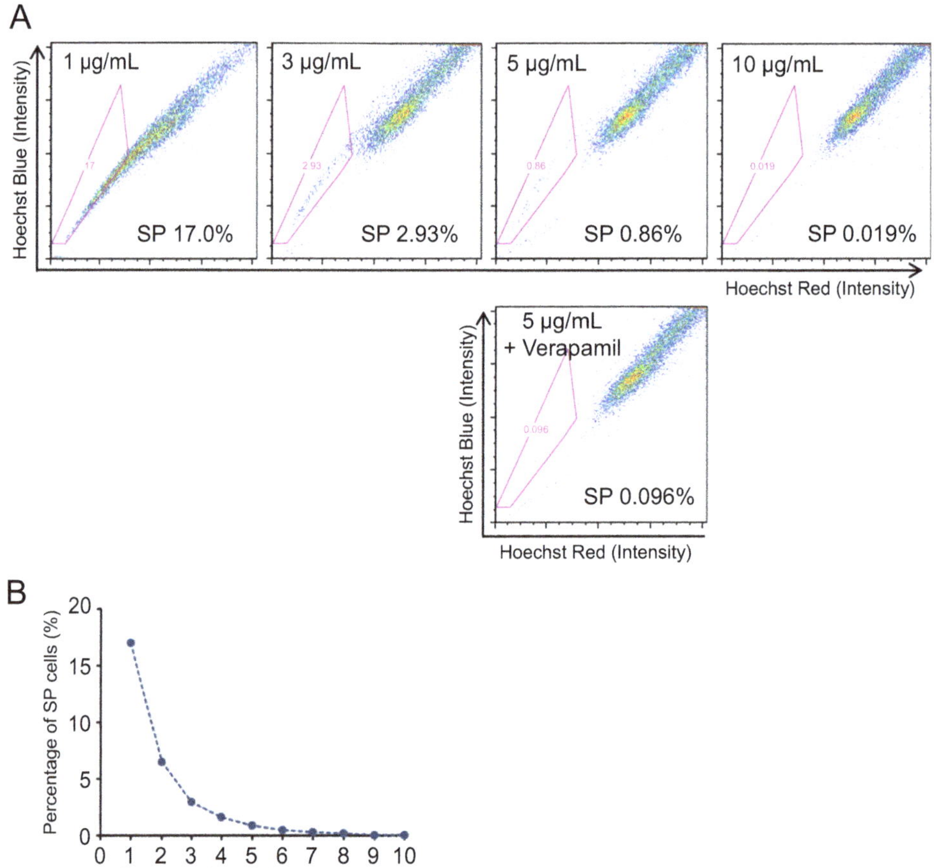

Fig. 3 Determination of a concentration of Hoechst 33342 appropriate for obtaining SP cell fraction by flow cytometric analysis. (**A**) Representative flow cytometric profiles after staining H1650 cells with different concentrations of Hoechst 33342. Percentages of SP cell fractions, which disappear in the presence of 100 μM verapamil (data not shown for cells treated with 1, 3, or 10 μg/mL Hoechst), depend on concentrations of Hoechst. Low concentrations of Hoechst such as 1 μg/mL lead to an unsaturated Hoechst profile, where MP cells are introduced in the SP gate. On the other hand, cells treated with high concentrations of Hoechst such as 10 μg/mL result in failure to obtain SP cell fraction, probably because the cells exposed to high concentrations of Hoechst may not completely efflux the dye out of the cells or suffer from cell damage. (**B**) Titration curve for SP cell fractions of H1650 cells treated with different concentrations of Hoechst 33342. Note that the optimal Hoechst dye concentration lies within a plateau region as the percentage of SP cells is considered to be stable, i.e., 5 μg/mL Hoechst in H1650 cells, which gives 0.86% of SP cell fraction

Importantly, to confirm the specificity of the dye efflux, the ABC transporter inhibition assay using verapamil is necessary besides the Hoechst concentration curve.

5. Verapamil has been used at various concentrations ranging from 50 to 200 μM in previous studies, but 100 μM verapamil is suitable for the inhibition of the ABC transporters without cell toxicity in human lung carcinoma cell lines.
6. The location of the SP in histograms is determined by identifying the putative SP population that disappears by treatment with verapamil (Figs. 1 and 3).
7. Because the tubes in a FACS machine are usually not sterile, the collected cells by the FACS analysis should be washed twice or more before being subjected to cell culture.
8. It takes a long time to propagate SP cells. Thus, the isolated SP cells sometimes cannot help being stored in liquid nitrogen. This step does not affect the percentage of the SP cell fraction very much. However, repeated passages of the SP cells under culture result in a decrease in percentage of SP cells.

Acknowledgments

This work was supported by Adaptable and Seamless Technology Transfer Program Through Target-driven R&G from the Japan Science and Technology Agency (AS2614150Q).
All the authors in this manuscript certify (1) that the paper has not been previously published or submitted elsewhere for publication; (2) that this study does not have financial or other relationships that might lead to a conflict of interest; (3) that all the authors have read and approved the manuscript, and also agreed with the authorship; (4) that Dr. Yasunori Okada is the corresponding author of this paper.

References

1. Goodell MA, Brose K, Paradis G, Conner AS, Mulligan RC (1996) Isolation and functional properties of murine hematopoietic stem cells that are replicating in vivo. J Exp Med 183 (4):1797–1806
2. Zhou S, Schuetz JD, Bunting KD, Colapietro AM, Sampath J, Morris JJ, Lagutina I, Grosveld GC, Osawa M, Nakauchi H, Sorrentino BP (2001) The ABC transporter Bcrp1/ABCG2 is expressed in a wide variety of stem cells and is a molecular determinant of the side-population phenotype. Nat Med 7 (9):1028–1034. doi:10.1038/nm0901-1028
3. Camargo FD, Chambers SM, Drew E, McNagny KM, Goodell MA (2006) Hematopoietic stem cells do not engraft with absolute efficiencies. Blood 107(2):501–507. doi:10.1182/blood-2005-02-0655
4. Challen GA, Boles NC, Chambers SM, Goodell MA (2010) Distinct hematopoietic stem cell subtypes are differentially regulated by TGF-beta1. Cell Stem Cell 6(3):265–278. doi:10.1016/j.stem.2010.02.002
5. Storms RW, Goodell MA, Fisher A, Mulligan RC, Smith C (2000) Hoechst dye efflux reveals a novel CD7(+)CD34(−) lymphoid

progenitor in human umbilical cord blood. Blood 96(6):2125–2133
6. Asakura A, Seale P, Girgis-Gabardo A, Rudnicki MA (2002) Myogenic specification of side population cells in skeletal muscle. J Cell Biol 159(1):123–134. doi:10.1083/jcb.200202092
7. Iwatani H, Ito T, Imai E, Matsuzaki Y, Suzuki A, Yamato M, Okabe M, Hori M (2004) Hematopoietic and nonhematopoietic potentials of Hoechst(low)/side population cells isolated from adult rat kidney. Kidney Int 65 (5):1604–1614. doi:10.1111/j.1523-1755.2004.00561.x
8. Shimano K, Satake M, Okaya A, Kitanaka J, Kitanaka N, Takemura M, Sakagami M, Terada N, Tsujimura T (2003) Hepatic oval cells have the side population phenotype defined by expression of ATP-binding cassette transporter ABCG2/BCRP1. Am J Pathol 163(1):3–9. doi:10.1016/S0002-9440(10)63624-3
9. Clayton H, Titley I, Vivanco M (2004) Growth and differentiation of progenitor/stem cells derived from the human mammary gland. Exp Cell Res 297(2):444–460. doi:10.1016/j.yexcr.2004.03.029
10. Summer R, Kotton DN, Sun X, Ma B, Fitzsimmons K, Fine A (2003) Side population cells and Bcrp1 expression in lung. Am J Physiol Lung Cell Mol Physiol 285(1):L97–104. doi:10.1152/ajplung.00009.2003
11. Kim M, Morshead CM (2003) Distinct populations of forebrain neural stem and progenitor cells can be isolated using side-population analysis. J Neurosci 23(33):10703–10709
12. Reya T, Morrison SJ, Clarke MF, Weissman IL (2001) Stem cells, cancer, and cancer stem cells. Nature 414(6859):105–111. doi:10.1038/35102167
13. Lapidot T, Sirard C, Vormoor J, Murdoch B, Hoang T, Caceres-Cortes J, Minden M, Paterson B, Caligiuri MA, Dick JE (1994) A cell initiating human acute myeloid leukaemia after transplantation into SCID mice. Nature 367(6464):645–648. doi:10.1038/367645a0
14. Collins AT, Berry PA, Hyde C, Stower MJ, Maitland NJ (2005) Prospective identification of tumorigenic prostate cancer stem cells. Cancer Res 65(23):10946–10951. doi:10.1158/0008-5472.CAN-05-2018
15. Bapat SA, Mali AM, Koppikar CB, Kurrey NK (2005) Stem and progenitor-like cells contribute to the aggressive behavior of human epithelial ovarian cancer. Cancer Res 65(8):3025–3029. doi:10.1158/0008-5472.CAN-04-3931
16. Takaishi S, Okumura T, Tu S, Wang SS, Shibata W, Vigneshwaran R, Gordon SA, Shimada Y, Wang TC (2009) Identification of gastric cancer stem cells using the cell surface marker CD44. Stem Cells 27(5):1006–1020. doi:10.1002/stem.30
17. Al-Hajj M, Wicha MS, Benito-Hernandez A, Morrison SJ, Clarke MF (2003) Prospective identification of tumorigenic breast cancer cells. Proc Natl Acad Sci U S A 100 (7):3983–3988. doi:10.1073/pnas.0530291100
18. Eramo A, Lotti F, Sette G, Pilozzi E, Biffoni M, Di Virgilio A, Conticello C, Ruco L, Peschle C, De Maria R (2008) Identification and expansion of the tumorigenic lung cancer stem cell population. Cell Death Differ 15 (3):504–514. doi:10.1038/sj.cdd.4402283
19. Tirino V, Desiderio V, Paino F, Papaccio G, De Rosa M (2012) Methods for cancer stem cell detection and isolation. Methods Mol Biol 879:513–529. doi:10.1007/978-1-61779-815-3_32
20. Bleau AM, Hambardzumyan D, Ozawa T, Fomchenko EI, Huse JT, Brennan CW, Holland EC (2009) PTEN/PI3K/Akt pathway regulates the side population phenotype and ABCG2 activity in glioma tumor stem-like cells. Cell Stem Cell 4(3):226–235. doi:10.1016/j.stem.2009.01.007
21. Chiba T, Kita K, Zheng YW, Yokosuka O, Saisho H, Iwama A, Nakauchi H, Taniguchi H (2006) Side population purified from hepatocellular carcinoma cells harbors cancer stem cell-like properties. Hepatology 44 (1):240–251. doi:10.1002/hep.21227
22. Chua C, Zaiden N, Chong KH, See SJ, Wong MC, Ang BT, Tang C (2008) Characterization of a side population of astrocytoma cells in response to temozolomide. J Neurosurg 109 (5):856–866. doi:10.3171/JNS/2008/109/11/0856
23. Haraguchi N, Utsunomiya T, Inoue H, Tanaka F, Mimori K, Barnard GF, Mori M (2006) Characterization of a side population of cancer cells from human gastrointestinal system. Stem Cells 24(3):506–513. doi:10.1634/stemcells.2005-0282
24. Ho MM, Ng AV, Lam S, Hung JY (2007) Side population in human lung cancer cell lines and tumors is enriched with stem-like cancer cells. Cancer Res 67(10):4827–4833. doi:10.1158/0008-5472.CAN-06-3557
25. Mitsutake N, Iwao A, Nagai K, Namba H, Ohtsuru A, Saenko V, Yamashita S (2007) Characterization of side population in thyroid cancer cell lines: cancer stem-like cells are enriched partly but not exclusively. Endocrinology 148(4):1797–1803. doi:10.1210/en.2006-1553

26. Patrawala L, Calhoun T, Schneider-Broussard R, Zhou J, Claypool K, Tang DG (2005) Side population is enriched in tumorigenic, stem-like cancer cells, whereas ABCG2+ and ABCG2- cancer cells are similarly tumorigenic. Cancer Res 65(14):6207–6219. doi:10.1158/0008-5472.CAN-05-0592
27. Wu C, Alman BA (2008) Side population cells in human cancers. Cancer Lett 268(1):1–9. doi:10.1016/j.canlet.2008.03.048
28. Wu C, Wei Q, Utomo V, Nadesan P, Whetstone H, Kandel R, Wunder JS, Alman BA (2007) Side population cells isolated from mesenchymal neoplasms have tumor initiating potential. Cancer Res 67(17):8216–8222. doi:10.1158/0008-5472.CAN-07-0999
29. Zhou J, Wulfkuhle J, Zhang H, Gu P, Yang Y, Deng J, Margolick JB, Liotta LA, Petricoin E 3rd, Zhang Y (2007) Activation of the PTEN/mTOR/STAT3 pathway in breast cancer stem-like cells is required for viability and maintenance. Proc Natl Acad Sci U S A 104(41):16158–16163. doi:10.1073/pnas.0702596104
30. Ota M, Mochizuki S, Shimoda M, Abe H, Miyamae Y, Ishii K, Kimura H, Okada Y (2016) ADAM23 is downregulated in side population and suppresses lung metastasis of lung carcinoma cells. Cancer Sci 107(4):433–443. doi:10.1111/cas.12895

Chapter 6

Self-Renewal and CSCs In Vitro Enrichment: Growth as Floating Spheres

Pooja Mehta, Caymen Novak, Shreya Raghavan, Maria Ward, and Geeta Mehta

Abstract

Cancer stem cells (CSC) are a vital component to the progression and reoccurrence of cancers, making them a primary target of study for both fundamental understanding of cancer biology and the development of effective and targeted treatments. CSCs reside in a complex 3D microenvironment, and the 3D spheroids are an indispensable tool in tumor biology due to their 3D structure and replication of the tumor microenvironment. Within this chapter the methodology for CSC isolation, suspension culture in hanging drop model, and characterization assays for CSC are described. First, the methodology for identifying and isolating CSCs from patient tumors, ascites, or cancer cell lines is described through the use of FACS analysis. Next, a detailed description of 3D hanging drop model for generating CSC spheroids is provided, followed by maintenance and monitoring techniques for extended 3D culture. Analysis methods are described for the quantification of CSC spheroid proliferation and viability tracking, throughout culture by on-plate alamarBlue fluorescence. Additional viability assays are described utilizing confocal microscopy with Live/Dead Viability/Cytotoxicity Kit. The characterization of CSCs populations within spheroids is described through FACS analysis. Further, an immunohistochemistry procedure is described for cell-cell and cell-matrix interaction assessment. Finally, several notes and tips for successful experiments with 3D CSC spheroids on the hanging drop model are provided. These methods are not only applicable to CSCs within a variety of tumor cell types, for not only understanding the fundamental tumor biology, but also for drug screening and development of preclinical chemotherapeutic strategies.

Key words Spheroid, Cancer stem cells, Ovarian cancer, Hanging drop, Proliferation, Viability, Drug sensitivity

1 Introduction

Cancer stem cells (CSC) are classified as the subpopulation of tumor cells capable of tumor initiation, self-renewal, and differentiation [1, 2]. CSCs maintain a level of pluripotency which drives tumor heterogeneity [1, 3, 4]. Through heterogeneity, adaptations

Pooja Mehta, Caymen Novak, Shreya Raghavan and Maria Ward contributed equally to this work.

Gianpaolo Papaccio and Vincenzo Desiderio (eds.), *Cancer Stem Cells: Methods and Protocols*, Methods in Molecular Biology, vol. 1692, DOI 10.1007/978-1-4939-7401-6_6, © Springer Science+Business Media LLC 2018

arise that enable better survival of cancer cells when confronted with chemotherapy drugs or other treatments such as radiation and inhibitors [1, 5]. These treatments act akin to natural selection process targeting only a select group of cells and leaving behind those resistant to the treatment because cells with different characteristics respond differently to treatment [6]. CSCs are often more difficult to kill and thus are predicted to survive despite apparent reduction in the primary tumor. This resistance to treatment is attributed to characteristics such as overexpression of ABC transporters, enhanced aldehyde dehydrogenase activity, specific signaling pathways, response to DNA damage, epithelial to mesenchymal transition, and dormancy [6, 7]. They can make up small fractions of the bulk tumor, as little as 0.1% [8]. CSC populations thus provide the tumor with a source of not only constant bulk renewal but continued survival for a small subpopulation despite drug treatment. These CSC traits harbor poor outcomes for patients so long as CSC populations are retained. In order to improve patient outcomes, CSCs are a prime target for developing effective treatment strategies.

In vivo, tumor cells reside in a three-dimensional (3D) environment with complex structural and environmental signaling. The complexity of this habitat is difficult to mimic in traditional 2D monolayer cultures. We have previously demonstrated that by utilizing hanging drop plates, which provide a 3D environment to culture few to single cells at a time, we can recapitulate the key features of the innate tumor microenvironment. The hanging drop method has been found to more closely mimic the outcomes of drug success in vivo, providing a more accurate representation of effectiveness and patient response [9–11].

The hanging drop method provides a 3D isolated suspension environment where a small number of cells, such as rare patient-derived CSCs, can be maintained and propagated into spheroids originating from the same stem or progenitor cells. This allows for the propagation of selected cell populations over several weeks and thus is useful for the study of predicted CSC markers and treatment. Here, we demonstrate the hanging drop method to produce CSC spheroids from malignant ascites or primary tumors that have been isolated using desired CSC markers. We detail the preparation and care required for CSC spheroid plating in 384 hanging drop plates, maintenance through feeding and image tracking of spheroid formation, as well as proliferation and viability analysis. Finally, use of spheroids for quantifying drug sensitivity response is described, as well as proper embedding and sectioning techniques for immunohistochemistry analysis of CSC spheroids. We have chosen ovarian cancer as the model system for these demonstrations; however, this approach can be applied to CSCs from any cancers. Beyond ovarian cancers, we believe that this platform developed in this proposal has a wide appeal to a variety of other cancer cells and CSCs, and will prove useful for both tumor biology, as well as drug-screening studies.

2 Materials

Prepare all the solutions using ultrapure deionized water and analytical research grade reagents. Commercial antibody sources are indicated within the methods.

Following materials are required for the protocols:

DMEM and Ham's F12 basal cell culture medium, fetal bovine serum (FBS) 10%, Antibiotic/Antimycotic solution, PBS, Ammonium-Chloride-Potassium (ACK) lysis buffer, alamarblue reagent, Live/Dead Cytotoxicity kit, 4′,6-diamidino-2-phenylindole (DAPI), low melting agarose, CD133 antibody, Pluronic acid, cisplatin, ALDH1A antibody, secondary antibodies, and ALDEFLUOR assay kit (StemCell Technologies, Vancouver, BC).

2.1 CSC Spheroids Cell Culture Medium (See Note 1)

In order to promote the formation of spheroids, and the maintenance of the CSC population, the cell culture growth medium composition is the key. For spheroids initiated with CSCs, use of a serum-free medium is strongly recommended. 50 mL of a common medium composition can be made in the manner outlined below, though this will not work for all spheroids, and some composition adjustment may be necessary for CSCs of a specific tumor. The composition noted below applies to CSCs from ovarian cancers.

1. Form a 1:1 mixture of DMEM and Ham's F12 medium in a 50 mL conical tube.
2. Place 47.150 mL of the DMEM/F12 mixture into a separate tube.
3. Add 1 mL of 50× B-27 Supplement without Vitamin A to the same tube for a 1× mixture.
4. Add 25 μL of 10 μg EGF to the tube to form a 5 ng/mL Solution.
5. Add 25 μL of 10 μg bFGF to the tube to form a 5 ng/mL Solution.
6. Add 500 μL of 100× Antibiotic-Antimycotic for a 1× Solution.
7. Add 500 μL of 100× MEM Non-Essential Amino Acids for a 1× Solution.
8. Add 500 μL of 100× Insulin-Transferrin-Selenium for a 1× Solution.

9. Add 300 μL of 200 mM L-Glutamine to the tube, to form a 1.2 mM Solution.
10. Mix all reagents together and store this serum-free CSC medium in a 4 °C fridge.

3 Methods

3.1 Isolation of CSCs Using Fluorescent-Activated Cell Sorting (FACS) from Primary Patient Malignant Ascites or Ovarian Cancer Cell Lines

Our lab isolates ovarian cancer CSCs based on a concurrent elevated activity in Aldehyde dehydrogenase (ALDH) and expression of CD133, based on previously published protocols [12], nevertheless Subheading 3.2 and following, apply to CSCs independent of tumor type and isolation method. We routinely isolate ovarian CSCs from patient ascites, primary or metastatic tumors and from several ovarian cancer cell lines. The following outlined protocol is used to isolate ovarian CSCs.

1. Centrifuge the malignant ascites, primary, or metastatic tumor sample collected under IRB approved protocols at 1000 × *g* for 5 min (*see* **Note 2**).
2. Lyse the red blood cells using the ACK lysis buffer following the manufacturer's protocol. Briefly, incubate the cell pellet for 3–5 min with ACK buffer, and centrifuge at 300 × *g* for 5 min. Discard the supernatant and resuspend cell pellet with neutral phosphate-buffered saline pH 7.4.
3. Filter cell suspension through 40 μm nylon filters twice, washing in between filtration and recovering cells using centrifugation.
4. Triturate cell suspension by pipetting to obtain single-cell suspensions (*see* **Note 3**).
5. Stain and sort by flow cytometry cell population that express both ALDH+ (Aldefluor Kit, following manufacture instruction) and CD133+. A representative FACS sorting of ovarian CSCs from patietn ascites is shown in Fig. 1.

The following methods can be performed on CSCs from different tumors that have been selected with other methods and markers.

3.2 Generating Spheroids from CSCs Using the 384-Well Hanging Drop Array Plate

1. Sonicate the new hanging drop plate in a water bath for 20 min to dislodge any debris on the surface or within the wells.
2. Using gloves, rinse the plate in running DI water, periodically shaking the plate out vigorously—to remove debris incurred from injection molding and manufacture of plates.
3. Place the plate in a 0.1% Pluronic acid bath for 24 h and cover bath. Pluronic applies an amphiphilic surfactant coating to the plate preventing cell adhesion and thus promoting proper spheroid formation [13, 14].

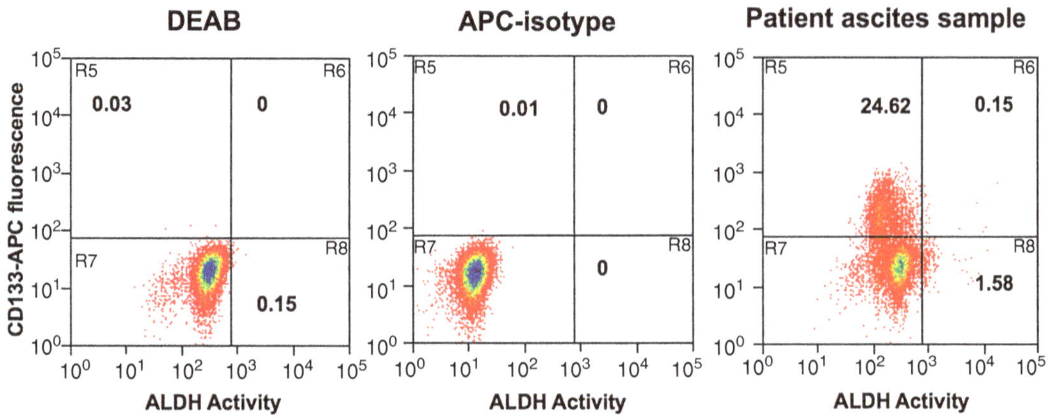

Fig. 1 ALDH+ CD133+ ovarian cancer stem cells are sorted from patient ascites via fluorescent-activated cell sorting (FACS). Malignant ascites samples were filtered to remove debris, and labeled with DEAB (a negative control for Aldehyde dehydrogenase), an isotype-control for the APC antibody, or double labeled with ALDH and CD133-APC. The *Y*-axis indicates APC fluorescence, while the *X*-axis indicated ALDH activity. By gating based on the negative control samples (DEAB and APC-isotype), we can identify distinct populations within malignant ascites (derived from patient sample) that are CD133+ ALDH+ (0.15%), CD133+ ALDH– (24.62%), ALDH+ CD133– (1.58%), or ALDH– CD133– (73.65%). Ovarian cancer stem cells or OvCSCs are isolated based on ALDH+ CD133+ expression

4. Remove the plate with gloved hands from the bath and rinse the plate again in DI water, making sure to remove all water from wells.
5. Place the plate under UV light for sterilization for at least 30 min on each side. The plate is now ready to use (*see* **Note 4**).
6. Prepare a sterile 6-well plate to act as a humidity chamber by adding 4–5 mL of filtered DI water into each of the 6 wells. This will provide the humidity necessary to maintain the hanging drops over extended periods of time. Without proper humidification excessive evaporation of the drops is observed leading to cell death.
7. Next, place the 384 hanging drop plate atop the prepared 6-well plate and pipet 800 μL of filtered DI water into each of the border reservoirs for further humidity control.
8. Each hanging drop will contain 20 μL of volume. Plan out plate design before proceeding to plating. Be sure to leave a 2-well border around the outside edges of the plate in order to avoid contact with the hydration wells. Schematic of optimal design of hanging drop plate is shown in Fig. 2.
9. Trypsinize cells as per a regular passage, and count cells using a hemocytometer or any other automated cell counter. Dilute cell concentration appropriately to the desired concentration (i.e., 100 cells in a 20 μL drop). It is suggested that 100 cell spheroids are attempted first and working down to smaller concentrations (and even as low as 1 cell per hanging drop).

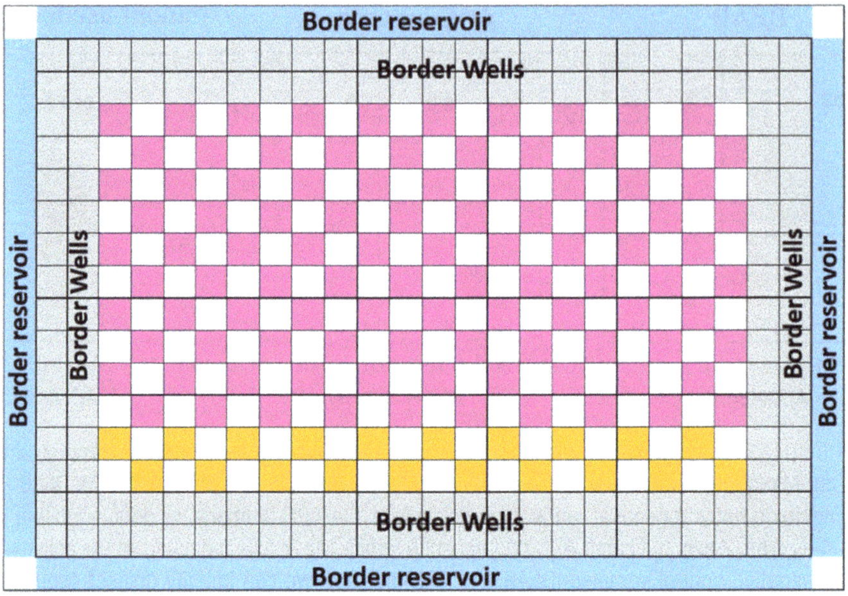

Fig. 2 Ideal plate layout for spheroid generation in 384-well hanging drop array plates. This experimental design features hanging drops (illustrated in *pink color*) that are staggered from each other in order to avoid droplet merging. The open access holes are represented as *white*. The experiments can be designed to have specific groups across the same row. At least two rows are recommended for use for any specific experimental group, to serve as technical replicates (20 spheroids in 2 rows)

10. Mix the working cell solution using a 1000 μL pipet before plating (*see* **Note 5**).
11. Pipet 20 μL of the cell solution into desired well (Fig. 2; *see* **Note 6**).
12. Once all desired wells are filled, place the lid of the 6-well plate, atop the hanging drops effectively sandwiching the 384-well plate.
13. Use parafilm® to carefully seal all outside edges of plates in order to prevent additional evaporation of droplets.
14. Place the entire sandwiched plate carefully into a standard CO_2 humidified incubator (5% CO_2, 37 °C). The hanging drops will need to be fed once every other day for cell maintenance.

3.3 Maintenance and Monitoring of Ovarian CSC Spheroids in Hanging Drop Arrays

1. Carefully remove the plate from the incubator and place into sterilized space in a biological safety cabinet.
2. Remove parafilm from plate edges, being careful not to disturb the droplets (*see* **Note 7**).
3. Carefully carry only the 384-well plate from the biological safety cabinet to the imaging location and lower into microscope tray for live-cell imaging using the right plate adapter

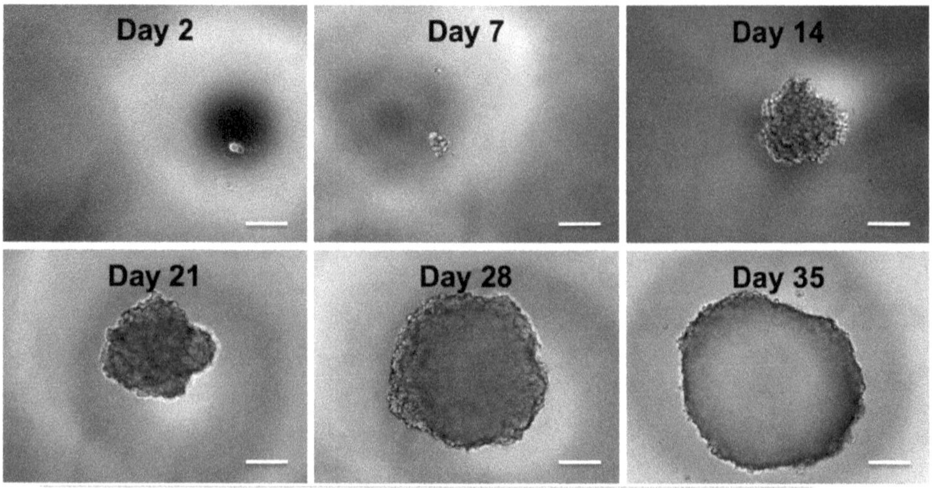

Fig. 3 Patient OvCSC spheroids can be grown from 1 cell/drop over 35 days in hanging drop culture. Spheroids were initiated with 1 OvCSC (isolated from patient ascites) per drop on 384-well hanging drop arrays, and monitored using phase contrast microscopy over 35 days. Cells within spheroids proliferate and aggregate, and form tight compact spherical structures. Spheroids can be maintained for over 1 month in culture. Scale bar = 100 μm

(standard multiwall plate adapters for microscope stages will fit the 384-well hanging drop array plate).

4. Using the scanning option at either 10× or 20× magnification, hanging drops can be observed and imaged on an inverted microscope (e.g., Olympus IX81, Japan, equipped with an ORCA R2 cooled CCD camera and CellSens software). Figure 3 demonstrates phase images of a patient-derived CSC spheroid developing from day 1 through day 35, initiated from a single ALDH+ CD133+ cell, isolated using flow cytometry (*see* **Note 8**). Figure 4a illustrates increase in spheroid size over 5 days, when initiated with 100 cells per drop.
5. Remove the plate from imaging stage and place back into the laminar flow biological safety cabinet, atop the hydration plate.
6. Add 2 or 3 μL of medium to each well containing a droplet. 2 μL is advised for every other day. These volumes can be adjusted according to the observed droplet size as some may evaporate more than others (*see* **Note 9**).
7. Place the lid back on the 384-well plate and 6-well plate stack
8. Reseal edges of stack with parafilm and carefully place in an incubator.

3.4 Quantification of CSC Spheroids' Proliferation and Viability

Alamarblue is a cell viability indicator that uses the natural reducing power of living cells to convert resazurin to the fluorescent molecule, resorufin. The resazurin is a nontoxic, cell permeable compound that is blue in color and nonfluorescent [15, 16]. Upon

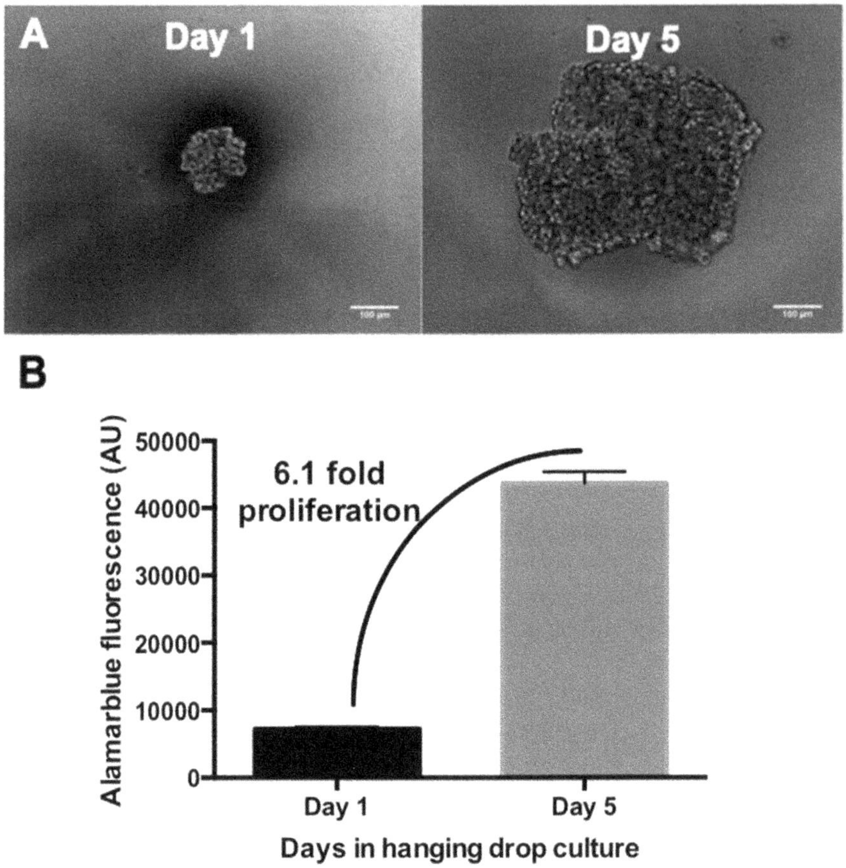

Fig. 4 Proliferation within OvCSC spheroids is quantified with on-plate alamarblue fluorescence detection. (**a**) Phase contrast images are depicted for ovarian cancer spheroids initiated with 100 cells/drop. Representative images are shown for Day 1 and Day 5, where spheroids increase in size owing to proliferation and compaction. (**b**) Alamarblue fluorescence was measured at Day 1 and Day 5, and represented graphically. A comparison of fluorescence at Day 5 with fluorescence at Day 1 indicated that there was a 6.1 fold proliferation within spheroids. Scale bar = 100 μm

entering cells, resazurin is reduced to resorufin, which produces very bright red fluorescence. Viable cells continuously convert resazurin to resorufin, thereby generating a quantitative measure of viability and cytotoxicity [17]. Alamarblue can be used in both 2D and 3D cell culture platforms [14, 15, 17]. Typically, alamarblue is added in a 1–10 dilution, with altered incubation times based on cell number. For wells with very low cell number (less than 500), alamarblue can be added and incubated overnight, reading the following day after 12–18 h of incubation. Higher cell densities can be read within a few hours or less. Some optimization may be needed to find the ideal incubation time for the experiment type. After incubation, fluorescence readings are collected at 560 nm excitation, and 590 nm emission within a fluorescence plate reader.

Proliferation Assay: In order to examine proliferation, alamarblue fluorescence is collected at Day 1 of plating, and at a further day upon which the data is desired, such as Day 7. The fluorescence from the end time point day, such as Day 7, is normalized to Day 1, giving a value of change in fold proliferation (*see* Fig. 4b).

Viability Assay: Cell viability after drug treatment is evaluated at the end of the time point. The values obtained for the drug-treated group are normalized to the control group that did not receive treatment. Refer to Subheading 3.7 for more detailed protocols.

The following steps describe the addition of the alamarblue reagent and quantification of the hanging drops plates on a microplate reader.

1. Remove the plate from the incubator and carefully remove parafilm.
2. Add 2 μL of filtered alamarblue solution to each well desired for analysis. The same methodology as feeding is recommended for this step. Once alamarblue is added to a hanging drop it is not recommended for use in future analysis, due to possible degradation products; therefore, this should be taken into account when planning analysis. Often one or two rows of spheroids will be analyzed at a time to maintain the rest of the plate for further culture.
3. Place cover back atop hanging drop plate and 6-well plate stack. There is no need to reapply the parafilm the edges as the plate will need to be read on the microplate reader within a few hours.
4. Place hanging drop stack back in an incubator for 4 h. This incubation time may need to be adjusted depending on the experiment as it depends on several factors such as cell number, pH of the solution, and cell type. Specific incubation times should be experimentally determined for each case.
5. Remove the plate from the incubator and place in a sterilized biological safety cabinet.
6. Remove the lid of hanging drop stack and place face down in a biological safety cabinet.
7. Carefully remove the 384-well plate from the humidifying 6-well bottom plate and place the 384-well plate into the prepared plate reader.
8. Read the plate at 560 nm excitation and 590 nm emission within a fluorescence plate reader (e.g., Synergy HT, BioTek Instruments, Winooski, VT).
9. Once finished remove the plate from the reader and carefully place back into the biological safety cabinet atop the 6-well hydration plate.

10. Place the lid back onto the hanging drop stack and reapply the parafilm edges of the stacked plates.
11. Place the plate in an incubator for further analysis.

3.5 Confocal Microscopy to Assay Viability of the Ovarian CSC Spheroids

Our lab uses the Live/Dead Viability/Cytotoxicity Kit to assess the presence of live and dead cells in the spheroids. It is a simple and quick method for imaging and quantifying the amount of cell death within a spheroid.

1. Prepare a solution of 8 μM Calcein AM and 16 μM Ethidium Homodimer-1 in 1× PBS. This should be prepared fresh each time, as Calcein AM is not stable for long periods of time when exposed to moisture.
2. Add 5 μL of this solution to the 20 μL drop on the hanging drop plate, and let it incubate for 1 h. Longer incubations may be needed for spheroids over 1000 cells. We recommend incubating on the same day as the fluorescent imaging.
3. Use a 1000 μL pipette to carefully pull the spheroid out of the hanging drop, and place on a glass coverslip.
4. Set the z-stack parameters on a confocal microscope (Olympus IX81, equipped with a Yokogawa CSU-X1 confocal scanning laser unit, Andor iXon x3 CCD camera, and Metamorph 7.8 software) to image the entirety of the spheroid, marking the top and bottom of the spheroid, and set the step size as per recommendations from the microscope software.
5. Select the wavelengths of 488 nm (green), and 561 nm (red), to image live and dead cells, respectively.
6. Adjust the gain and the exposure to avoid saturation of the image. Keep these settings constant throughout all spheroids.
7. Collect fluorescent images readout of the entire spheroid over the z-stack at these two wavelengths.
8. Save images from each wavelength separately to allow for more accurate quantification, and as a 16-bit TIFF image to reserve picture quality.

Figure 5 demonstrates that majority of the cells within patient-derived CSC spheroids are alive (green), with a few dead cells (red).

3.6 Characterization of Ovarian CSC Populations Within Spheroids by FACS

In order to determine ovarian CSC populations, patient-derived spheroids are harvested from 384-well hanging drop array plates, and collected in a tube. We typically assay for $ALDH^+$, $CD133^+$ status, but additional markers like CD44, CD117, etc. can be utilized to assay for other ovarian CSC markers using this method as well.

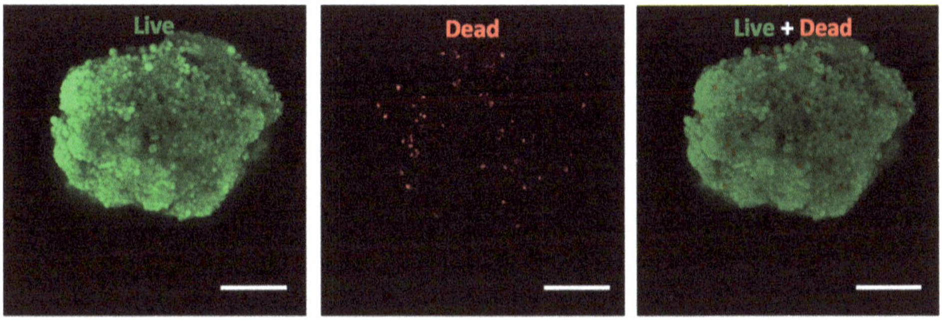

Fig. 5 Ovarian CSC spheroids contain majority of viable cells. Live/Dead staining was performed using the Live/Dead Cytotoxicity kit. Patient-derived CSC spheroids were incubated with calcein-AM (*green*) and ethidium homodimer (*red*) for 60 min, and fluorescence was visualized using a confocal microscope. *Green* fluorescence indicates live cells within the spheroid, while *red* fluorescence indicates dead cells within spheroids. The balance of live/dead cells indicates good viability of cells within patient CSC spheroids. Scale bar = 100 μm

1. Harvest spheroids from 384-well hanging drop array plates, triturate to generate single-cell suspensions, filter through a 40 μm nylon filter and count cells.
2. Centrifuge suspension to recover cells, and follow protocols established for FACS analysis of CSCs within the spheroids (for example, as noted in Subheading 3.1).

3.7 Assessment of Drug Sensitivity and the Use of Ovarian CSC Spheroids for Preclinical Drug Testing

Screening of novel effective anti-neoplastic therapeutics is a nontrivial problem. The activity of anticancer drugs has been conventionally evaluated in 2D-cultured isogenic cancer cell lines, which fail to identify promising drugs that exhibit potency in vivo [18]. Physiological 3D models, such as the spheroids, have now been firmly established to more accurately mimic the drug sensitivity/resistance behavior of cancer cells found in solid tumors in vivo than the cancer cells cultured under conventional 2D monolayer conditions [19, 20]. Spheroids possess several in vivo features of tumors such as cell-cell interaction, hypoxia, drug penetration, response and resistance, and production/deposition of extracellular matrix [21]. Therefore, our lab utilizes spheroids to screen for novel drugs that could be effective against targeting CSCs and chemoresistant cells.

The following steps outline the treatment of the spheroids with a conventional clinically relevant chemotherapy drug for ovarian cancers, cisplatin. However, the same steps can be used for the screening of any drug compounds.

1. Seed CSCs in hanging drop plates at a seeding density of 50cells per well as outlined in Subheading 3.3.
2. Monitor cells for spheroid formation for 3 days—using live-cell microscopy as outlined in Subheading 3.4.

3. To a 20 μL-hanging drop we typically add 2 μL drug, so the drug to cells ratio is 1:10. For example, weigh 1 mg Cisplatin and dissolve in 1 mL of DI water to get a 1 mg/mL concentration of Cisplatin. Dilute the stock to make a final drug concentration, of 50 μM in each hanging drop.
4. After uniform spheroids are observed under the microscope at Day 3, add 2 μL drug to the hanging drops (*see* **Note 10**).
5. A standard 384-well plate can house 140 spheroids, with spheroids in alternate wells, and staggered rows. Apart from adding the drugs to majority of the wells of the hanging drop plate, 20–30 spheroids remain untreated with the drug, these wells act as a negative control. Add 2 μL of the cell culture growth medium to the negative control spheroids.
6. Seventy two hours the addition of the drug, image the spheroids (both negative control and drug treated) on the inverted microscope.
7. Perform the alamarblue metabolic assay as described in Subheading 3.4 and normalize the fluorescence intensity of the drug-treated spheroids with the negative control.

Figure 6 shows the results of cisplatin treatment on ovarian cancer spheroids initiated with 50 cells/drop of the OVCAR3 cell line. Two different concentrations of cisplatin were dosed, 30 μM and 50 μM. Compared to control untreated spheroids (normalized to 100%), cisplatin-treated spheroids had reduced viabilities (60–80%).

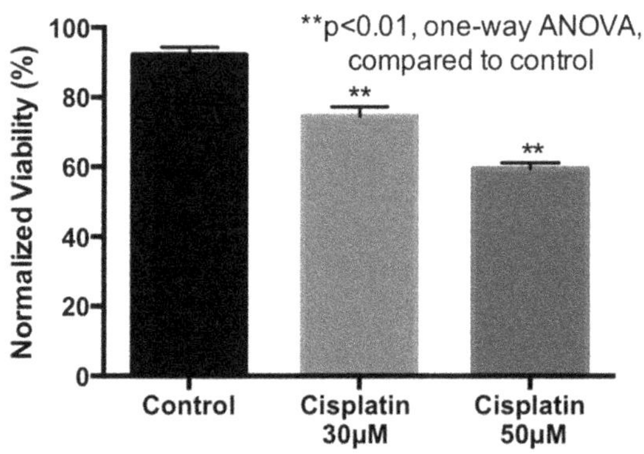

Fig. 6 Hanging drop ovarian CSC spheroids can be successfully utilized for drug screening or treatment using alamarblue fluorescence quantification. Ovarian cancer cells (50 cells per drop) were treated with Cisplatin (30 μM and 50 μM) on day 3, after confirming the formation of spheroids. On day 7, spheroids were incubated with alamarblue and the fluorescence intensity was quantified 4 h after incubation. The drug-treated values were normalized to control. Drug-treated spheroids are less viable than control untreated spheroids

3.8 Histological Assessment of Spheroid 3D Structure and Cell-Cell and Cell-Matrix Interactions

Given that the spheroids are 3D microtissues, confocal microscopy enabled by immunostaining and immunohistochemistry are key to study specific cell-cell and cell-matrix interactions within spheroids [22]. Embedding 3D spheroids in agarose is relatively inexpensive and easy to perform. We use low melting point agarose to envelop the spheroids to provide a stable mold for spheroids once it cools down and solidifies.

1. Make a 2%w/v low melting point agarose solution in deionized water.
2. Pipette out 50 μL warm (40–45 °C) 2% agarose on a sterile non-reactive surface, making an agarose drop.
3. Using a pipette, harvest spheroids from their respective wells on the hanging drop array plate and embed in the agarose drop.
4. Fix the samples in 4% formalin overnight.
5. Remove the biopsy cassette containing samples from formalin and place in 70% ethanol. If paraffin processing for microtomy, place cassettes in 70% ethanol, and run through a tissue processor and embed in paraffin blocks.
6. If staining agarose embedded spheroids, perform a quick Glycine buffer pH 7 wash, and wash with 1× PBS.
7. Add appropriate permeabilization, blocking buffer, primary and secondary antibodies including careful wash steps in between, to visualize proteins within spheroids using confocal microscopy.

Figure 7 shows an ovarian cancer spheroid generated from 100 cells/drop. Spheroids were embedded in agarose at Day 7, fixed and stained with a primary antibody directed against ALDH1A1. The red fluorescence indicates the presence of ALDH1A1, and the nuclei are counterstained blue with DAPI.

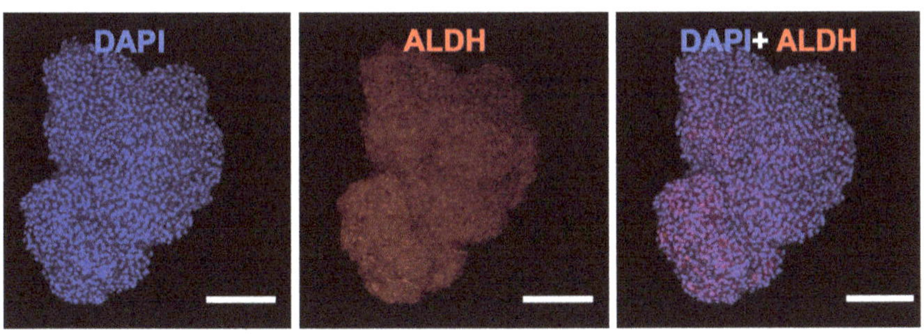

Fig. 7 OvCSC spheroids can be histologically analyzed for CSC markers. Ovarian cancer spheroids were embedded in agarose, and stained with a rabbit polyclonal antibody directed against ALDH1A1 and a TRITC-conjugated secondary antibody. The *red* fluorescence within spheroids indicates the presence and expression of the stem cell marker, ALDH1A1. The nuclei are counterstained *blue* with DAPI, and the images were acquired on a spinning disk confocal microscope. Scale bar = 100 μm

4 Notes

1. We recommend making fresh serum-free medium every week for the CSC spheroids.
2. For cell lines, trypsinize cell lines from a regular tissue culture plate and omit the ACK lysing buffer step, and proceed with the staining. For primary tissues, mechanically dissociate tissues following dissection until single-cell suspensions are obtained. The Miltenyi MACS human Tumor Cell Dissociation and Isolation Kit can also be used.
3. A standard hub pipetting needle can also be used to break cell pellets into single-cell suspensions. Use up to gauge 23.
4. It is important to sterilize both the faces of the hanging drop plate.
5. It is recommended to mix the cell suspension often in order to achieve consistent cell counts per drop, as cells tend to aggregate in solution over time, which changes the cell density in the suspension.
6. It is recommended that the pipet tip rests on the well at an angle, since the vertical positioning tends to cause the droplet to fall. Also, it is advised to use every other well, staggering each row to avoid the unintentional merging of droplets.
7. Be sure all parafilm is removed before attempting to take off lid as remnants of parafilm can cause sticking and disturbance of hanging drops. It is advised to hold the plate stable for this process by placing pressure on the lid.
8. Keep the imaging time under 10–15 min, as prolonged exposure to the microscope light will cause evaporation leading to cell death, as well as increased likelihood of acquiring debris.
9. When adding medium to the hanging drop, place the pipet tip at an angle to the well to prevent unnecessary disruption of the hanging drop.
10. It may take longer than 3 days for cells to form spheroids depending on the patient sample, in which case monitor spheroid formation using live-cell microscopy before drug treatment.

References

1. Magee JA, Piskounova E, Morrison SJ (2012) Cancer stem cells: impact, heterogeneity, and uncertainty. Cancer Cell 21:283–296
2. Wang HJ, Guo YQ, Tan G et al (2013) miR-125b regulates side population in breast cancer and confers a chemoresistant phenotype. J Cell Biochem 114:2248–2257
3. Korkaya H, Wicha MS (2010) Cancer stem cells: nature versus nurture. Nat Cell Biol 12:419–421

4. Wang A, Chen L, Li C, Zhu Y (2015) Heterogeneity in cancer stem cells. Cancer Lett 357:63–68
5. Hanai JI, Doro N, Seth P, Sukhatme VP (2013) ATP citrate lyase knockdown impacts cancer stem cells in vitro. Cell Death Dis 4: e696
6. Singh A, Settleman J (2010) EMT, cancer stem cells and drug resistance: an emerging axis of evil in the war on cancer. Oncogene 29:4741–4751
7. Alison MR, Lin WR, Lim SM, Nicholson LJ (2012) Cancer stem cells: in the line of fire. Cancer Treat Rev 38:589–598
8. Kase M, Minajeva A, Niinepuu K et al (2013) Impact of CD133 positive stem cell proportion on survival in patients with glioblastoma multiforme. Radiol Oncol 47:405–410
9. Longati P, Jia X, Eimer J et al (2013) 3D pancreatic carcinoma spheroids induce a matrix-rich, chemoresistant phenotype offering a better model for drug testing. BMC Cancer 13:95
10. Raghavan S, Mehta P, Horst EN, Ward MR, Rowley KR, Mehta G (2016) Comparative analysis of tumor spheroid generation techniques for differential in vitro drug toxicity. Oncotarget 7:16948–16961
11. Raghavan S, Ward MR, Rowley KR et al (2015) Formation of stable small cell number three-dimensional ovarian cancer spheroids using hanging drop arrays for preclinical drug sensitivity assays. Gynecol Oncol 138:181–189
12. Silva IA, Bai S, McLean K et al (2011) Aldehyde dehydrogenase in combination with CD133 defines angiogenic ovarian cancer stem cells that portend poor patient survival. Cancer Res 71:3991–4001
13. Futrega K, Palmer JS, Kinney M et al (2015) The microwell-mesh: a novel device and protocol for the high throughput manufacturing of cartilage microtissues. Biomaterials 62:1–12
14. Tung YC, Hsiao AY, Allen SG, Torisawa YS, Ho M, Takayama S (2011) High-throughput 3D spheroid culture and drug testing using a 384 hanging drop array. Analyst 136:473–478
15. Zhou X, Holsbeeks I, Impens S et al (2013) Noninvasive real-time monitoring by alamarBlue((R)) during in vitro culture of three-dimensional tissue-engineered bone constructs. Tissue Eng Part C Methods 19:720–729
16. Rampersad SN (2012) Multiple applications of Alamar blue as an indicator of metabolic function and cellular health in cell viability bioassays. Sensors (Basel) 12:12347–12360
17. O'Brien J, Wilson I, Orton T, Pognan F (2000) Investigation of the Alamar blue (resazurin) fluorescent dye for the assessment of mammalian cell cytotoxicity. Eur J Biochem 267:5421–5426
18. Imamura Y, Mukohara T, Shimono Y et al (2015) Comparison of 2D- and 3D-culture models as drug-testing platforms in breast cancer. Oncol Rep 33:1837–1843
19. Weiswald LB, Bellet D, Dangles-Marie V (2015) Spherical cancer models in tumor biology. Neoplasia 17:1–15
20. Zanoni M, Piccinini F, Arienti C et al (2016) 3D tumor spheroid models for in vitro therapeutic screening: a systematic approach to enhance the biological relevance of data obtained. Sci Rep 6:19103
21. Mehta G, Hsiao AY, Ingram M, Luker GD, Takayama S (2012) Opportunities and challenges for use of tumor spheroids as models to test drug delivery and efficacy. J Control Release 164:192–204
22. Weiswald LB, Guinebretiere JM, Richon S, Bellet D, Saubamea B, Dangles-Marie V (2010) In situ protein expression in tumour spheres: development of an immunostaining protocol for confocal microscopy. BMC Cancer 10:106

Chapter 7

In Vitro Tumorigenic Assay: The Tumor Spheres Assay

Hui Wang, Anna M. Paczulla, Martina Konantz, and Claudia Lengerke

Abstract

Cancer stem cells (CSCs) are a subpopulation of cells within cancer tissues that are thought to mediate tumor initiation. CSCs are furthermore considered the cause of tumor progression and recurrence after conventional therapies, based on their enhanced therapy resistance properties. A method commonly used to assess CSC potential in vitro is the so-called tumor spheres assay in which cells are plated under non-adherent culture conditions in serum-free medium supplemented with growth factors. Tumor spheres assays have been used in cancer research as an intermediate in vitro cell culture model to be explored before performing more laborious in vivo tumor xenograft assays.

Key words Cancer stem cell, Tumor spheres assay, In vitro

1 Introduction

Years of research indicate pronounced cellular heterogeneity within individual tumor samples, with only a subpopulation of tumor cells—the CSCs—being able to both self-renew and differentiate giving rise to more differentiated tumor cell types. Given this definition, putative CSC populations need to be analyzed in functional assays. In the past two decades, the identification of CSCs able to establish tumors following experimental implantation in immunosuppressed murine hosts [1] (versus non-tumorigenic non-CSC tumor cells derived from the same sample) brought CSCs to the spotlight in cancer research.

The tumor spheres assay has been developed as an in vitro surrogate method to study CSC potential, next to the more time-consuming and laborious in vivo tumorigenicity assays. When cultured under certain conditions (with low nutrients but specific growth factor exposure) and in a suspension environment, CSCs can survive and clonally expand building so-called tumor spheres, whereas non-CSCs undergo programmed cell death presumably due to anchorage loss to substrates from the surrounding extracellular matrix [2]. Of note, while tumor spheres are enriched for

Gianpaolo Papaccio and Vincenzo Desiderio (eds.), *Cancer Stem Cells: Methods and Protocols*, Methods in Molecular Biology, vol. 1692, DOI 10.1007/978-1-4939-7401-6_7,

CSCs, these also contain more differentiated tumor cells that emerge from CSCs. Tumor spheres assays are reported to enrich CSCs from bulk cells in various types of cancers and are here widely used to analyze self-renewal.

Spheres assays allowing quantification and characterization of floating spherical aggregates were first developed in the neural system, where healthy neural stem cells were demonstrated to undergo clonal expansion and form neurospheres on a single-cell basis under specific culture conditions [3, 4]. Shortly after, free-floating sphere cultures were reported to identify brain tumor CSCs [5]. Dontu and colleagues later adapted and confirmed the suitability of this assay for the evaluation of stem cells in healthy and malignant breast tissues [6, 7]. Human mammary epithelial cells plated in different numbers in serum-free medium supplemented with epidermal growth factor (EGF), basic fibroblast growth factor (bFGF), B-27, and heparin were cultured under non-adherent conditions for 7–14 days before sphere formation was scored microscopically. Following this protocol with some adjustments in cell numbers, growth medium, and supplements, several groups have explored in vitro stem cell potential from several cancer types such as breast [8, 9], brain [10], ovarian [11, 12], pancreas [13], colon [14], and prostate carcinoma [15].

Traditionally, spheres assays are performed by plating multiple cells per well, and thus, as we and others have shown, are easily influenced by cell density [12]. Single cell-based sphere formation assays are an attractive alternative to identify CSCs. Figure 1 shows schematic experimental steps for single cell-based spheres assays.

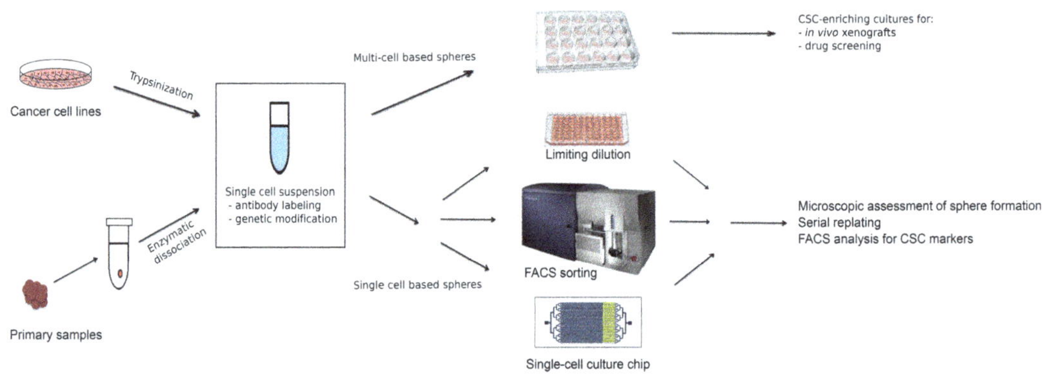

Fig. 1 Workflow of tumor spheres assay. After cell preparation (stem cell marker positive) tumor cells are sorted by FACS into individual wells of a 96-well plate in spheres medium; alternatively, suitable cell populations are plated into individual wells or through a single-cell chip. For multi cell-based spheres assays, 100–1000 cells are placed into one well. Plating efficiency is assessed by microscopy performed after sorting or plating. Spheres were scored by microscopy after 1–2 weeks, then dissociated into single cells and if applicable analyzed for surface expression of CSC markers via flow cytometry. At this stage, collected cells can be also replated into secondary spheres assays or used for other assays

Performing in vitro single cell-based spheres assays, however, is technically more challenging than the traditional multi cell-based assays.

2 Materials

2.1 Preparation of Primary Tumor Single-Cell Suspensions (Here for Example: Ovarian Tumor Tissue)

1. Washing solution: Phosphate-buffered saline (PBS), 2% Penicillin/streptomycin.
2. Digestion solution: Collagenase (Biochrom, CI-22) 2 mg/ml in RPMI (NO FBS) or other medium according to tumor origin.
3. Trypan blue.

2.2 Preparation of Cancer Cell Line Single-Cell Suspensions

1. Phosphate-buffered saline (PBS).
2. 0.05% Trypsin-EDTA.
3. Basic Medium: cell culture medium (according to the origin of tumor, e.g., for ovarian cancer cell lines normally RPMI is used) supplemented with FBS 10% and 2% penicillin/streptomycin.

2.3 Preparation of Spheres Culture Medium (see Table 1)

Spheres culture medium was prepared as shown in Table 1.

2.4 Equipment

1. Ultra-low attachment plates (6, 24, 48, 96, or 384 wells, Corning).
2. Petri dishes.
3. 25 ml, 10 ml, 5 ml serological pipettes.
4. Surgery tools (scalpels, scissors).
5. Cell strainer (40 and 70 μm).
6. 37 °C water bath.
7. Incubator (37 °C and 5% CO_2).
8. Microscope.
9. Fluorescence Activated Cell Sorter (FACS).
10. Centrifuge.

3 Methods

3.1 Medium Preparation

For conventional 2D cell cultures and generation of single-cell suspensions from cell lines a medium is generated according to the protocol of ATCC. The same medium is used, where applicable,

Table 1
Spheres culture medium for different sources of cells (basic medium + supplements)

Human cancer cell source	Basic medium	Supplements
Ovarian carcinoma cell lines (OVCAR-3, Caov-3) and primary cells [11, 12]	MEGM	20 ng/ml rEGF, 20 ng/ml bFGF, B-27, 4 μg/ml heparin, hydrocortisone, insulin (SingleQuot kit)
Breast carcinoma cell lines (MCF7, T47D) and primary cells [8]	DMEM	30% F12, 20 ng/ml rEGF, 20 ng/ml bFGF, 2% B-27, 1% penicillin/streptomycin, 1% L-glutamine
Colon carcinoma cell lines (Colo205) and primary cells [14]	DMEM/ F12	20 ng/ml rEGF, 10 ng/ml bFGF, 2% B-27, 10 ng/ml LIF, 2 mM L-glutamine
Lung carcinoma, primary cells (lung) [16]	DMEM/ F12	50 μg/ml insulin, 20 μg/ml rEGF, 10 μg/ml bFGF, 0.4% BSA, 100 mg/ml apo-transferrin, 10 mg/ml putrescine, 0.03 mM sodium selenite, 2 mM progesterone, 0.6% glucose, 5 mM HEPES, 0.1% sodium bicarbonate,
Glioblastoma, primary cells [10]	Stem cell media	20 ng/ml rEGF, 20 ng/ml bFGF, 2% B-27, Neurobasal A, 1% penicillin/streptomycin, non-essential amino acids, sodium pyruvate, vitamin A,
Pancreas carcinoma, primary cells [13]	DMEM/ F12	3% FBS, 20 ng/ml rEGF, 20 ng/ml bFGF, 2% B-27, 10 ng/ ml LIF, 1% N2 supplement, 1% penicillin/streptomycin, non-essential amino acids, 100 μM Beta-mercaptoethanol
Prostate carcinoma cell lines (PC3) [15]	DMEM/ F12	20 ng/ml rEGF, 20 ng/ml bFGF, B-27, 4 μg/ml heparin, insulin (SingleQuot kit)

for 2D cultures and generation of single-cell suspensions from primary tumor specimens. For tumor spheres assays/cultures, the tumor spheres medium is generated by the addition of specific supplements to basic medium as indicated in Table 1 (*see* **Note 1**). Carry out all the procedures in a sterile hood to minimize chances of culture contaminations.

3.2 Preparation of Single-Cell Suspensions from Primary Tumor Samples (Here for Example: Ovarian Carcinoma Tissue)

1. Wash fresh tumor samples washing solution.
2. Place tumor samples in a petri dish.
3. Cut the tumor samples into small pieces using autoclaved scissors and mince completely using a scalpel.
4. Digest tumor pieces enzymatically with a digestion solution and incubate at 37 °C for 3 h, mix occasionally.
5. Mix digested tumor samples sequentially with a 25 ml, 10 ml, and finally 5 ml pipette to separate the cells.
6. Filter the digested sample through a 70 μm cell strainer cap filter twice.

7. Centrifuge cells at 1500 × *g* at room temperature (15–25 °C) for 7 min, wash once with PBS, and resuspend the pellet in the spheres medium.

3.3 Preparation of Single-Cell Suspensions from Cell Lines

1. Aspirate media from flask, wash cells once with PBS, and trypsinize cells for 3 min.
2. Inactivate trypsin by using basic medium (see above, containing FBS and penicillin/streptomycin), centrifuge cells at 1500 × *g* at room temperature (15–25 °C) for 5 min, and resuspend the pellet in the spheres medium.
3. Use a 40 μm cell strainer cap filter to obtain single-cell suspension.

3.4 Plating Multi-Cell Tumor Spheres Assays

For multi cell-based spheres assays, adjust cells to a proper concentration in the spheres medium, e.g., plate 100 cells per well in a 100 μl spheres medium in a 96-well plate. For this, test different concentrations side by side to identify the concentration window introducing minimal bias [12].

For a methylcellulose-based spheres assay, prepare first a twofold concentrated spheres medium and 2% methylcellulose (Sigma-Aldrich, M-0387). Resuspend cells in a 1/2 volume (e.g., for 96-well plate is 50 μl, for 24-well plate is 250 μl) with twofold concentrated medium, mix the cells in a 1:1 ratio in 2% methylcellulose, and plate in each well (*see* **Notes 2** and **3**).

3.5 Plating Single-Cell Tumor Spheres Assays

3.5.1 Limiting Dilution

Adjust cell number to 1000 cells per 100 μl, dilute every sample 1:2 to access one cell per 100 μl, and plate 100 μl per well in ultra low-attachment 96-well plates.

3.5.2 Single-Cell Sorting

1. Prepare an ultra low-attachment 96-well plate with a 100 μl spheres medium (Table 1). (Penicillin/streptomycin may be added to the medium at a concentration of 1:1000 to minimize the risk of putative contamination.)
2. Stain cells with stem cell markers (e.g., CD24, CD44, CD133, etc.) if required.
3. Sort (stem cell marker positive) cells (using, e.g., FACS Aria II, BD Biosciences) into each well of a medium-filled 96-well plate (*see* **Note 4**). Check sort success and respectively numbers of sorted cells in each well after sorting (Fig. 2 top).
4. Incubate cells under standard conditions at 37 °C and 5% CO_2.
5. After 10 days, total tumor spheres counts and, if applicable, fluorescence signal intensities are quantified on a fluorescence microscope (e.g., Olympus IX50 Osiris, Fig. 2 bottom) (*see* **Notes 5–7**).

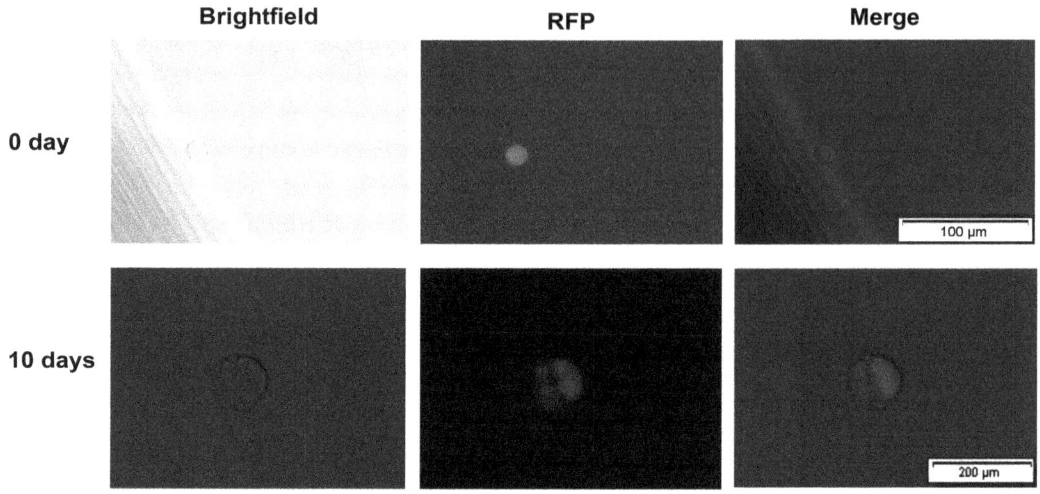

Fig. 2 Imaging of sorted single cells after plating and after 10 days of tumor spheres formation. Single fluorescence marked cells (here RFP+, ref. 12) are sorted into each well of a 96-well plate and analyzed for correct plating by using a (fluorescence) microscope. Tumor spheres are assessed by microscopy performed after 10 days (adapted from ref. 12)

6. Calculate spheres-forming capacity (*see* **Note 8**) in the 96-well plate according to the following formula:

$$\text{Tumor spheres efficiency}(\%) = (\text{number of spheres})/(\text{number of wells seeded}) \times 100$$

3.6 Serial Passaging of Spheres

1. Place the content of each well in an appropriate sterile tube and centrifuge at 1000 × *g* for 5 min at room temperature.
2. Remove the supernatant and resuspend the pellet in 200 μl of 0.05% Trypsin-EDTA.
3. In order to achieve optimal cell separation, incubate the cell suspension at 37 °C for 5–8 min on a soft shaker and then triturate gently using a 100 μl pipette tip.
4. Wash the cells by adding 500 μl sterile PBS and centrifuge at 1500 × *g* for 5 min.
5. Remove the supernatant and resuspend in the spheres medium. Use a 40 μm cell strainer cap filter to obtain a single-cell suspension.
6. Seed 1 cell per well manually into a new ultra low-attachment 96-well plate. For 100 cells per well, seed as described in Subheading 3.4 and count the number of cells after plating.
7. Assess spheres-forming efficiency in secondary, tertiary, and quaternary passages using the formula described above (Subheading 3.5.2, **step 6**).

4 Notes

1. The activity of the growth factors may decrease over time. Make new spheres medium after 7 days when stored at 4 °C. In addition, it is speculated that EGF and FGF may quickly degrade. In some protocols, these growth factors are added daily to the growing spheres. We tested daily EGF and FGF addition versus initial supplementation only in OVCAR-3 cells, but achieved similar results with both the methods [12]. Since individual cancer types might be differentially affected by EGF and FGF concentrations, we recommend upfront testing of the requirement for daily versus one-time growth factor supplementation for the specific tissues, if feasible.
2. Initial cell density can influence the numbers of scored spheres. In some cases, wells seeded with lower cell numbers paradoxically showed higher spheres numbers than those seeded with higher cell numbers (Fig. 3a left, Fig. 3b). We hypothesize that cell clumping and/or sphere fusion or disaggregation can occur, modifying sphere numbers and leading to inaccurate results especially in multi cell-based spheres assays. To reduce this bias, we propose to use addition of1% methylcellulose to the sphere culture to limit cell mobility. Indeed, methylcellulose addition improved accuracy of results that were more comparable to those obtained in single-cell assays [12]. Nevertheless, also in the presence of methylcellulose, sphere disaggregation or fusion might occur, latter for example at particularly high densities. Furthermore, semi-solid methylcellulose, collagen, or matrigel, which have been also previously used to limit cell mobility and aggregation, have limitations: not all cell types can form spheres in semi-solid medium, and medium exchange is challenging.

   Therefore, if multi-cell-based sphere assays are used, upfront investigation of the proper cell concentration will be performed [12] and supplementation with methylcellulose evaluated additionally.
3. Rapid movement of plates (e.g., when the medium is changed or spheres are analyzed under the microscope) should be avoided especially for multi-cell-based spheres assays since they can lead to aggregation or disruption of cells and respectively spheres.
4. Most accurate results are obtained with single-cell-based spheres. However, to reliably quantify rare CSCs, thousands of such single-cell suspension cultures are required. If the limiting dilution method is used without a robotic system, this method is labor intensive.

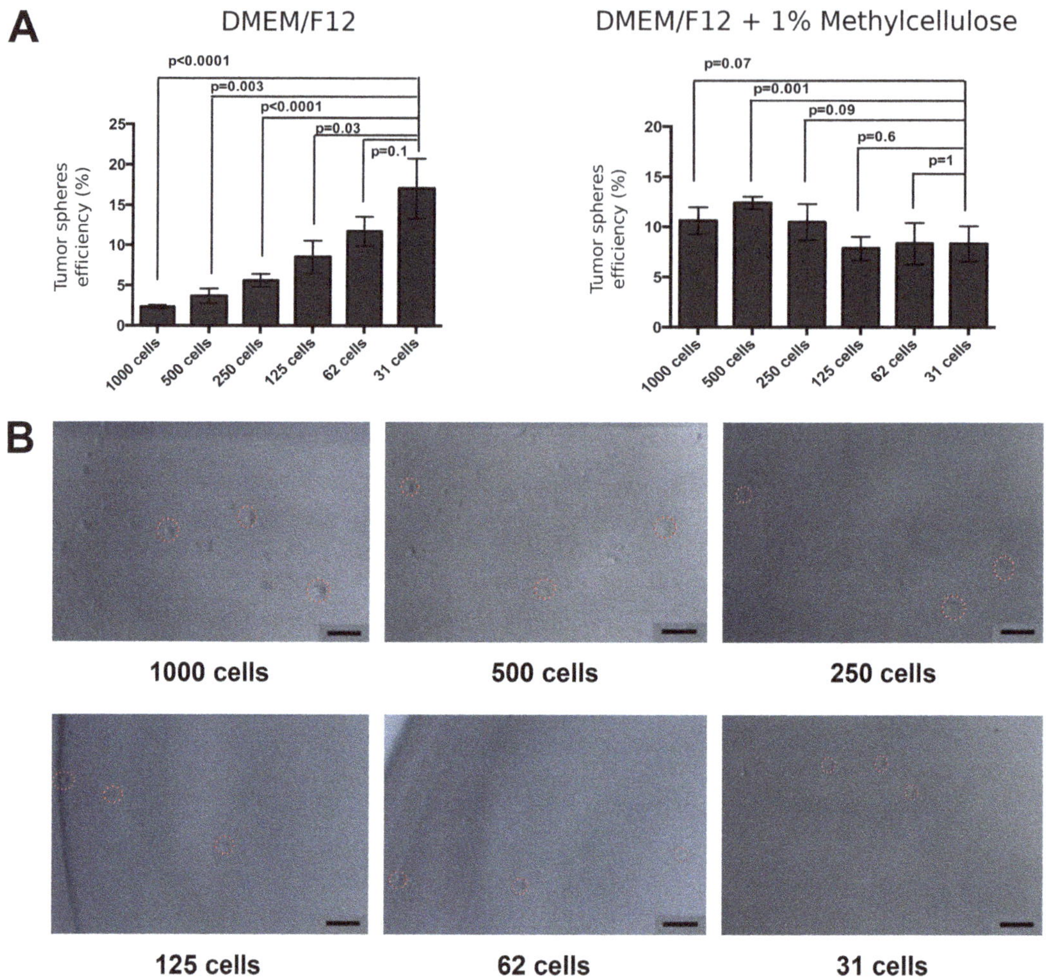

Fig. 3 Cell plating density strongly impacts sphere counts from ovarian carcinoma cell line (OVCAR-3) derived cells in the multi cell-based spheres assay performed in liquid but not in methylcellulose supplemented cultures. Use of different cell densities to analyze possible biases introduced by these variables. Therefore, cells plated at different densities in 200 μl of different spheres culture media (DMEM/F12 with all supplements as detailed in the protocol section, or DMEM/F12 with all supplements and containing 1% methylcellulose) and sphere formation is scored after 7 days (**a**). Shown in (**b**) are microscopy pictures of cells plated at different densities taken 1 day after plating in DMEM/F12 spheres culture medium without methylcellulose. Note the cell clusters emerging at high cellular density as opposed to single cells seen in low-density plates. Scale bar for pictures: 50 μm (adapted from ref. 12)

Fluorescence-activated cell sorting (FACS) can automate the single-cell dispensing process and achieve higher single-cell seeding rate; however, high shear stress during sorting can potentially affect cell viability and also influence results [17]. Moreover, single plated cells may display different growth properties in the absence of supportive signals provided by neighboring cells, thus perhaps lowering sensitivity of this assay.

The microfluidic culture system is a newly established method for single-cell studies. Single-cell capture chips were developed for single-cell-derived sphere assays in combination with a non-adherent culture substrate [18].

5. Typically, a spheres assay would require 7–14 days of culture. For some tumor cell types, spheres formation might require longer time, especially if emerging from single cells. Thus, when establishing spheres assays with a new tumor type longer observation times should be included.
6. Tumor spheres from CSCs should reach a diameter of >50 μm to be scored as such.
7. The prolonged time for imaging over large areas limits the assay throughput and could potentially affect cell viability if no environmental chamber is used during image capture under the microscope.
8. Side-by-side analyses of tumor cells of the same source indicate that not every sphere-forming cell has in vivo tumorigenic properties upon transplantation in immunosuppressed mice [11]. The frequency of sphere initiating cells was higher than the frequency of tumor initiating cells measured in vivo [11], suggesting that either the tumor spheres assay may lead also to false positive results (e.g., due to co-recognition of more differentiated progenitor cells) or, alternatively, the in vivo assay may be inefficient and results in false negative results (perhaps due to technical reasons). Recently, our laboratory has performed further side-by-side investigations of in vivo tumorigenicity using zebrafish as an alternative animal model [19]. Indeed, this model, which allows highly sensitive detection of tumor formation via in vivo microscopy, revealed much higher frequencies of tumor initiating cells when compared to the murine model (Fig. 4). While the results obtained in zebrafish suggest that indeed murine xenotransplant studies might underestimate the frequency of CSC, this model has its own caveats (as reviewed in [19]) and requires further investigation. Of note, the zebrafish environment might be more supportive for the outgrowth of some xenotransplanted tumor types and less of others (e.g., of tumor cells that heavily rely on cytokines or growth factors that are perhaps not fully conserved cross-species between fish and human).

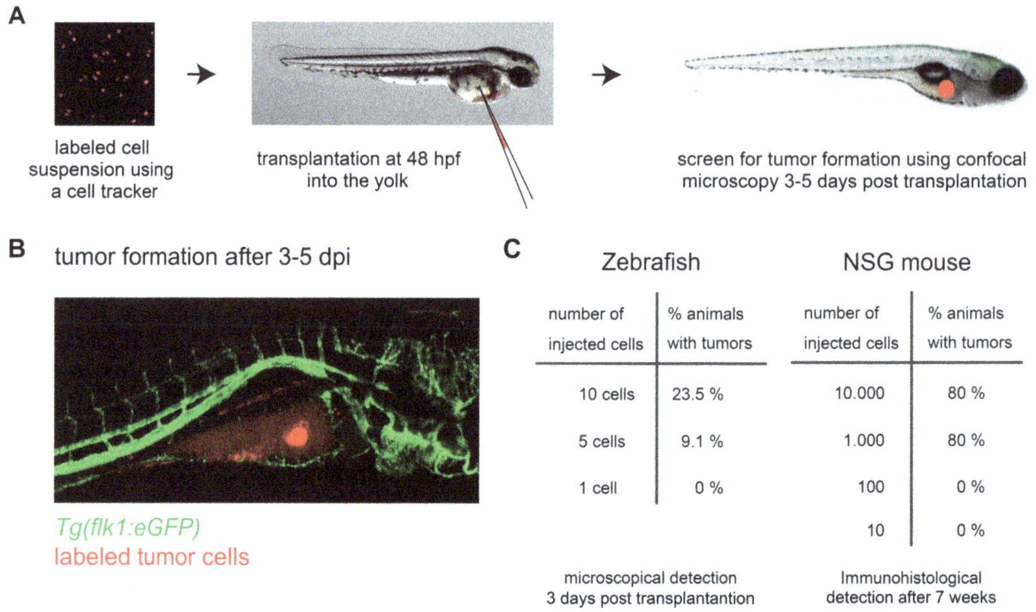

Fig. 4 Human OVCAR-3 cells harboring GFP as a selection marker were xenotransplanted at different numbers into zebrafish embryos or via subcutaneous injection into NSG mice. Note the low numbers of human cells (down to single cells) that can be transplanted and visualized by in vivo microscopy into the yolk of 48 hpf zebrafish embryos (**a**) and that tumor development can be scored—due to the transparency of the zebrafish—already 3 days post injection (**b**). Note that the zebrafish xenotransplant assays indicate a much higher frequency of tumor initiating cells as the murine assay (**c**)

Acknowledgment

This work was supported by grants from the Deutsche Forschungsgemeinschaft to C. Lengerke (Project C6, SFB773) and the Schweizer Nationalfonds to C. Lengerke (SNF 310030E_164200).

References

1. Hermann PC et al (2010) Cancer stem cells in solid tumors. Semin Cancer Biol 20(2):77–84
2. Kruyt FA, Schuringa JJ (2010) Apoptosis and cancer stem cells: implications for apoptosis targeted therapy. Biochem Pharmacol 80 (4):423–430
3. Reynolds BA, Weiss S (1992) Generation of neurons and astrocytes from isolated cells of the adult mammalian central nervous system. Science 255(5052):1707–1710
4. Uchida N et al (2000) Direct isolation of human central nervous system stem cells. Proc Natl Acad Sci U S A 97(26):14720–14725
5. Singh SK et al (2003) Identification of a cancer stem cell in human brain tumors. Cancer Res 63(18):5821–5828
6. Dontu G et al (2003) In vitro propagation and transcriptional profiling of human mammary stem/progenitor cells. Genes Dev 17 (10):1253–1270
7. Shaw FL et al (2012) A detailed mammosphere assay protocol for the quantification of breast stem cell activity. J Mammary Gland Biol Neoplasia 17(2):111–117
8. Leis O et al (2012) Sox2 expression in breast tumours and activation in breast cancer stem cells. Oncogene 31(11):1354–1365

9. Schaefer T et al (2015) Molecular and functional interactions between AKT and SOX2 in breast carcinoma. Oncotarget 6 (41):43540–43556
10. Higgins DM et al (2013) Brain tumor stem cell multipotency correlates with nanog expression and extent of passaging in human glioblastoma xenografts. Oncotarget 4(5):792–801
11. Bareiss PM et al (2013) SOX2 expression associates with stem cell state in human ovarian carcinoma. Cancer Res 73(17):5544–5555
12. Wang H, Paczulla A, Lengerke C (2015) Evaluation of stem cell properties in human ovarian carcinoma cells using multi and single cell-based spheres assays. J Vis Exp 95:e52259
13. Wang YJ et al (2013) Sphere-forming assays for assessment of benign and malignant pancreatic stem cells. Methods Mol Biol 980:281–290
14. Li YF et al (2012) Cultivation and identification of colon cancer stem cell-derived spheres from the Colo205 cell line. Braz J Med Biol Res 45(3):197–204
15. Queisser A et al (2016) Ecotropic viral integration site 1, a novel oncogene in prostate cancer. Oncogene 36(11):1573–1584
16. Eramo A et al (2008) Identification and expansion of the tumorigenic lung cancer stem cell population. Cell Death Differ 15(3):504–514
17. Shapiro E, Biezuner T, Linnarsson S (2013) Single-cell sequencing-based technologies will revolutionize whole-organism science. Nat Rev Genet 14(9):618–630
18. Cheng YH et al (2016) Scaling and automation of a high-throughput single-cell-derived tumor sphere assay chip. Lab Chip 16 (19):3708–3717
19. Konantz M et al (2012) Zebrafish xenografts as a tool for in vivo studies on human cancer. Ann N Y Acad Sci 1266:124–137

Chapter 8

In Vitro Tumorigenic Assay: Colony Forming Assay for Cancer Stem Cells

Vijayalakshmi Rajendran and Mayur Vilas Jain

Abstract

Colony forming or clonogenic assay is an in vitro quantitative technique to examine the capability of a single cell to grow into a large colony through clonal expansion. Clonogenic activity is a sensitive indicator of undifferentiated cancer stem cells. Here, we described the colony forming ability of the isolated breast cancer stem cells from the total population of cancer cells using double-layered, soft agarose-based assay. This method demonstrates that cancer stem cells can survive and generate colony growth in an anchorage-independent culture model. The 0.005% crystal violet solution is used in this assay to visualize the generated colonies.

Key words Clonogenic assay, Agarose, Cancer stem cell, Colony growth, Crystal violet

1 Introduction

Colony forming (or clonogenic) assay is the commonly used in vitro technique to determine the capacity of a single cell to self-renew into colony of 50 or more cells [1]. Initially, in 1956, Puck and Marcus have developed a quantitative technique to assess the survival rate of cancer cell line (HeLa) in response to high-energy radiation of X-rays [2]. This study has revealed a marked decrease in the reproductive ability, growth rate, and colony forming ability of the cancer cells due to increased radiosensitivity [2]. Although the clonogenic assay has initially been developed as a tool to test the efficacy of radiation effect on mammalian cancer cell survival and proliferation, later it has been widely used to evaluate the effects of different cytotoxic, anti-angiogenic agents, genetic modifications, and screening of novel chemotherapeutic drugs that target the reproductive integrity of cancer cells in a dose-dependent manner [1]. Furthermore, this assay has also been developed to detect the stemness of the cancer cells isolated from tumors [3] and cancer cell lines [4]. In a tumor, only a few cells retain stemness those have the potency to undergo epigenetic alterations leading to asymmetric

Gianpaolo Papaccio and Vincenzo Desiderio (eds.), *Cancer Stem Cells: Methods and Protocols*, Methods in Molecular Biology, vol. 1692, DOI 10.1007/978-1-4939-7401-6_8, © Springer Science+Business Media LLC 2018

cell division and initiate tumorogenesis [5, 6]. This method helps to assess the ability of the in vitro propagated tumor-derived cells or cancer stem-like cells from cell lines to develop into a new tumor upon transplantation into a naive recipient in vitro [7]. However, testing the clonogenic potency in vitro reduces use of animals for in vitro studies.

Additionally, this method has been used to evaluate the efficacy of stem cells isolated from various tissues to undergo "unlimited" cell division and generate colonies of single-cell-derived clonal population [8–10]. Clonogenecity is an important characteristic feature of stem cells to ensure their proliferation and differentiation patterns [9]. In regenerative medicine, to determine the efficacy of stem cell-based treatment applications, the attributed properties of stem cells such as high proliferative rate, self-renewal nature, and multi-lineage differentiation potential have to be essentially tested [11]. However, the clonogenic nature of the stem cells is effectively represented at a restricted plating efficiency, i.e., at an appropriate limiting dilution to produce progeny consists pool of clonogenic progenitors [9].

The optimal method to perform colony forming assay for all types of cells is the soft agar method as the agarose helps to hold the colony together and prevent dispersed colony formation [12]. Generally, adherent cell populations are widely evaluated by colony forming assay [13], but the soft agar technique provides a platform to assess the colony forming efficiency of anchorage-independent tumor cells and hematopoietic progenitors. Although various techniques are currently available to detect very precisely the survival fractions of cancer cells after different treatment protocols, the advantage in colony forming assay is that the potency of a single cell to grow into a large colony can be visualized microscopically [14].

The main aim of this chapter is to go through the steps involved in performing colony forming assay in an established cancer cell line in detail using the soft agar method.

2 Materials

2.1 Agar Preparation

1. 2× DMEM complete medium—100 ml: In screw top glass bottle, add 95 ml of sterile water (add close to the final volume as possible). Add 2.76 gm of DMEM powder to room temperature water with gentle stirring. Add 0.74 gm of sodium bicarbonate powder to the above solution. Adjust the pH —7.0 by slowly adding and mixing, 1 N NaOH or 1 N HCL (*see* **Note 1**). Adjust the final volume to 100 ml. Supplemented with 20% FBS and 2× antibiotics. Process the DMEM medium through the 0.2 microns filter using a 20 ml syringe. Prepare aliquots of

25 ml sterile medium in sterile 50 ml tubes and store at 4 °C (*see* **Note 2**).

2. 1× DMEM complete medium: 1× DMEM supplemented with 10% FBS and 1× antibiotics. Store at 4 °C.
3. Agarose solutions: In a 250 ml screw top glass bottle, add 1 gm of agarose to 100 ml sterile water to make 1% agarose. Autoclave the screw top glass bottle. Use a similar procedure to obtain a 0.7% agarose solution by adding 0.7 gm to 100 ml sterile water (*see* **Note 3**).
4. Water bath: Prepare the water bath using a 1000 ml glass beaker filled with adequate amount of sterile water and maintain the temperature at 40 °C using a heat plate.
5. Phosphate-buffered saline (PBS).
6. Fetal bovine serum (FBS).
7. Antibiotics (penstrep).
8. Trypsin/EDTA.
9. Syringe 20 ml.
10. Light Microscope.
11. Fluorescent-activated cell sorting (FACS) when necessary.

2.2 Fixing and Staining the Colonies

1. Crystal violet solution: 0.005 gm of crystal violet in 100 ml of 25% methanol (75% distilled water, 25% methanol) (*see* **Note 4**).
2. Image J software.

3 Methods

3.1 Preparation of Base Agar Layer

1. Place the water bath inside the cell culture hood which makes the handling easier (*see* **Note 5**).
2. Equilibrate the 2× DMEM complete medium and agarose (*see* **Note 3**) bottle in a 40 °C water bath for 30 min (*see* **Note 6**).
3. Mix equal volume of agarose and 2× DMEM complete medium to make final 0.5% agarose and 1× DMEM complete medium (*see* **Note 7**).
4. Quickly add 1 ml of mixture to a 6-well cell culture plate and spread evenly. Allow agarose to solidify which takes 5–10 min (*see* **Note 8**).

3.2 Preparation of Top Agar Layer

1. Keep ready the base layer agar plates at room temperature.
2. Place 0.7% agarose solution in 40 °C in a water bath (*see* **Note 3**).
3. Prepare the cells (*see* **Note 9**).

(a) Collect the suspension of breast cancer mammosphere cells in a 15 ml tube and centrifuge 300 × *g* for 5 min, discard the supernatant.

(b) Wash the breast cancer mammosphere cells with PBS and centrifuge 300 × *g* for 5 min, discard the supernatant.

(c) Add required volume of trypsin and incubate all cells at 37 °C for 10–15 min. Add desired volume of complete media to neutralize.

(d) Wash the cells with PBS and centrifuge 300 × *g* for 5 min, discard the supernatant.

(e) Count the cells and stain with desired cancer stem cells (CSC) markers following the manufacturer's instructions. (Optional—otherwise move to step h).

(f) Sort the CSC markers positive cells by using FACS and centrifuge 300 × *g* for 5 min, discard the supernatant (Optional).

(g) Wash the sorted CSC cells with PBS and centrifuge 300 × *g* for 5 min, discard the supernatant (Optional).

(h) Resuspend the cells in the 2× DMEM complete medium and count the cells.

(i) Prepare 2× concentration of desired number of cells and use at least three different concentrations of cells (*see* **Note 10**).

4. Keep different concentrations of cells with 2× DMEM complete medium in different tubes with proper labeling.
5. Mix 0.7% agarose and 2× DMEM with cells in a 1:1 ratio to obtain a final 0.35% agarose, 1× concentration of cells, and 1× DMEM complete medium (*see* **Note 11**).
6. Quickly add 1 ml of mixture on the base agar layer in a 6-well cell culture plate and spread evenly. Allow the agarose to solidify which takes 5–10 min (*see* **Note 12**).
7. Add 2 ml of 1× DMEM complete medium in each well of a 6-well cell culture plate. Keep the plates in 37 °C with 5% CO_2 in a humidified atmosphere.
8. Incubate the cells for 2–3 weeks and change the media twice a week. Observe the colony growth under a light microscope.

3.3 Fixing and Staining the Colonies

1. Add 0.5 ml of 0.005% crystal violet solution in each 6-well plate for 1 h at room temperature (*see* **Note 13**).
2. Wash crystal violet off by adding 2 ml of water to the soft agar plate and keep it on a shaker, repeat the process several times to get clear transparent background as shown in Fig. 1 (*see* **Note 14**).

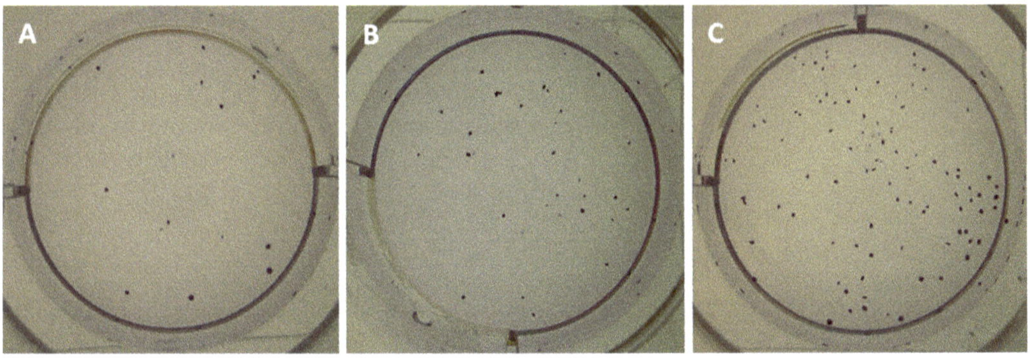

Fig. 1 Images were taken 14 days after the initiation of colony forming assay. Colonies generated when different concentrations of breast cancer cell line (SKBR3); (**a**) 5000, (**b**) 25,000 and (**c**) 50,000 were seeded in each well

3. Image on the dissecting microscope and count the colonies (*see* **Note 15**).
4. If you have lot of colonies, you can use Image J software for quantification.

3.4 Analyze Stained Colonies

1. Open the desired image by using Image J software.
2. Adjust the picture by using a crop tool to see only well image.
3. Image–adjust–threshold–adjust threshold to include colonies and exclude the dazzle. Use the same setting for all the colony populations.
4. Analyze–analyze particle. Set circularity to 0.2–0.8. Select bare outline from drop down menu to visualize the colonies and adjust the parameters.
5. Graph average of colony numbers.

4 Notes

1. The pH may rise 0.2–0.3 unit upon filtration, therefore adjust accordingly.
2. Perform the sterilization work in Class II cell culture hood. Apply constant pressure on syringe during filtration, high pressure will damage the membrane in the filter.
3. Agarose solutions can be prepared the day before the experiment and store in a sterile place. Make sure before using it should be in a solution form (after heating at 40 °C in a water bath).
4. Follow the safety regulation and work under the fume hood. Crystal violet gives strong color and hazardous to body, pay extra attention while weighing and preparing the solution.

5. Use tissue and 70% ethanol to wipe the water bath from outside to avoid any kind of contamination.
6. Fill with sufficient water to submerge the agarose bottle and media bottle. Excess water can cause contamination while working in next steps. Keep stirring occasionally to keep agarose in the solution state.
7. While mixing, avoid contact with water from the beaker and work as fast as possible and mix gently.
8. If you see any bubble in 6-well plates, remove using a pipette tip before solidification of agarose. Plates can be prepared advance and stored in a sterile environment up to 1 week at 4 °C.
9. Cell sorting and subsequent steps need to be done as fast as possible. Extra hands from a colleague will be helpful.
10. Proper labeling on the tubes as well as on 6-well plate save time and prevent confusion. Using different concentrations of cells provide more reliable results.
11. While mixing avoid contact with water from the beaker and work as fast as possible and mix gently to avoid damage to the cells.
12. If you see any bubble in 6-well plates remove using pipet tip before solidification of agarose.
13. Collect the waste in a specific waste container and dispose according to the safety regulation.
14. Replace water and keep it on a shaker four to five times, if you do not see clear background, keep it on a shaker with water overnight. Sometimes, it takes longer to get clear.
15. If a dissecting microscope is not available, you can take a picture using a digital camera. Use light background below the soft agar plate.

Acknowledgment

This work was supported by the startup support from Linkoping University and Cancerfonden.

References

1. Munshi A, Hobbs M, Meyn RE (2005) Clonogenic cell survival assay. Methods Mol Med 110:21–28
2. Puck TT, Marcus PI (1956) Action of x-rays on mammalian cells. J Exp Med 103(5):653–666
3. Li P et al (2013) Hypoxia enhances stemness of cancer stem cells in glioblastoma: an in vitro study. Int J Med Sci 10(4):399–407
4. Jain MV et al (2015) Nuclear localized Akt enhances breast cancer stem-like cells through counter-regulation of p21(Waf1/Cip1) and p27(kip1). Cell Cycle 14(13):2109–2120

5. Reya T et al (2001) Stem cells, cancer, and cancer stem cells. Nature 414(6859):105–111
6. Polyak K, Hahn WC (2006) Roots and stems: stem cells in cancer. Nat Med 12(3):296–300
7. Neering SJ et al (2007) Leukemia stem cells in a genetically defined murine model of blast-crisis CML. Blood 110(7):2578–2585
8. Friedenstein AJ et al (1974) Precursors for fibroblasts in different populations of hematopoietic cells as detected by the in vitro colony assay method. Exp Hematol 2(2):83–92
9. Sarugaser R et al (2009) Human mesenchymal stem cells self-renew and differentiate according to a deterministic hierarchy. PLoS One 4 (8):e6498
10. O'Connor MD et al (2008) Alkaline phosphatase positive colony formation is a sensitive, specific, and quantitative indicator of undifferentiated human embryonic stem cells. Stem Cells 26(5):1109–1116
11. Ponnaiyan D, Jegadeesan V (2014) Comparison of phenotype and differentiation marker gene expression profiles in human dental pulp and bone marrow mesenchymal stem cells. Eur J Dent 8(3):307–313
12. Franken NA et al (2006) Clonogenic assay of cells in vitro. Nat Protoc 1(5):2315–2319
13. Rafehi H et al (2011) Clonogenic assay: adherent cells. J Vis Exp 49:2573
14. Buch K et al (2012) Determination of cell survival after irradiation via clonogenic assay versus multiple MTT assay–a comparative study. Radiat Oncol 7(1):1

Chapter 9

Xenograft as In Vivo Experimental Model

Manuela Porru, Luca Pompili, Carla Caruso, and Carlo Leonetti

Abstract

The identification of experimental models that recapitulate human cancers designed to predict patient clinical response to therapies is a major break in oncology. Cancer stem cells (CSCs) represent a small tumor cell population responsible for drug resistance, where their effective killing may lead to identifying better treatment options. While the CSCs hypothesis highlights the need for a specific tumor target, patient-derived xenografts (PDXs) should also be considered for drug development as they better represent tumor heterogeneity and the environment in which a tumor develops.

Key words Immunosuppressed mice, Patient-derived xenografts, Transplantation assay, Predictive model, Tumorigenicity, Heterogeneity, Stroma

1 Introduction

Advances in the molecular understanding of human tumors have provided a solid ground for the development of a great number of new antineoplastic compounds that have exhibited remarkable tumor responses in preclinical studies. Unfortunately, less than 5% of these therapeutic treatments showed efficacy when tested in clinical trials, thus highlighting that our ability to translate cancer research into clinical success is extremely low. Many factors are responsible for this high failure rate including the inherent complexity of the disease and the need for new clinical trial approaches to improve the selection of the best dose, as well as the application of a biomarker-driven patient sub-selection strategy to better identify responsive patients [1]. Unquestionably, a major reason for this high failure rate is the lack of preclinical models ability in recapitulating this human disease; thus the identification of appropriate mouse cancer models remains a major challenge in improving drug development.

Manuela Porru and Luca Pompili are co-authors to this work.

Gianpaolo Papaccio and Vincenzo Desiderio (eds.), *Cancer Stem Cells: Methods and Protocols*, Methods in Molecular Biology, vol. 1692, DOI 10.1007/978-1-4939-7401-6_9, © Springer Science+Business Media LLC 2018

The first reports using in vivo murine tumor models for drug efficacy studies were published in the 1950s [2] and since then researchers dedicated great efforts toward developing animal models of cancer in order to predict the response of chemotherapeutic agents in humans. Later, the use of immune-deficient mice in which human tumor cell lines could be implanted by ectopic or orthotopic injection of cells, was instrumental in accelerating drug discovery. However, knowledge that these xenografts derived from the implantation of in vitro long-term established cell lines showed little resemblance to the original tumors, in terms of molecular complexity, tumor heterogeneity, and response to treatments, has limited the relevance of these models and has frequently been cited as one of the most important reasons for the high failure rate of new agents in oncology [3].

The hypothesis of the existence of small-cell populations called cancer stem cells (CSCs), possessing a self-renewal capacity, differentiation abilities, and resistance to therapy within a heterogeneous tumor, had great expectations in the development of new therapeutic strategies where targeting this cell subpopulation could eradicate and definitively cure cancer. Consequently, in the last 10–15 years CSCs have become a highly prioritized task for many labs throughout the world but unfortunately these enormous efforts offered very little concrete improvement in treating cancer [4].

It had long been accepted that only the CSCs could initiate tumor formation and that the eradication of CSCs would be sufficient to eliminate the disease and prevent subsequent relapse [5]. Following this hypothesis, cell-surface markers have been proposed as determinants for the identification of CSCs in contrast to the non-tumor initiating and non-tumor propagating cells, as for example $CD34^{+}$ $CD38^{neg}$ and $CD90^{neg}$ for acute myeloid leukemia [6, 7], $CD44^{+}$ $CD24^{-/low}$ for breast cancer [8], or CD133 for brain tumors [9]. The studies in animals by transplantation assay showed that few cells expressing these markers were able to initiate and propagate tumors in immunosuppressed mice, while cells not expressing these markers were not tumorigenic. In addition, the phenotype of tumors resembles the tumors from which CSCs were isolated.

Based on observations from different studies, the CSCs paradigm should be revisited as much of the evidence representing the basis for the CSCs theory is difficult to reproduce and debate [4]. In particular, in some cases, a high percentage of cells and not only very few cells showed tumorigenic ability depending on the experimental conditions. In fact, Quintana et al. [10] demonstrated that the number of tumor initiating melanoma cells dramatically increased by changing the animal models, just like when cells were injected in NOD/SCID mice the average frequency of tumor-forming cells was 1 in 837,000 cells. In contrast, after the injection in the more immunocompromised mice NOD/SCID interleukin-2 receptor gamma chain null (Il2rg(−/−) mice, the percentage of tumorigenic cells had significantly increased to 1 in 5–1 in 15 cells, thus suggesting that changing the mouse model number of detectable tumorigenic cells is dramatically higher. This has opened the door to an important question, since tumorigenic cells represent a great part of the tumor, focusing our attention on a small cell population following the CSCs hypothesis is not a right track to identify an effective anticancer therapy.

The same markers used to identify CSCs such as CD133, CD44, EpCAM, and ALDH activity or in the case of human leukemia a combination of CD34, CD38, and IL3Rα are not universal for the different tumor histotypes and sometimes for the same tumor type [4]. Moreover, these markers are not exclusively expressed by CSCs [11].

An important aspect to consider is the emergence of CSC differentiation and the observation that under the dominance of the tumor micro-environment non-CSCs could acquire CSCs characteristics [4, 12]. This cell plasticity puts into question the concept that CSCs, as the only tumorigenic cells, need to be targeted for curative purposes. So, while we consider that CSCs still represent an important area in preclinical oncology research, we believe that in addition to CSCs as they are now identified, efficient tumor treatment requires the eradication of the entire tumor cell population including the seemingly non-tumorigenic cells that could have a key role in tumor progression and resistance to therapy.

From this perspective, a relevant approach is represented by the patient-derived xenografts (PDXs) obtained by the fresh implantation of tumor tissue from patient to immunosuppressed mice and individual tumors expanded to generate tumor-bearing mice for anticancer treatment testing. The advantage of the PDXs model is that during propagation PDXs maintain the pathological structure and the heterogeneity of patient tumors [13]. A key point is that these tumors include critical stromal elements, which provide sustenance under periods of extensive growth, thus PDX tumors more closely recapitulate the cancers from which they are derived. Moreover, analysis of tumors revealed that PDXs preserve the overall genomic and gene expression profile and fidelity in transcriptome of the corresponding patient tumors [14, 15], thus highlighting that PDXs have the potential to provide a more predictive experimental model for evaluating therapeutic responses. Interestingly, the response/resistance of PDXs to standard chemotherapeutic or targeted compounds strictly correlated with clinical data in patients from which PDXs have been derived [16, 17].

Our opinion is that the identification of CSCs remains a key challenge in experimental oncology, but PDXs, which include CSCs, seem to be a more suitable xenograft model. Based on these considerations, we will describe both the methods to develop in vivo xenografts, either from CSCs or from PDXs.

1.1 CSCs Xenografts

A fundamental problem in cancer research is the identification of the cell type capable of initiating and sustaining the growth of neoplastic clones. There is overwhelming evidence showing that virtually all cancers are clonal and represent the progeny of a single cell. What is less clear for most cancers is which cells within the tumor clone possess self-renewal activity and are capable of maintaining tumor growth [18].

To evaluate the tumor formation ability in vivo of CSCs a *limiting dilution assay* needs to be performed [5, 19]. This functional assay is useful for the quantitative analysis of cells with repopulating capacity.

The basic principle of a limiting-dilution assay is that one cell is required to produce 50 percent takes in recipient mice. To apply the limiting-dilution assay is necessary to determine the number of cells that give 50 percent takes in mice (TD_{50} cell number). If it is assumed that a positive take depends only upon the presence of one clonogenic cell in the injection, the possibility that a given implant will contain one cell with a repopulating potential will follow a Poisson distribution [20]. A limiting-dilution assay will normally use different concentrations of cells injected to identify the lowest CSCs cell concentration capable of forming a tumor.

2 Materials

2.1 CSCs

1. Medium for in vitro culture is different for CSCs of different origin, prepare it accordingly.
2. PBS 1×.
3. Trypsin.
4. NOD scid IL2Rgamma^{null} (NSG) mice (*see* **Note 1**).
5. BD Matrigel™ Basement Membrane Matrix.
6. Insulin syringe with a 22G needle.
7. Vernier caliper.

2.2 PDX

The tumor fragment is obtained directly from the patient biopsy in the surgical room. The fragment is immediately placed in a sterile tube containing Culture Medium [21].

1. Culture medium: DMEM Dulbecco's Modified Eagle's Medium (DMEM/HIGH Glucose), Penicillin/Streptomycin from 100× solution, Fetal Bovine Serum (FBS) 10%.
2. Freezing solution: FBS supplemented with 10% Dimethyl Sulfoxide (DMSO).
3. Anesthetic: Tiletamine-Zolazepam (Telazol) and Xylazine (xylazine) given intramuscularly at 2 mg/kg.
4. BD Matrigel™ Basement Membrane Matrix.

5. Steril tweezers and scalpels. Vernier caliper.
6. SCID (severe combined immunodeficiency mice) mice (*see* **Note 2**).
7. NOD (non-obese diabetes)/SCID mice (*see* **Note 3**) [22].
8. NSG (NOD/SCID interleukin-2 receptor gamma chain null) mice.

3 Methods

3.1 CSCs

1. Tripsinize CSCs cells previously identified and selected for the expression of stemness-related markers and count in Trypan blue by a Thoma camera to evaluate cell viability.
2. Wash the cell suspension two times with PBS 1× by centrifuging cells at 1000 × *g* for 5 min and divide them into different groups for each cell concentration.
3. Dissolve each cell concentration in cold Matrigel (*see* **Note 4**).
4. Inject five mice (*see* **Note 5**) in each group using an insulin syringe with a 22G needle (*see* **Note 6**) subcutaneously into the flanks (*see* **Note 7**). Based on the *limiting dilution assay,* inject the cells at logarithmic concentrations from 10, 100, 1000 to 1×10^5 CSC cells/mouse in 200 μl of Matrigel. In parallel perform the same experiment by using cells from the bulk population of the same tumor from which CSCs are derived.
5. Monitor the tumor appearance by tumor palpation.
6. Measure the tumor sizes three times a week, starting at least 1 week after tumor cell injection, in two dimensions by a vernier caliper and calculate tumor weight or volume (*see* **Note 8**) using the following formula: $a \times b^2/2$, where a and b are the long and short diameters of the tumor, respectively.
7. To perform immunohistochemistry analysis, euthanize the animals and maintain tumor samples in formalin or immediately frozen in liquid nitrogen and store at −80 °C.

3.2 PDX

3.2.1 Tumor Collection

1. Under sterile laminar flow cabinet transfer the tumor to a sterile Petri dish using sterile tweezers.
2. Dice the tumor into 15–20 mm^3 long pieces with a sterile scalpel. After this step, the tumor can be implanted in mice or frozen in the Freezing solution and stored at −80 °C.

3.2.2 Implantation

1. Anesthetize immunosuppressed mice with the Anesthetic solution. The non-obese diabetic/severe combined immunodeficiency (NOD/SCID) or NOD/SCID/IL2λ-receptor null (NSG) models are better suited for PDX generation due to higher engraftment rates [23] (*see* **Note 9**). Make a small

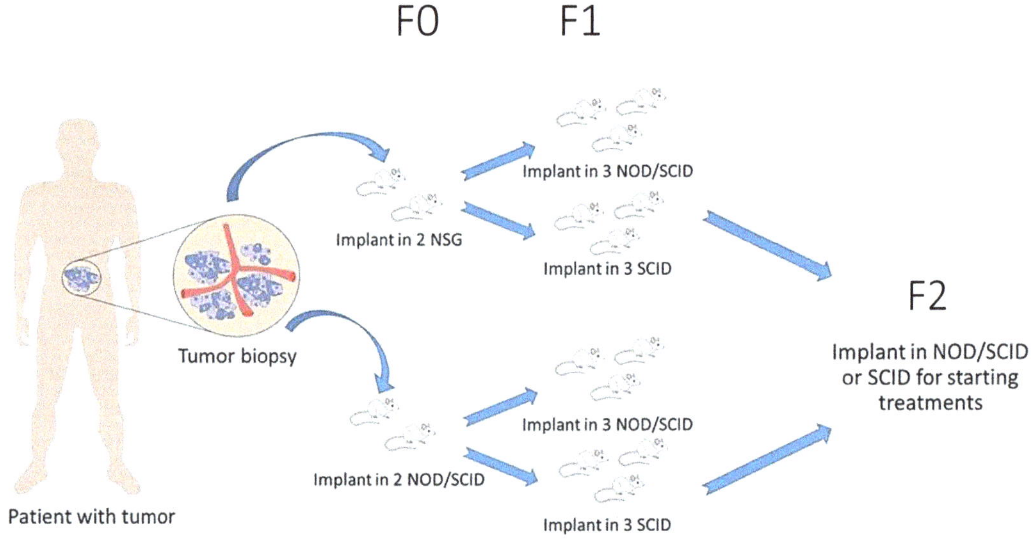

Fig. 1 Generation of PDX from colorectal cancer

incision on the lower back of each animal and place the tumor specimen of about 15–20 mm^3 into the subcutaneous pocket with one drop of Matrigel [24] to facilitate the engraftment. The incision will be closed in two layers using non-absorbable sutures. This generation harboring the patient-derived material is termed F0 [13].

2. Determine the appearance of the tumor by palpation and then follow the tumor growth by measuring the tumor size three times a week in two dimensions by a vernier caliper. The tumor volume is calculated in the same manner as the CSCs xenografts.
3. When the PDX tumor reaches a volume of approximately 500 mm^3, it can be harvested for the serial transplantation [25]. Thus, sacrifice the tumor-bearing animals and dice the tumor into fragments of about 15–20 mm^3 for implanting, as described above, in no less than three mice to elicit a larger number of tumor-bearing animals. This generation harboring the patient-derived material is termed F1 (Fig. 1).
4. Pass the tumors another time. Thus, at the generation F2 the tumors are allowed to grow to 250–300 mm^3 where the mice are divided into homogeneous groups (*see* **Note 10**) in order to start treatments for chemosensitivity testing.
5. Sacrifice the animals at the end of the treatments when the tumor reaches a mean of 2.5–3.0 cm^3 or when the animals become moribund during the observation period. Record the time of euthanization as the time of death. Store the tumors at −80 °C as described above (*see* **Note 11**).

3.2.3 Immunohistochemical Analysis

Paraffin-embedded 4 μm thick sections from major organs or tumors will be stained with Hematoxylin-Eosin (H&E) and analyzed by an optical microscope.

1. Analyze the stability of expression of clinically relevant biomarkers [26] by the histological analysis. It is important to verify the identity of the PDX tumors with the tumor of patient after serial passages in mice.
2. Evaluate by immunohistochemistry analysis on untreated and treated tumors the expression levels of markers of proliferation, apoptosis, necrosis, and DNA damage to verify the efficacy of the treatments.

4 Notes

1. Use mice 4 weeks old and weighing 22–24 g, in a barrier facility on high-efficiency particulate air HEPA-filtered racks. Feed the animals with autoclaved laboratory rodent diet.
2. SCID (severe combined immunodeficiency) mice lack T- and B- lymphocytes. Matrigel is liquid at 4 °C and at room temperature is solid.
3. NOD (non-obese diabetes)/SCID mice have an additional mutation-causing Beta-2-Microglobulin Deficiency and lack of NK-cell activity.
4. Matrigel is liquid at 4 °C and at room temperature is solid. Before use, thaw Matrigel by submerging the bottle in ice and storing in the 4 °C overnight.
5. We suggest using NSG mice that are the more immunosuppressed mice and could give better information on the tumorigenic potential of CSCs.
6. Use a 22G needle because the smaller size can cause cell stress.
7. CSCs cells of different histotypes can be also injected orthotopically into the organ of origin.
8. Tumor mass could be expressed in mg or mm^3.
9. In general, at least for the first implants in the F0 generation, we suggest using the non-obese diabetic/severe combined immunodeficiency (NOD/SCID) or NOD/SCID IL2λ-receptor null (NSG) to achieve the best engraftment rate. In our experience, in the case of colorectal cancer, we obtained a full engraftment at F1 generation using the SCID mice, that are cheaper than the NOD/SCID or NSG mice. Therefore, we suggest implanting the PDX tumor from colorectal cancer in SCID and/or NOD/SCID mice at the F1 generation (Fig. 1). Nevertheless, based on our own experience, the best mice model to use will be in accordance with the rate take on the tumor histotype.

10. It is possible that not all tumors will reach the volume of about 250–300 mm^3 at the same time [27]. In our experience, we observed that the PDX tumors can reach that size between 30 and 60 days. For every single mouse, treatment starts when the tumor has reached this size. Each animal will be considered a single patient.
11. Freezing the PDX tumors can also occur in the harvesting of the F0 and F1 generation to store subsequent implants and/or immunohistochemical analysis.

Acknowledgment

This work was supported by a grant from Italian Association for Cancer Research AIRC IG #18637 to C. Leonetti.

References

1. Rubin EH, Gilliland DG (2012) Drug development and clinical trials-the path to an approved cancer drug. Nat Rev Clin Oncol 9:215–222
2. Kirschbaum A, Geisse NC, Sister T J, Meyer LM (1950) Effect of certain folic acid antagonists on transplanted myeloid and lymphoid leukemias of the F strain of mice. Cancer Res 10(12):762–768
3. Hutchinson L, Kirk R (2011) High drug attrition rates–where are we going wrong? Nat Rev Clin Oncol 8(4):189–190. doi:10.1038/nrclinonc.2011.34
4. Skrbo N, Tenstad E, Mælandsmo GM, Sørlie T, Andersen K (2015) From autonomy to community; new perspectives on tumorigenicity and therapy resistance. Cancer Treat Rev 41 (10):809–813. doi:10.1016/j.ctrv.2015.10.004. Epub 2015 Oct 20
5. Reya T, Morrison SJ, Clarke MF, Weissman IL (2001) Stem cells, cancer, and cancer stem cells. Nature 414:105–111
6. Bonnet D, Dick JE (1997) Human acute myeloid leukemia is organized as a hierarchy that originates from a primitive hematopoietic cell. Nat Med 3:730–737
7. Blair A, Hogge DE, Ailles LE, Lansdorp PM, Sutherland HJ (1997) Lack of expression of Thy-1 (CD90) on acute myeloid leukemia cells with long-term proliferative ability in vitro and in vivo. Blood 89:3104–3112
8. Al-Hajj M, Wicha MS, Benito-Hernandez A, Morrison SJ, Clarke MF (2003) Prospective identification of tumorigenic breast cancer cells. Proc Natl Acad Sci U S A 100:3983–3988
9. Galli R, Binda E, Orfanelli U, Cipelletti B, Gritti A, De Vitis S, Fiocco R, Foroni C, Dimeco F, Vescovi A (2004) Isolation and characterization of tumorigenic, stem-like neural precursors from human glioblastoma. Cancer Res 64:7011. doi:10.1158/0008-5472.CAN-04-1364
10. Quintana E, Shackleton M, Sabel MS, Fullen DR, Johnson TM, Morrison SJ (2008) Efficient tumour formation by single human melanoma cells. Nature 456:593–598. doi:10.1038/nature07567. [nature07567 [pii]]
11. Visvader JE, Lindeman GJ (2012) Cancer stem cells: current status and evolving complexities. Cell Stem Cell 10(6):717–728. doi:10.1016/j.stem.2012.05.007
12. Rycaj K, Tang DG (2015) Cell-of-origin of cancer versus cancer stem cells: assays and interpretations. Cancer Res 75(19):4003–4011. doi:10.1158/0008-5472.CAN-15-0798. Epub 2015 Aug 19
13. Tentler JJ, Tan AC, Weekes CD, Jimeno A, Leong S, Pitts TM, Arcaroli JJ, Messersmith WA, Eckhardt SG (2012) Patient-derived tumour xenografts as models for oncology drug development. Nat Rev Clin Oncol 9 (6):338–350
14. Reyal F, Guyader C, Decraene C, Lucchesi C, Auger N, Assayag F, De Plater L, Gentien D, Poupon MF, Cottu P, De Cremoux P, Gestraud P, Vincent-Salomon A, Fontaine JJ, Roman-Roman S, Delattre O, Decaudin D, Marangoni E (2012) Molecular profiling of

patient-derived breast cancer xenografts. Breast Cancer Res 14(1):R11

15. Zhao X, Liu Z, Yu L, Zhang Y, Baxter P, Voicu H, Gurusiddappa S, Luan J, Su JM, Leung HC, Li XN (2012) Global gene expression profiling confirms the molecular fidelity of primary tumor-based orthotopic xenograft mouse models of medulloblastoma. Neuro Oncol 14 (5):574–583. doi:10.1093/neuonc/nos061
16. Topp MD, Hartley L, Cook M, Heong V, Boehm E, McShane L, Pyman J, McNally O, Ananda S, Harrell M, Etemadmoghadam D, Galletta L, Alsop K, Mitchell G, Fox SB, Kerr JB, Hutt KJ, Kaufmann SH, Swisher EM, Bowtell DD, Wakefield MJ, Scott CL, Australian Ovarian Cancer Study (2014) Molecular correlates of platinum response in human high-grade serous ovarian cancer patient-derived xenografts. Mol Oncol 8(3):656–668. doi:10.1016/j.molonc.2014.01.008
17. Nunes M, Vrignaud P, Vacher S, Richon S, Lievre A, Cacheux W, Weiswald LB, Massonnet G, Chatean-Joubert S, Nicolas A, Dib C, Zhang W, Watters J, Bergstrom D, Roman-Roman S, Bieche I, Dangles-Marie V (2015) Evaluating patient-derived colorectal cancer-xenografts as preclinical models by comparison with patient clinical data. Cancer Res 75 (8):1560–1566. pii: canres.1590.201
18. Wang JC, Dick JE (2005) Cancer stem cells: lessons from leukemia. Trends Cell Biol 15:494–501
19. O'Brien CA, Pollett A, Gallinger S, Dick JE (2007) A human colon cancer cell capable of initiating tumour growth in immunodeficient mice. Nature 445:106–110
20. Porter EH, Berry RJ (1964) The efficient design of transplantable tumour assays. Br J Cancer 17:583–595
21. Jin K, Teng L, Shen Y, He K, Xu Z, Li G (2010) Patient-derived human tissue xenografts in immunodeficient mice: a systematic review. Clin Transl Oncol 12:473–480
22. Wartha K, Herting F, Hasmann M (2014) Fit-for purpose use of mouse models to improve predictivity of cancer therapeutics evaluation. Pharmacol Ther 142:351–361
23. Hidalgo M, Amant F, Biankin AV, Budinská E, Byrne AT, Caldas C, Clarke RB, de Jong S, Jonkers J, Mælandsmo GM, Roman-Roman S, Seoane J, Trusolino L, Villanueva A, EurOPDX Consortium (2014) Patient-derived xenografts models: an emerging platform for translational cancer research. AACR J 4 (9):998–1013
24. Porru M, Artuso S, Salvati E, Bianco A, Franceschin M, Diodoro MG, Passeri D, Orlandi A, Savorani F, D'Incalci M, Biroccio A, Leonetti C (2015) Targeting G-Quadruplex DNA structures by EMICORON has a strong antitumor efficacy against advanced models of human colon cancer. Mol Cancer Ther 14 (11):2541–2551
25. Damhofer H, Ebbing EA, Steins A, Welling L, Tol JA, Krishnadath KK, van Leusden T, van de Vijver M, Besselink MG, Bush OR, van Berge Henegouwen MI, van Delden O, Meijer SL, Dijk F, Medema JP, van Laarhoven HW, Bijlsma MF (2015) Establishment of patient-derived xenograft models and cell lines for malignancies of the upper gastrointestinal tract. J Transl Med 13:115
26. Zhang X, Claerhout S, Prat A, Dobrolecki LE, Petrovic I, Lai Q, Landis MD, Wiechmann L, Schiff R, Giuliano M, Wong H, Fuqua SW, Contreras A, Gutierrez C, Huang J, Mao S, Pavlick AC, Froehlich AM, Wu MF, Tsimelzon A, Hilsenbeck SG, Chen ES, Zuloaga P, Shaw CA, Rimawi MF, Perou CM, Mills GB, Chang JC, Lewis MT (2013) A renewable tissue of phenotipycally stable, biologically and ethnically diverse, patient-derived human breast cancer Xenograft models. Cancer Res 73:4885–4897
27. Morton CL, Houghton PJ (2007) Establishment of human tumor xenografts in immunodeficient mice. Nat Protoc 2(2):247–225

Chapter 10

How to Assess Drug Resistance in Cancer Stem Cells

Maria Laura De Angelis, Ruggero De Maria, and Marta Baiocchi

Abstract

Banks of genetically characterized cancer stem cells (CSCs) isolated from individual patients and grown as spheroids offer an invaluable approach to identify genetic determinants of drug resistance versus sensitivity, and to study new stem cell-directed therapies. Here, we describe our standardized procedure for in vitro drug screening on colorectal CSCs, taking irinotecan as an example.

Key words CSC, Cancer stem cell culture, Drug screening, Drug resistance, In vitro assays, Colorectal cancer

1 Introduction

Colorectal CSCs are a small population of self-renewing cells that initiate and sustain tumor and metastasis development [1, 2]. As shown by ours and other groups, CSCs are particularly resistant to chemotherapeutics [3–7], this explaining the relapse that in most cases follows treatment with such agents: In fact, even a strong reduction of the tumor burden may spare some CSCs, few of which would be sufficient to re-initiate the tumor at later time. Therefore, therapeutic approaches able to hit CSCs are presently the focus of intense research effort, with the hope to achieve long-lasting tumor remission [8–12].

Recently, we have been able to generate a biobank of colorectal CSCs isolated from fresh tumor samples, upon tissue dissociation and cell expansion in serum-free media [7]. In these conditions, CSCs grow as spheroids, which we routinely validate for: (1) STR (short tandem repeats) matching with original patient's normal tissue; (2) expression of stem cell markers; (3) capability to generate differentiated xenografts phenotypically compatible with the original patient's tumor [13]. CSCs are then analyzed by whole exome sequencing (WES), and finally frozen and banked. By testing the effect of chemotherapeutics and targeted agents on panels of genetically defined spheroid cultures, in conjunction with proteomic

Gianpaolo Papaccio and Vincenzo Desiderio (eds.), *Cancer Stem Cells: Methods and Protocols*, Methods in Molecular Biology, vol. 1692, DOI 10.1007/978-1-4939-7401-6_10, © Springer Science+Business Media LLC 2018

analyses, we have shown that CSCs faithfully reproduce the main determinants of resistance to EGF-R pathway inhibitors of primary colon cancer [7]. Altogether CSCs have proved to constitute a sound model to investigate drug resistance determinants and novel therapeutic approaches, where the use of CSC defined media can also allow dissecting the impact of exogenous cytokines and stromal factors. As compared to other experimental systems recently developed for cancer drug screening, such as patient-derived xenografts (PDX) [10] and organoids [11], CSC spheroid cultures are easier, faster, and less expensive to expand, manipulate, and analyze.

To screen therapeutic agents on CSCs in vitro, we have established a standard luminescence viability test in 96-well plates, which can be easily adapted to high-throughput automated systems. Here, we describe a typical dose-response assay of irinotecan on CSCs.

2 Materials

2.1 Medium and Supplements

CSC medium composition was formulated by modification of [14, 15], as follows.

CSC medium: Advanced DMEM F12 (ADF) added with 100 units/mL of penicillin, 100 μg/mL of streptomycin, 0.29 mg/mL glutamine, 6 g/L glucose, 5 mM HEPES, 3.6 g/L BSA, 0.1% $NaHCO_3$, 4 mg/L (≥700 U/L) heparin,10 mM nicotinamide, 10% Hormone Mix 10×, 20 ng/mL human recombinant EGF, 10 ng/mL human recombinant bFGF (*see* **Note 1**).

Hormone Mix (10×): ADF added with 1 g/L apo-transferrin, 250 mg/L insulin, 161 mg/L putrescine, 52 μg/L sodium selenite, 62 μg/L progesterone, 10 mM HEPES (*see* **Note 2**).

2.2 Spheroid Dissociation and Counting

1. PBS.
2. TrypLE™ Express 1×, Thermo Fisher Scientific.
3. Trypan Blue 0.4% in PBS.

2.3 CSC Plating

1. 96-well clear-bottom white polystyrene microplates, Corning.

2.4 Cell Viability Assay

1. CellTiter-Glo® Luminescent Cell Viability Assay, Promega.
2. Microplate luminescence reader.

2.5 Miscellaneous Laboratory Equipment

1. Sterile hood, humidified thermostated incubator, microscope, centrifuge, thermostated water bath, cell count chamber, pipet-aid, disposable serological pipets, multichannel pipette, Gilson pipettes and tips, Falcon tubes, Eppendorf micro tubes.

3 Methods

Handle cells and all the supplements under a sterile hood, in order to avoid microbial contamination. Use cell culture-grade sterile, disposable plasticware at all the steps. Avoid glass or metal tools in manipulating medium or medium reagents, to avoid contamination with toxic elements. Incubate cultures in a humidified incubator at 37 °C, 5% CO_2.

3.1 Preliminary Assessment of Running Culture Quality

Quality and log growth phase of running cultures from which spheroids are harvested is essential for reliable drug testing on CSCs. Use CSCs from cultures passed 3–5 days before, depending on the strain and on the actual health of the cells (*see* **Note 3**). Check spheroid quality the day before beginning the test as follows:

1. Observe cultures under a microscope: irregular borders and dark centers indicate spheroid overgrowth, presence of dead cells within the clusters, and in general a poor-quality culture. Since single CSC strains have different optimal spheroid size, it is quite common that some cultures are healthy and growing when spheroid size is relatively larger, while other stop to grow and need to be dissociated when spheroids are still relatively small.
2. Harvest, dissociate by TrypLE (*see* Subheading 3.2), and count a small culture sample (about 1 mL out of a 10 mL flask): This allows verifying not only whether enough cells will be available the following day for the test, but also the percentage of dead cells in the culture. In our experience, up to 10–15% of dead cells in the starting culture are acceptable (*see* **Note 4**).

3.2 CSC Dissociation and Counting

According to our standard procedure, we dissociate spheroids into single cells by enzymatic treatment with TrypLE. Spheroid dissociation is a critical step for a good quality test, because both incomplete dissociation and excessive presence of dead cells will negatively affect the results. Indeed, cell death is induced by dissociation itself, and the sensitivity to TrypLE differs in individual strains, both in terms of the propensity of spheroids to dissociate, and in terms of cell death following the dissociation. Therefore, general instructions given here may need to be adapted to individual CSC. Perform all the operations at room temperature, unless otherwise stated.

1. Collect desired volume (here for example, 10 mL) of CSC suspension from running flask in a 15 mL Falcon tube. Centrifuge for 5 min at 150 × *g* to remove CSC medium, discard the supernatant, resuspend the cell pellet in PBS. Centrifuge 5 min at 150 × *g* then discard the supernatant: at this step, accurately remove PBS, to ensure that TrypLE will not end up diluted during the following step. Aspirate the most of the volume by a 10 mL pipet, and then remove residual PBS by a Gilson.

2. Add TrypLE to cell pellet. Grossly adjust TrypLE volume to the expected number of cells in the pellet: the ratio we use is 0.5 mL for about 2×10^6 cells.
3. Incubate the tube in a thermostated water bath at 37 °C for 3 min, then retrieve the tube and, upon gently shaking, observe whether spheroids are disappeared or reduced in size. If big clusters are still visible in the tube, incubate for further 3 min. A maximum of three incubations of 3 min each are usually sufficient to obtain a suspension, in which few or no clusters are evident. Further incubation would damage the cells excessively; therefore, it is not recommended even in the case spheroids are still visible.
4. At the end of the incubation(s), gently pass cell suspension through a yellow Gilson tip mounted on a 2 mL serological pipet. Depending on the CSC strain, 5–20 passages should be sufficient to dissociate residual clusters, if any was still present, and to obtain a single-cell suspension.
5. Add 10 mL of CSC medium: this will inactivate TrypLE. Centrifuge at $150 \times g$ for 5 min. Discard the supernatant and suspend the cell pellet in a volume suitable for counting; for example, if starting from 10^6 expected cells, suspend the pellet in 1 mL medium. Calculate proportionally for different expected cell numbers.
6. Collect 50 μL of suspension by Gilson pipette from the tube; mix with an equal volume of Trypan Blue 0.4% in PBS. Count cell suspension by a cell count chamber under a microscope.

This procedure should ensure to obtain a single-cell suspension, containing no more than 15% of dead cells, ready to be plated (*see* **Notes 5** and **6** for troubleshoot).

3.3 CSC Plating

Calculate the number of plates and wells needed on the base of the assay to be run. Figure 1 shows our standard plating scheme, which includes untreated cell control at plating (Plate A, Day^{-1}) and drug testing plate (Plate B, Day 4). We routinely test irinotecan in tenfold serial dilutions, starting from 1 mM to 0.01 μM, and plate six replicates per experimental point, including untreated controls, as in the figure.

1. On the base of the cell count obtained as in Subheading 3.2, **step 6**, dilute cells with CSC medium, to obtain a suspension of $3.3\text{x}10^4$ cells/mL.
2. Dispense 90 μL/well in white 96-well plates, according to the scheme in Fig. 1, by a multichannel pipette. This results in plating 3000 cells/well (*see* **Note 7**).
3. Place plates B in a humidified incubator until the following day.

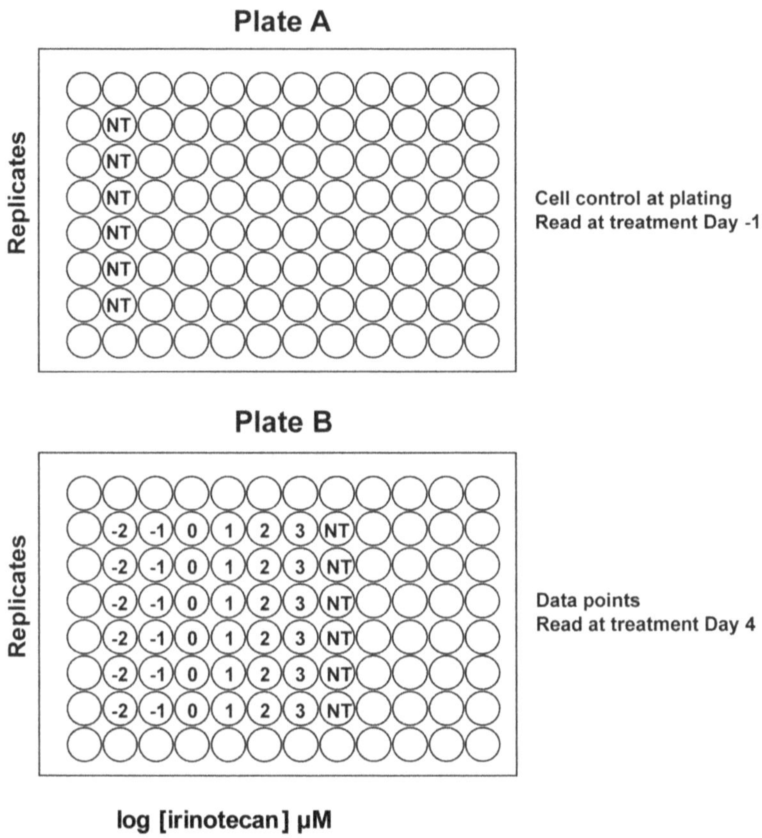

Fig. 1 Scheme of well plating for drug testing on CSCs. Final concentrations are indicated as logarithms

4. Immediately analyze cell viability in control plate A by CellTiter-Glo, according to the procedure in Subheading 3.5. This value represents the luminescence of the cells plated, i.e., 3000 cells.

3.4 Starting the Treatment

We add the drug dilutions to the cells, 24 h after plating. In plate B, we dispense 10 μL of drug/well, containing cells in 90 μL of medium; therefore, for every drug dose we wish to test, we prepare a drug solution ten times more concentrated, by serially diluting a starting solution of 10 mM irinotecan down to 0.01 μM (*see* **Note 8**).

1. Recover plate B from incubator, transfer 10 μL of appropriate drug solutions in corresponding wells containing CSCs, according to the scheme in Fig. 1. Dispense 10 μL of medium in untreated control wells.
2. Incubate cells in a humidified incubator for 96 h.

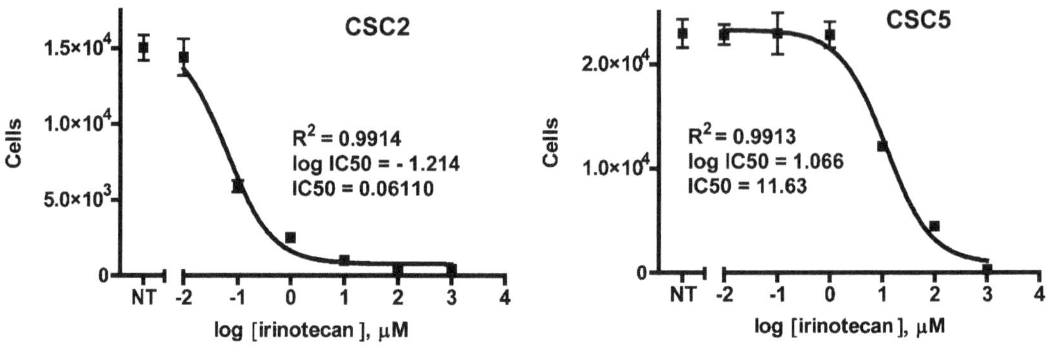

Fig. 2 Dose-response assay of irinotecan on two different colorectal CSC strains. Data points were expressed as absolute cell numbers using the average luminescence at Treatment Day^{-1} (3000 cells) as a conversion factor, and average luminescence of controls at Treatment Day^{-1} was subtracted from all the data points. Data represent the average of six replicate/point $\pm$ SEM. Calculations and nonlinear regressions were done by GraphPad Prism software. The equation of fitting curve is: $Y = \text{Bottom} + \frac{(\text{Top-Bottom})}{1+10^{\text{LogEC50}-X}}$

3.5 CSC Viability Assessment by CellTiter-Glo kit

We detect cell viability after 4 days of incubation with the drug, by CellTiter-Glo kit, with minor modifications to the instructions of the manufacturer.

1. To each well, add 50 microliters of CellTiter-Glo reagent by multichannel pipette. Allow the reaction to proceed 5–10 min. Detect luminescence by microplate luminometer.

3.6 Assay Analysis and Graphing

We use GraphPad Prism software for data graph and analysis. Figure 2 shows the dose-response assay to irinotecan on two different CSCs (*see* **Notes 9** and **10**). The difference in IC50 observed between the two CSCs (CSC2, IC50 = 0.06110; CSC5, IC50 = 11.63) depicts the wide variability in drug response of different strains.

4 Notes

1. To prepare 1 L of CSC medium: to 803.6 mL of ADF add 10 mL of Penicillin/Streptomycin/Glutamine solution 100×, 40 mL BSA 90 g/L, 13.4 mL glucose 45%, 14 mL sodium bicarbonate 7.5%, 2 mL heparin 2 mg/mL, 5 mL HEPES 1 M, 10 mL nicotinamide 1 M, 100 mL Hormone Mix 10×. This medium can be stored at +4 °C for 2 weeks. We supplement CSC medium with 1000× growth factor stock solutions just before use; growth factor complete medium should be used within the day.

   For Penicillin/Streptomycin/Glutamine, glucose, sodium bicarbonate, and HEPES, we use commercial cell grade solutions. We prepare nicotinamide 1 M stock solution by dissolving nicotinamide powder (Sigma-Aldrich, N3376) at 122 mg/mL in ADF; Aliquots of this solution can be stored at −20 °C for 1 year. We prepare 1000× stock solutions of human recombinant EGF and bFGF by dissolving lyophilized powder in ADF, at 20 μg/mL and 10 μg/mL respectively. Aliquots of growth factors can be stored at −80 °C for 6 months.

2. To prepare 1 L of Hormone Mix 10×: to 963 mL of ADF add 1 g apo-transferrin (Sigma-Aldrich T2252 1-G) pouring the powder directly from the bottle, and rinsing the bottle with 2.5 mL ADF. Dissolve 250 mg of insulin (Sigma-Aldrich I5500) in 5 mL HCl 0.1 N, then mix with 22.5 mL sterile H_2O, and add the whole solution (27.5 mL) to the mix. Prepare a 6.2 μg/mL solution of progesterone (Sigma-Aldrich P8783) in ethanol, and then add 100 μL of it to the mix. For putrescine dihydrochloride (Sigma-Aldrich P5780) and sodium selenite (Sigma-Aldrich S5261), we prepare 1000× concentrated stock solutions in ADF (161 mg/mL and 52 μg/mL, respectively), and add 1 mL of each to the mix. These stock solutions can be stored at −20 °c for 1 year. Finally, add 5 mL of HEPES 1 M to the mix after all the other reagents. Hormone Mix can be split into 50 mL aliquots and stored at −20 °C for 6 months.

3. We pass CSC running cultures weekly, seeding about 5×10^4 dissociated CSCs/mL, in 25 cm^2 ultra-low attachment flasks (Corning). Most of the strains duplicate in about 2–3 days, so after 6 days of culture CSC density is about $2–4 \times 10^5$/mL.

4. If running cultures look poor, re-starting the culture, by dissociating and passing the cells in fresh medium and flask should be considered.

5. In the event that at the end of the procedure residual clusters are observed, three steps can be taken, alternatively or sequentially:
   - Filter the suspension through a 100 μm nylon mesh.
   - Leave the tube standing in vertical position for 5–10 min, checking until residual clusters sediment on the bottom by gravity. Harvest the supernatant.
   - Centrifuge suspension for 1 min at 50 × *g*, collect the supernatant, and discard the pellet containing non-dissociated clusters.

6. In the event that too many dead cells are present in the suspension, wash cells with ADF by centrifuging at 150 × *g* for 3 min, discard and replace the medium in order to remove cell debris. This step may be repeated up to three times. Further washing would damage the cells.

7. In order to avoid medium evaporation during the test, we fill with sterile distilled water the frame of wells that surrounds those that contain cells, in plate B.
8. To make a tenfold serial dilution of irinotecan prepare a starting solution of irinotecan 10 mM in CSC. Prepare five Eppendorf micro tubes, and dispense 900 μL of CSC medium in each. With a Gilson pipette, transfer 100 μL of starting solution in the first Eppendorf tube of the series, mix well, collect 100 μL of this solution and transfer to the following Eppendorf tube. Repeat this passage from tube to tube until the last. This will give six solutions, each ten times diluted than the previous, which in this case are 10 mM (starting solution), 1 mM, 100 μM, 10 μM, 1 μM, 0.1 μM. By diluting each of these 1:10 into the cell wells, the final concentrations indicated in Fig. 1 will result.
9. If analyzing proliferation inhibition, verify that untreated control cells have replicated during the assay. To assess this, check that the luminescence of untreated control cells at Day 4 is at least twofolds that of untreated control cells at Day^{-1}. For all the CSC we tested, upon plating 3000 cells/well, the untreated controls at Day 4 had at least duplicated. In some cases, however, particularly slow CSCs may not grow enough to give reliable data on proliferation inhibition. In this case, the number of cells plated may be increased up to 5000/well. In addition, longer incubations up to a maximum of 6 days may allow increasing overall cell growth at the end of the assay. Conversely, for particularly fast-growing CSCs drug treatment may be reduced to 3 days.
10. Luminescence values can be transformed in absolute cell numbers, by using as a conversion factor the values of the controls at Treatment Day^{-1}, i.e., the luminescence of 3000 cells (or any other number of cells plated). Graph baseline can be reduced to zero by subtracting the luminescence of control cells at Treatment Day^{-1}, from all the values registered at Treatment Day 4.

Acknowledgments

This work was financially supported by the Italian Association for Cancer Research (AIRC) 5 per Mille 9979 grant to RDM.

References

1. Oskarsson T, Batlle E, Massague J (2014) Metastatic stem cells: sources, niches, and vital pathways. Cell Stem Cell 14(3):306–321. doi:10.1016/j.stem.2014.02.002
2. Zeuner A, Todaro M, Stassi G, De Maria R (2014) Colorectal cancer stem cells: from the crypt to the clinic. Cell Stem Cell 15 (6):692–705. doi:10.1016/j.stem.2014.11.012
3. Todaro M, Alea MP, Di Stefano AB, Cammareri P, Vermeulen L, Iovino F, Tripodo C, Russo A, Gulotta G, Medema JP, Stassi G (2007)

Colon Cancer stem cells dictate tumor growth and resist cell death by production of interleukin-4. Cell Stem Cell 1(4):389–402. doi:10.1016/j.stem.2007.08.001

4. Cammareri P, Scopelliti A, Todaro M, Eterno V, Francescangeli F, Moyer MP, Agrusa A, Dieli F, Zeuner A, Stassi G (2010) Aurora-A is essential for the tumorigenic capacity and chemoresistance of colorectal cancer stem cells. Cancer Res 70(11):4655–4665. doi:10.1158/0008-5472.Can-09-3953
5. Kreso A, O'Brien CA, van Galen P, Gan OI, Notta F, Brown AM, Ng K, Ma J, Wienholds E, Dunant C, Pollett A, Gallinger S, McPherson J, Mullighan CG, Shibata D, Dick JE (2013) Variable clonal repopulation dynamics influence chemotherapy response in colorectal cancer. Science 339(6119):543–548. doi:10.1126/science.1227670
6. Colak S, Zimberlin CD, Fessler E, Hogdal L, Prasetyanti PR, Grandela CM, Letai A, Medema JP (2014) Decreased mitochondrial priming determines chemoresistance of colon cancer stem cells. Cell Death Differ 21(7):1170–1177. doi:10.1038/cdd.2014.37
7. De Angelis ML, Zeuner A, Policicchio E, Russo G, Bruselles A, Signore M, Vitale S, De Luca G, Pilozzi E, Boe A, Stassi G, Ricci-Vitiani L, Amoreo CA, Pagliuca A, Francescangeli F, Tartaglia M, De Maria R, Baiocchi M (2016) Cancer stem cell-based models of colorectal cancer reveal molecular determinants of therapy resistance. Stem Cells Transl Med 5(4):511–523. doi:10.5966/sctm.2015-0214
8. Gupta PB, Onder TT, Jiang G, Tao K, Kuperwasser C, Weinberg RA, Lander ES (2009) Identification of selective inhibitors of cancer stem cells by high-throughput screening. Cell 138(4):645–659. doi:10.1016/j.cell.2009.06.034
9. Kreso A, van Galen P, Pedley NM, Lima-Fernandes E, Frelin C, Davis T, Cao L, Baiazitov R, Du W, Sydorenko N, Moon YC, Gibson L, Wang Y, Leung C, Iscove NN, Arrowsmith CH, Szentgyorgyi E, Gallinger S, Dick JE, O'Brien CA (2014) Self-renewal as a therapeutic target in human colorectal cancer. Nat Med 20(1):29–36. doi:10.1038/nm.3418
10. Gao H, Korn JM, Ferretti S, Monahan JE, Wang Y, Singh M, Zhang C, Schnell C, Yang G, Zhang Y, Balbin OA, Barbe S, Cai H, Casey F, Chatterjee S, Chiang DY, Chuai S, Cogan SM, Collins SD, Dammassa E, Ebel N, Embry M, Green J, Kauffmann A, Kowal C, Leary RJ, Lehar J, Liang Y, Loo A, Lorenzana E, Robert McDonald E 3rd, ME ML, Merkin J, Meyer R, Naylor TL, Patawaran M, Reddy A, Roelli C, Ruddy DA, Salangsang F, Santacroce F, Singh AP, Tang Y, Tinetto W, Tobler S, Velazquez R, Venkatesan K, Von Arx F, Wang HQ, Wang Z, Wiesmann M, Wyss D, Xu F, Bitter H, Atadja P, Lees E, Hofmann F, Li E, Keen N, Cozens R, Jensen MR, Pryer NK, Williams JA, Sellers WR (2015) High-throughput screening using patient-derived tumor xenografts to predict clinical trial drug response. Nat Med 21(11):1318–1325. doi:10.1038/nm.3954
11. van de Wetering M, Francies HE, Francis JM, Bounova G, Iorio F, Pronk A, van Houdt W, van Gorp J, Taylor-Weiner A, Kester L, McLaren-Douglas A, Blokker J, Jaksani S, Bartfeld S, Volckman R, van Sluis P, Li VSW, Seepo S, Pedamallu CS, Cibulskis K, Carter SL, McKenna A, Lawrence MS, Lichtenstein L, Stewart C, Koster J, Versteeg R, van Oudenaarden A, Saez-Rodriguez J, Vries RGJ, Getz G, Wessels L, Stratton MR, McDermott U, Meyerson M, Garnett MJ, Clevers H (2015) Prospective derivation of a living organoid biobank of colorectal cancer patients. Cell 161(4):933–945. doi:10.1016/j.cell.2015.03.053
12. Marcucci F, Stassi G, De Maria R (2016) Epithelial-mesenchymal transition: a new target in anticancer drug discovery. Nat Rev Drug Discov 15(5):311–325. doi:10.1038/nrd.2015.13
13. Baiocchi M, Biffoni M, Ricci-Vitiani L, Pilozzi E, De Maria R (2010) New models for cancer research: human cancer stem cell xenografts. Curr Opin Pharmacol 10(4):380–384. doi:10.1016/j.coph.2010.05.002
14. Galli R, Gritti A, Vescovi AL (2008) Adult neural stem cells. Methods Mol Biol 438:67–84. doi:10.1007/978-1-59745-133-8_7
15. Sato T, Stange DE, Ferrante M, Vries RGJ, van Es JH, van den Brink S, van Houdt WJ, Pronk A, van Gorp J, Siersema PD, Clevers H (2011) Long-term expansion of epithelial organoids from human colon, adenoma, adenocarcinoma, and barrett's epithelium. Gastroenterology 141(5):1762–1772. doi:10.1053/j.gastro.2011.07.050

Chapter 11

Tumor Tissue Analogs for the Assessment of Radioresistance in Cancer Stem Cells

Meenakshi Upreti

Abstract

Over the years, radiotherapy-related research has been based on local tumor control as an experimental endpoint, yielding a wealth of data demonstrating the importance of cancer stem cells in tumor reoccurrence after radiotherapy. Literature is replete with experimental and clinical evidence that the cancer stem cell population in a tumor affects its radiocurability. An important consideration for radiotherapy is the microenvironmental stimuli in the CSC niche that results from factors such as hypoxia, extracellular matrix (ECM) elements and their intercellular interaction with non-stem cells and other cell types that prevail in the tumor milieu. In this chapter, we have described the methodology to develop in vitro 3D tumor models that incorporate these microenvironmental characteristics and design experiments that generate endpoints for understanding radioresistance in cancer stem cells.

Key words Tumor tissue analogs (TTA), Hypoxia, 3D co-cultures, Tumor microenvironment, Confocal microscopy, Immunohistochemistry

1 Introduction

Cancer stem cells (CSC) are characterized as tumor cells that have the enhanced ability to self-renew [1–3] and survive the current modalities of radiation and other curative anticancer treatments [4, 5]. Therefore, for a therapy to be effective in completely eradicating the tumor, it is of utmost importance to inactivate the CSC. The current treatment modalities target the bulk of the tumor volume without accounting for the CSC and the contribution of the tumor microenvironment. An understanding of how the tumor and its microenvironment protects or sensitizes the CSC from chemo-radiation therapies is critical for predicting the therapeutic response in cancer patients. The present chapter describes the method to develop an in vitro three-dimensional (3D) lung cancer model of color-coded tumor tissue analogs (TTA) comprised of human lung adenocarcinoma cells, fibroblasts, endothelial cells, and cancer stem cells (CSC) from Non-small cell lung cancer

Gianpaolo Papaccio and Vincenzo Desiderio (eds.), *Cancer Stem Cells: Methods and Protocols*, Methods in Molecular Biology, vol. 1692, DOI 10.1007/978-1-4939-7401-6_11, © Springer Science+Business Media LLC 2018

(NSCLC) patients maintained in (5% O_2) hypoxic conditions to recapitulate the physiologic conditions in tumors. Our studies have demonstrated that the inclusion of CSC in the 3D tumor model elucidates that radiation modifies the cell composition of the TTA in favor of a CSC-dominant phenotype. These findings closely correlate with the existing understanding that CSC are a key player in tumor radioresistance [4, 6, 7]. Previous reports including our own establish that the resistance observed in the CSC requires a hypoxic environment to adequately confer therapy resistance and the metastatic potential to the tumor cell population [6, 8, 9]. The experimental design requires the TTA to be maintained in hypoxic conditions to recapitulate the in situ environment that the tumor and tumor microenvironment would typically thrive in within the human body [10]. Thus, making the 3D co-culture tumor model physiologically relevant for investigating radiation response in CSC that co-exist in the tumor microenvironment. Tumor cells that survive the ionizing radiation express cancer stem cell markers and have an invasive phenotype with high levels of vimentin [11]. In this chapter, we discuss techniques to assess the expression of proteins involved in radioresistance such as vimentin in the TTA by intact immunoprobing or immunohistochemistry. Size and fluorescence intensity of contributing cell types has also been utilized to devise techniques for understanding radioresistance in CSC in the context of the tumor microenvironment. We expect that the methods described in this chapter will lay the foundation for the development of a new approach that utilizes physiologically representative tumor models to understand therapeutic response to existing and novel treatment modalities in cancer patients.

2 Materials

1. Monoclonal mouse anti-vimentin antibody (Dako, Carpinteria, CA).
2. Polyclonal rabbit anti-vimentin antibody (Bioss, Woburn, MA).
3. Quick coating solution to veneer flasks for human neonatal dermal fibroblasts (HNDF) cell culture (Angioproteomie, Shrewsbury, MA).

2.1 Cell Lines

We have used several cell lines that may or may not express fluorescent protein along with patient-derived primary cell types. These cell types and their origin are listed below:

1. Red fluorescence protein (RFP) expressing A549 human non-small cell lung cancer (NSCLC) epithelial cell line (A549-RFP) (AntiCancer Inc., San Diego, CA).

2. The human pulmonary artery endothelial cells (HPAEC) (Lonza, Walkersville, MD).
3. Green fluorescent protein (GFP) expressing human neonatal dermal fibroblast cells (HNDF-GFP) (Angioproteome, Shrewsbury, MA). The HNDF cells were isolated from normal neonatal forehead skin tissue samples and transfected with GFP-Lentiviral particles at passage one, selected using Puromycin (1 mg/ml) and maintained in DMEM containing 5% fetal bovine serum (FBS).
4. Human NSCLC cancer stem cells (CSC) prescreened for CD133, CD 44, SSEA ¾ and their ability to form tumors <1000 cells in mice (Celprogen, Inc., Torrance, CA).

2.2 Cell Culture

1. The A549 cells were cultured in DMEM high glucose medium, supplemented with 10% FBS, 1% penicillin-streptomycin, and 1% glutamax (Invitrogen, Carlsbad, CA).
2. The endothelial cells (HPAEC) were cultured in its recommended medium EGM™-2 BulletKit (Lonza, Walkersville, MD).
3. The human neonatal dermal fibroblasts (HNDF) were grown in flasks precoated with a quick coating solution and maintained in DMEM High Glucose containing 5% FBS, 1× Glutamax, and 1% Pen-Strep.
4. The human NSCLC stem cells (CSC) were incubated in the M36107-34S media and cultured on precoated ECM dishes (Celprogen, Inc., Torrance, CA) on flasks precoated with human lung cancer stem cell extracellular matrix also provided by Celprogen, Inc. at 5% Oxygen supply.
5. All cell lines were maintained at 37 °C and 5% CO_2 equilibrated with atmospheric O_2 in a humidified incubator that contains 20% O_2 unless otherwise mentioned.
6. The multicell 3D co-cultures were either maintained at 37 °C in a humidified atmosphere and either normoxic condition with 20% oxygen supply (hereafter referred to as normoxia) or in the Heracell™ Trigas hypoxia chamber (ThermoFischer Scientific, Waltham, MA) with 5% oxygen supply (hereafter referred to as hypoxia).

2.3 Clonogenic Cell Survival Assay

1. Plastic ware: T-25 flasks and 6-well culture plates.
2. Trypsin-EDTA.
3. Phosphate-buffered saline (PBS).
4. Deionized Water (18 MΩ-cm at 25 °C).
5. Isotone II Diluent for counting cells.
6. Coulter Counter (e.g., EZ2 Beckman Coulter, Inc., Brea, CA).

7. Crystal violet.
8. Methanol.

2.4 Tumor Tissue Analogs (TTA)

1. 48-well cell culture plate.
2. Optically clear cell repellent plates (Griener Cellstar, Kaysville, UT).
3. P20 pipette and tips (0.5–20 μl).
4. P1000 pipette tips (200–1000 μl).

2.5 X-Ray Irradiation

1. X-ray machine Varian 21 EX platinum TrueBeam System (Varian medical systems, Palo Alto, CA) or equivalent.

2.6 Microscopy and Image Processing

1. FV1000 laser scanning confocal fluorescence microscope (Olympus, Center Valley, PA) or equivalent.
2. Image analyses software.
3. ImageJv 1.47 (National Institute of Health, USA).

2.7 Immunoprobing Intact TTA

1. Paraformaldehyde.
2. PBS.
3. Bovine serum albumin (BSA).
4. Anti-vimentin polyclonal antibody.
5. Fluorescent labeled secondary antibody as appropriate for primary.
6. Nunc glass-bottom dishes (ThermoFisher Scientific, Waltham, MA).

2.8 Histogel Embedding and TTA Sections for Immunostaining

1. Formalin.
2. PBS.
3. Tissue-Tek® Cryomolds (Fisher Scientific, Waltham, MA).
4. Histogel (Thermoscientific, Kalamazoo, MI).
5. Ice.
6. Bio-wrap (Leica Biosystems, Buffalo Grove, IL).
7. Tissue biopsy cassette (Fisher Scientific, Waltham, MA).
8. Alcohol.
9. Xylene.
10. Paraffin.
11. Paraplast X-TRA [Wax] (Sigma-Aldrich, St. Louis, MO).
12. Leica microtome (Buffalo Grove, IL).

2.9 Immunohistochemistry on TTA Sections

1. Superfrost™ Plus Microscope slides (Fisher Scientific, Pittsburgh, PA).
2. Monoclonal mouse anti-vimentin V9 antibody (Dako #IR630).
3. EnVisioFLEX visualization System (Dako, Carpinteria, CA).
4. Xylene.
5. Alcihol.
6. Deionized Water (18 MΩ-cm at 25 °C).
7. EnVision FLEX high pH Target (antigen) retrieval buffer.
8. Decloaking Chamber (Biocare Medical, Concord, CA).
9. Dako Envision + Kit.
10. 3,3′-Diaminobenzidine **(DAB)**.
11. Hematoxylin.
12. Coverslip.
13. Permount Mounting Medium.
14. Axioskop 2 Plus Microscope (Carl Zeiss, Gottingen, Germany).
15. Axiocam Digital camera (Carl Zeiss, Gottingen, Germany).

3 Methods

3.1 Clonogenic Cell Survival Assay

Clonogenic survival assay is a technique to determine capability of cell in vitro to survive and proliferate by forming a large colony or a clone. This makes the cell clonogenic. The hypoxic microenvironment is a determinant of the cancer stem cell phenotype [12]. Clonogenic survival studies are therefore performed to understand the effect of physiological oxygen levels on the response of CSC to an increasing dose of radiation [9] (*see* **Note 1**). The Resistance of CSC to radiation exposure in hypoxia as assessed by colonogenic survival assay is demonstrated in Fig. 1.

1. **Preparation of CSC in culture flasks for irradiation**
   Label eight precoated ECM E36107-34-T25 flasks with 5 ml of medium as 0, 2.5, 5.0, and 10 Gy for the evaluation of the radiosensitivity of the CSC.
   Trypsinize the stock flask of CSC. Prepare a single-cell suspension and obtain an accurate cell count using Isotone II diluent and an automated Coulter counter.
   Seed 2.5×10^5 cells in each flask and allow them to adhere overnight in a hypoxic chamber maintained at 37 °C with 5% oxygen supply.

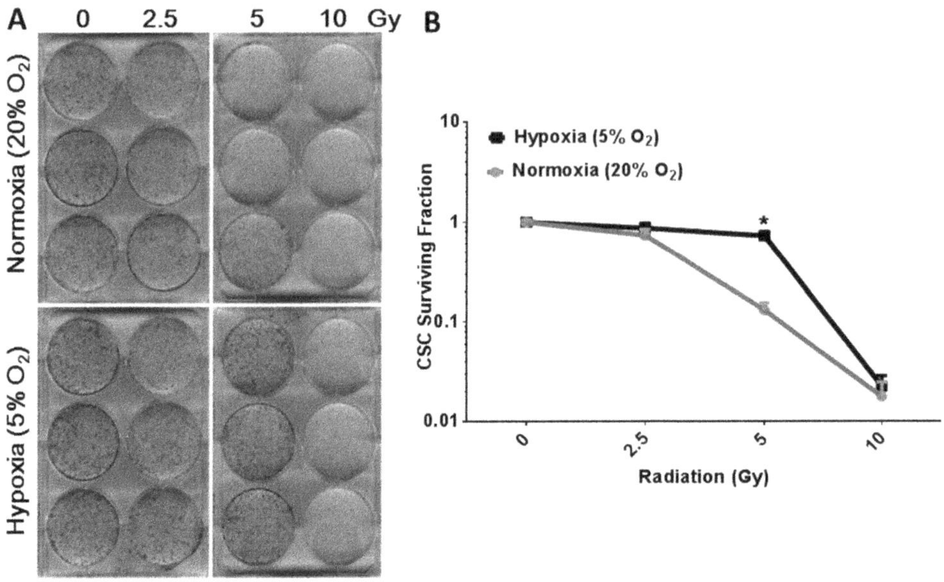

Fig. 1 Resistance of CSC to radiation exposure in hypoxia assessed by colonogenic survival assay. Colonies were stained with crystal violet and counted. Data representing mean ± SD ($n = 3$) was used to plot the surviving fraction of the CSC maintained in hypoxic and normoxic conditions after exposure to increasing dose of radiation as indicated. Figure courtesy Fig. 1 in [9]

2. **Irradiation of flasks and plating for Clonogenic Assay**

   Irradiate the flasks as per the experimental design. We used the X-ray machine Varian 21 EX platinum TrueBeam System.

   Keep the flasks on ice, trypsinize and prepare single-cell suspension.

   Count and plate 200 cells from control flask (0 Gy) and 500 cells from irradiated flasks (2.5, 5, and 10 Gy) in triplicate in ECM precoated 6-well plates in triplicate.

   Prepare two such sets of the 6-well plates.

   Incubate one set at 20% oxygen supply (normoxia) and the other in the hypoxia chamber with 5% oxygen supply (hypoxia). Maintain both the sets of culture plates for 10–12 days at 37 °C until large colonies (>1 mm or >50 cells) are formed.

3. **Fixing and staining of colonies**

   Fix and stain the colonies as described in [13] and let the plates dry overnight (*see* **Note 2**).

4. **Counting of colonies**

   Count the air-dried colonies in each dish under a magnified field using a dissecting microscope. A cluster of crystal violet stained cells with 25–50 cells is considered a colony.

   Average the colony counts from triplicates and determine the plating efficiency (PE) [13].

$$PE = \frac{\text{number of colonies formed}}{\text{number of cells seeded}} \times 100\%;$$

Following determination of PE, calculate the surviving fraction (SF)

$$SF = \frac{\text{number of colonies in teatment group}}{\text{number of cells seeded} \times PE}$$

Present the surviving fraction on a logarithmic scale plotted on the y-axis against the radiation dose on the x-axis.

3.2 Tumor Tissue Analogs (TTA)

3D tumor tissue analogs (TTA) were generated by co-culturing four different cell types: A549-RFP tumor cells, HPAEC endothelial cells, and HNDF-GFP cells with or without CSC in a "hanging drops" of medium as described [14]. The experiments to utilize 3D tumor TTA are designed to assess the impact of tumor microenvironment on the radioresistance in CSC. This involves analyses of several downstream endpoints such as biochemical assays, histology of intact TTA and their cryosections, high-throughput omics, and confocal imaging of the color-coded TTA (Fig. 2). In this chapter, we have described the techniques and methods used and modified in our laboratory to analyze some of these endpoints.

1. **Preparation of Single-cell suspension**
   Grow adherent cell cultures to 90% confluency, rinsed twice with PBS. Add 2 ml (for 100 mm plates) of 0.05% trypsin-1 mM EDTA, and incubate at 37 °C until cells detach. Block the trypsinization by adding 2 ml of complete medium.

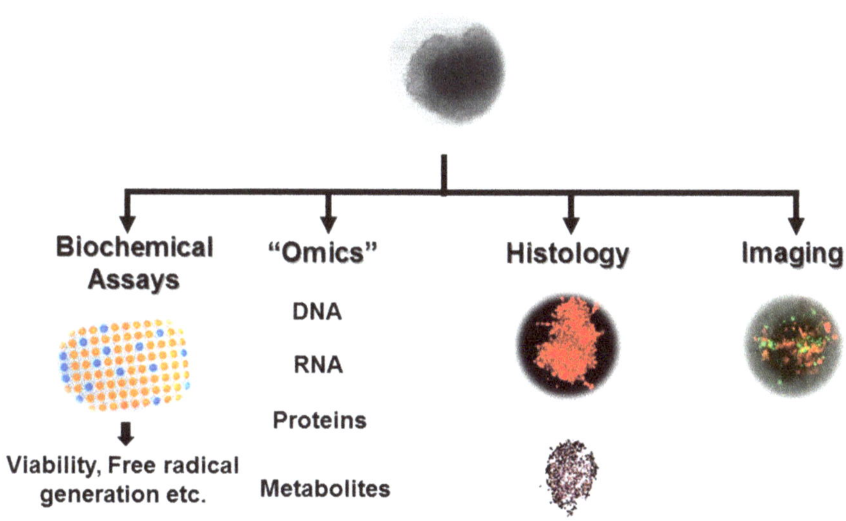

Fig. 2 The preparation of 3D Tumor tissue analogs (TTA) facilitates analysis of several downstream endpoints as indicated in the figure

Use a 5 ml pipette to triturate the mixture until cells are in suspension. Transfer cells to a 15 ml conical tube.

Vortex briefly and centrifuge at 200 × *g* for 5 min.

Discard the supernatant and wash the pellet with 1 ml complete tissue culture medium. Resuspend cells in 2 ml of culture medium.

Count the cells and adjust concentration to 1×10^6 cells/5 ml. Our studies were performed using an automated cell counter as described earlier (*see* **Note 3**).

Prepare a single-cell suspension mix of A549-RFP cells, HNDF-GFP cells, and HPAEC cells in the ratio of 1.2: 1: 1 (3200 cells/ 20 μl). For TTA + CSC (Tumor tissue analogs with cancer stem cells) the cell suspension mix of A549 -RFP cells, HNDF-GFP cells, HPAEC cells, and CSC was in the ratio of 1:1:1:0.2 (3200 cells/20 μl).

2. **Formation of TTA in "Hanging Drops" of medium**

   Remove the lid of a 48-well cell culture plate and fill each well with 1.5 ml of PBS in order to prevent the hanging drops on the lid from drying.

   Dispense 20 μl of each single-cell suspension mix onto the inverted lid of each well.

   Invert the lid gently onto the PBS-filled culture plate and incubate under the hypoxic condition (5% O_2), 37 °C and 95% humidity (*see* **Note 4**).

   Monitor the drops daily. Aggregates tend to form within 3–4 days. A stereo microscope can be used to assess the aggregates.

   Incubate for 10–12 days until an integrated morphology is observed. Use a confocal microscope for the observation of an integrated tissue-like morphology of the color-coded cell types in the TTA formed (*see* **Note 5**).

   The experiments to utilize 3D tumor TTA are designed to assess the impact of tumor microenvironment on the radioresistance in CSC by analyses of several downstream endpoints such as biochemical assays, histology of intact TTA and their cryosections, high-throughput omics, and confocal imaging of the color-coded TTA. The methods to analyze some of these endpoints have been described in this chapter (*see* **Note 6**). Figure 3 demonstrates the impact of CSC in TTA maintained in hypoxia condition to radiation exposure.

3. **Confocal imaging of the TTA**

   Analyze the captured images for sizing using an image analyses software and ImageJv 1.47 (National Institute of Health, USA).

   Graphically represent a comparison of the TTA size, green, and red fluorescence intensity of the contributing cell types analyzed in different environmental conditions of hypoxia and/or radiation (Fig. 4).

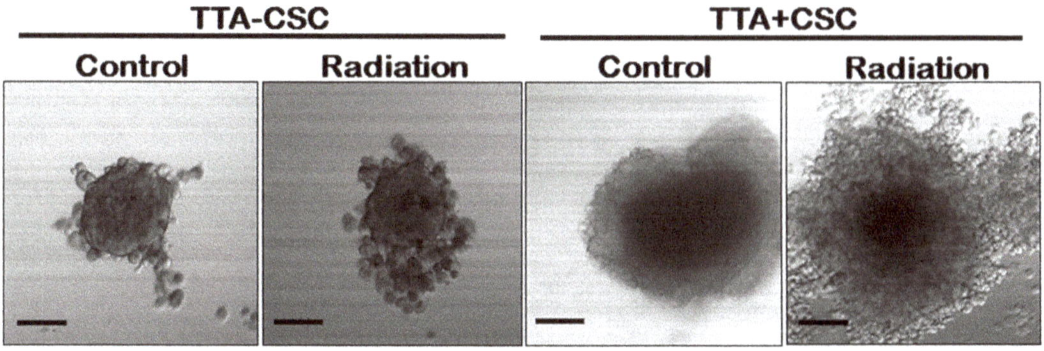

Fig. 3 Representative images of TTA with CSC (TTA+CSC) and without CSC (TTA−CSC) before and after radiation exposure maintained in hypoxic condition (5% O_2)

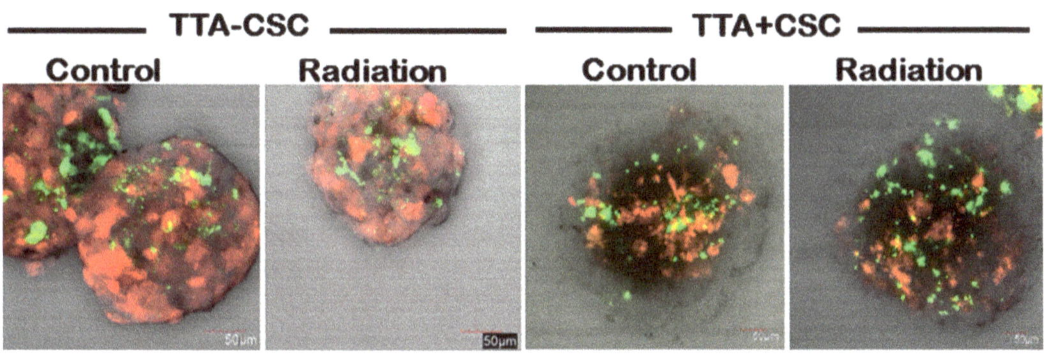

Fig. 4 An overlay of bright field red and green channels of representative images of the TTA with different cell compositions before and after radiation exposure in hypoxic condition (5% O_2). Figure modified courtesy Fig. 2 in [9]

3.3 Immunoprobing Intact TTA with Vimentin

Fix the intact TTA in 4% paraformaldehyde and wash with PBS.

Block the TTA in 5% BSA for 30 min.

Incubate with anti-vimentin polyclonal antibody for 1 h and wash with PBS twice.

Subsequently incubate with secondary antibody for 30 min and wash with PBS three times.

Transfer the TTA to glass-bottom plates for acquisition of confocal images.

Capture the images using a laser scanning confocal microscope at 10× and 20× magnifications.

Analyze and quantitate the vimentin staining as described as shown in Figs. 5 and 6 and represent graphically.

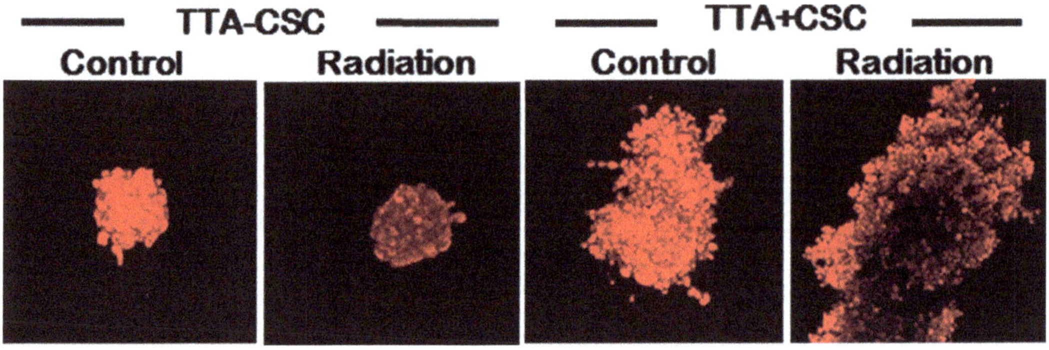

Fig. 5 Representative images after vimentin staining of TTA with different cell compositions before and after radiation exposure maintained in hypoxic condition (5% O_2). Figure modified courtesy Fig. 4 in [9]

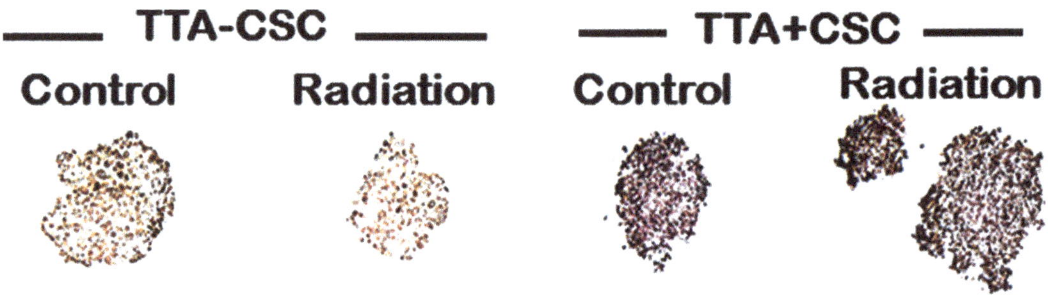

Fig. 6 Representative images after vimentin staining of TTA histogel embedded cryosections with different cell compositions before and after radiation exposure maintained in hypoxic condition (5% O_2)

3.4 Histogel Embedding and Immunohistochemistry of TTA Sections

1. **Histogel embedding of the TTA**

   Collected and fix the TTA in 10% formalin for 2 h and wash with PBS.

   Dehydrate twice with 50 and 70% ethanol for 15 min each.

   Transfer the dehydrated TTAs of each treatment group in one cryomold.

   Embed in Histogel liquefied by heating at 60° ± 5 °C (*see* **Note 7** and **8**).

   Subsequently solidify the TTA containing cryomolds in ice for 10 min.

   Dehydrate the Histogel plugs in increasing grades of alcohol.

   Clear the histogel plugs with xylene and impregnate with paraffin.

   Embedding the processed histogel plugs in paraffin wax.

   Cut 4–5 μm sections from the paraffin blocks with the help of a microtome.

4 Notes

1. All the experiments need to have appropriate controls. Dot not consider more than two variables for investigation in one experiment. Adequate replicates for the quantitative analysis for each treatment condition in an experiment should be considered.
2. Do not pour crystal violet stain used for clonogenic studies down the sink but collect in a bottle assigned for used stain.
3. If the cell type composition is being altered, the concentration of the single-cell suspension may be adjusted based on the cell size.
4. While incubating the TTA in 48-well culture plates humidity needs to be maintained by the addition of PBS (1.5 ml) in each well.
5. Each 48-well culture plate will provide up to 48 TTA. The TTA on the lids of the inner 24 wells tend to represent the best morphology. The TTA on the lid of the exterior wells tend to shrink owing to loss of moisture. They can be used after the verification of the integrated morphology and size by imaging.
6. For biochemical or molecular testing the 12–24 TTA per treatment condition can be grouped together. A minimum of three such sets will serve as replicates for quantitative analysis. Histogel is a solid at room temperature. It must be liquified for use by heating to ~60 °C. This can be achieved by placing the Histogel into a boiling water bath for 3–10 min.
7. Histogel is a solid at room temperature. It must be liquified for use by heating to ~60 °C. This can be achieved by placing the Histogel into a boiling water bath for 3–10 min.
8. After the histogel liquefies, the temperature may be lowered to ~50 °C where it will remain in the liquid state. The histogel at this temperature should be used to embed the TTA.

References

1. Clarke MF, Dick JE, Dirks PB, Eaves CJ, Jamieson CH, Jones DL, Visvader J, Weissman IL, Wahl GM (2006) Cancer stem cells–perspectives on current status and future directions: AACR workshop on cancer stem cells. Cancer Res 66(19):9339–9344
2. Clarke MF, Fuller M (2006) Stem cells and cancer: two faces of eve. Cell 124 (6):1111–1115
3. O'Brien CA, Kreso A, Jamieson CH (2010) Cancer stem cells and self-renewal. Clin Cancer Res 16(12):3113–3120
4. Diehn M, Clarke MF (2006) Cancer stem cells and radiotherapy: new insights into tumor radioresistance. J Natl Cancer Inst 98 (24):1755–1757
5. Kim Y, Joo KM, Jin J, Nam DH (2009) Cancer stem cells and their mechanism of chemo-radiation resistance. Int J Stem Cells 2 (2):109–114
6. Baumann M, Krause M, Hill R (2008) Exploring the role of cancer stem cells in radioresistance. Nat Rev Cancer 8(7):545–554
7. Desai A, Webb B, Gerson SL (2014) CD133+ cells contribute to radioresistance via altered

regulation of DNA repair genes in human lung cancer cells. Radiother Oncol 110(3):538–545
8. Zhao M, Zhang Y, Zhang H, Wang S, Zhang M, Chen X, Wang H, Zeng G, Chen X, Liu G, Zhou C (2015) Hypoxia-induced cell stemness leads to drug resistance and poor prognosis in lung adenocarcinoma. Lung Cancer 87 (2):98–106
9. Chan R, Sethi P, Jyoti A, McGarry R, Upreti M (2016) Investigating the radioresistant properties of lung cancer stem cells in the context of the tumor microenvironment. Radiat Res 185 (2):169–181
10. Ivanovic Z (2009) Hypoxia or in situ normoxia: the stem cell paradigm. J Cell Physiol 219(2):271–275
11. Gomez-Casal R, Bhattacharya C, Ganesh N, Bailey L, Basse P, Gibson M, Epperly M, Levina V (2013) Non-small cell lung cancer cells survived ionizing radiation treatment display cancer stem cell and epithelial-mesenchymal transition phenotypes. Mol Cancer 12(1):94
12. Plaks V, Kong N, Werb Z (2015) The cancer stem cell niche: how essential is the niche in regulating stemness of tumor cells? Cell Stem Cell 16(3):225–238
13. Franken NA, Rodermond HM, Stap J, Haveman J, van Bree C (2006) Clonogenic assay of cells in vitro. Nat Protoc 1(5):2315–2319
14. Upreti M, Jamshidi-Parsian A, Koonce NA, Webber JS, Sharma SK, Asea AA, Mader MJ, Griffin RJ (2011) Tumor-endothelial cell three-dimensional spheroids: new aspects to enhance radiation and drug therapeutics. Transl Oncol 4(6):365–376

Chapter 12

Generation of In Vitro Model of Epithelial Mesenchymal Transition (EMT) Via the Expression of a Cytoplasmic Mutant Form of Promylocytic Leukemia Protein (PML)

Anna Di Biase, Amanda K. Miles, and Tarik Regad

Abstract

Epithelial Mesenchymal Transition (EMT) is a key event in cancer progression. During this event, epithelial cancer cells undergo molecular and cellular changes leading to their trans-differentiation into mesenchymal cancer cells that are capable of migration, invasion, and metastasis to other tissues and organs. Here, we present a method for in vitro induction of EMT in prostate cancer cell lines using lentiviral expression of a PMLI isoform mutant construct.

Key words Epithelial mesenchymal transition (EMT), Prostate cancer (PCa), Mutagenesis, Promylocytic leukemia protein (PML), Lentiviral expression system, E-Cadherin, Vimentin, N-Cadherin, Epithelial cells, Mesenchymal cells

1 Introduction

EMT is an essential cellular event that is implicated in embryonic development, wound healing, and cancer progression [1]. Epithelial cells that are characterized by the presence of a baso-apical polarity start to transdifferentiate into mesenchymal cells. This cellular process, mediated by molecular changes, is accompanied by the loss of lateral cell–cell junctions, loss of cell polarity, and transformation into mesenchymal cells. These cells have the capacity to invade surrounding tissues and to metastasise to other organs. Several key cellular pathways have been shown to mediate EMT including TGF-β, WNT, HH, and Notch signaling.

The tumor suppressor PML regulate numerous cellular processes that are involved in cell proliferation, differentiation, and apoptosis. It plays an essential role in the formation of PML-nuclear bodies (PML-NBs), but is also found expressed in other cellular compartments including the nucleoplasm, the nucleolus, the nuclear envelope, and the cytoplasm where it plays different cellular

Gianpaolo Papaccio and Vincenzo Desiderio (eds.), *Cancer Stem Cells: Methods and Protocols*, Methods in Molecular Biology, vol. 1692, DOI 10.1007/978-1-4939-7401-6_12,

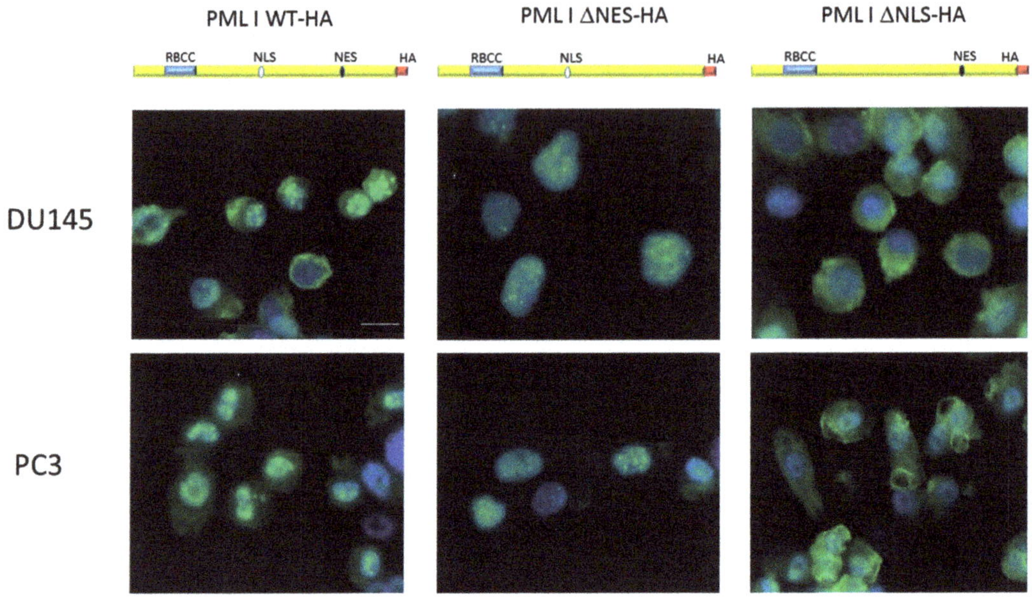

Fig. 1 Lentiviral expression of PML I mutant constructs in DU145 and PC3 prostate cancer cell lines. Immunofluorescence images of PML I wild-type (WT-HA), PML I ΔNES and PML I ΔNLS expression in DU145 and PC3 using anti-HA antibody. Scale bar = 20 μm

roles. In fact, these diverse patterns of expression within the cell are not due to the existence of a single molecule but to several isoforms (PML I-VII) which expression, cellular localization, and functions are dictated by physiologic and pathologic cellular events [2–6]. We have recently shown that cytoplasmic PML isoform I can induce EMT via the induction of TGF-β signaling [7]. We have generated prostate cancer cell lines that were infected with lentiviruses carrying a construct that expresses the mutant form of PML I and which has a deleted Nuclear Localization Signal (NLS) (Fig. 1). We show by immunofluorescence that this mutant is expressed in the cytoplasm where it promotes EMT. Cells that express this mutant form have low expression levels of the epithelial marker E-Cadherin and increased expression of the mesenchymal marker Vimentin (Fig. 2). As controls, we expressed the PML I wild-type and a PML I mutant form that lacks the Nuclear Export Signal (NES) and therefore is expressed in the nucleus. In summary, we provide here an in vitro method to induce EMT in prostate cancer cell lines via the expression of a cytoplasmic mutant of PML isoform I.

2 Materials

1. 14 mL BD Falcon polypropylene round-bottom tubes.
2. Petri dishes (100 mm plates).

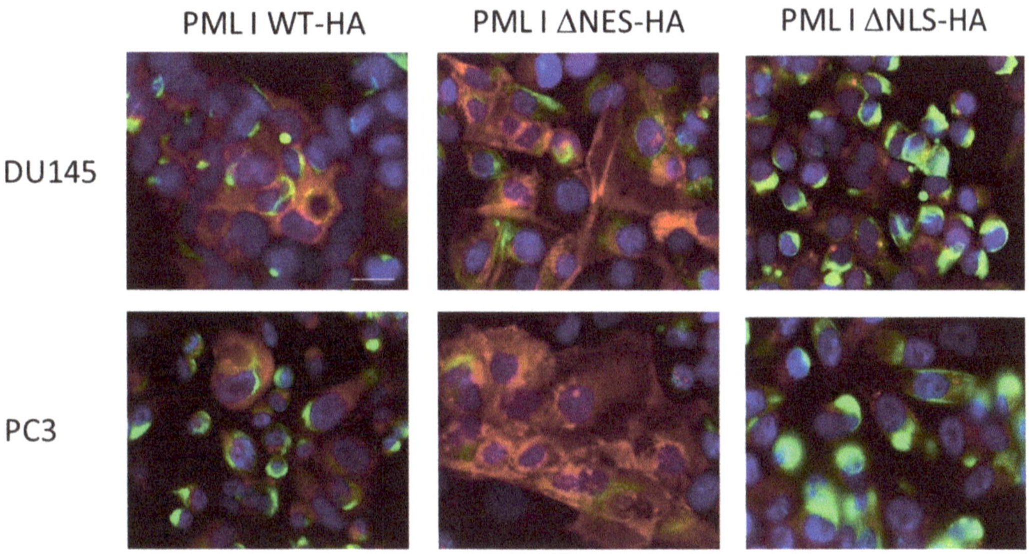

Fig. 2 Effect of expressing PML I mutant constructs in DU145 and PC3 prostate cancer cell lines. Immunofluorescence images from DU145 and PC3 prostate cancer cell lines stained with antibodies for E-Cadherin (*Red*) and Vimentin (*Green*) and expressing PML I wild type (WT-HA), PML I ΔNES and PML I ΔNLS. Scale bar = 20 μm

2.1 In Vitro Site-Directed Mutagenesis Reagents

3. *Pfu Turbo*® DNA polymerase (2.5 U/μL).
4. 10× reaction buffer.
5. *Dpn* I restriction enzyme (10 U/μL).
6. dNTP mix.
7. XL1-Blue supercompetent cells.
8. 10 mg/mL ampicillin.
9. 1 L glass flasks.
10. 0.1 mL thin-walled PCR tubes.

2.2 Inoue Method for Preparation of Competent Cells [8]

1. LB (Luria-Bertani) agar or LB-ampicillin agar (1 L)

   Dissolve *NaCl* (10 g/L), *Tryptone* (10 g/L), *Yeast extract* (5 g/L), and Agar (20 g/L) in pure H_2O (Milli-Q, or equivalent). Shake until dissolution of solutes. Adjust to pH 7.0 with 5 N NaOH. Autoclave the LB agar from 15 to 30 min at 15 psi (1.05 kg/cm^2) on liquid cycle. After cooling add Ampicillin (100 μg/mL) and mix the agar gently (*see* **Note 1**).
2. NZY+ broth:

   Dissolve *Casein hydrosylate* (10 g/L), *Yeast extract* (5 g/L), and *NaCl* (5 g/L) in pure H_2O. Shake until dissolution of solutes. Adjust to pH 7.0 with 5 N NaOH. Autoclave the LB agar from 15 to 30 min at 15 psi (1.05 kg/cm^2) on liquid cycle. Add the following filter sterilized supplements prior to use:

12.5 mL 1 M $MgCl_2$, 12.5 mL 1 M $MgSO_4$, 20 mL of 20% (w/v) glucose.
SELECTIVE PLATES: Pour the agar in polystyrene 100 mm cell culture dishes (*see* **Notes 2** and **3**) and then dry them in the laminar flow hood with the lid slightly off for 30 min.

3. TE buffer: Dissolve Tris–HCl (pH 7.5) 10 mM (1.57 g g/L) and EDTA 1 mM (0.292 g/L) in 1 L pure H_2O.
4. 10× Reaction Buffer: Dissolve KCl 100 mM (7.455 g/L), $(NH_4)_2SO_4$ 100 mM (13.214 g/L), Tris–HCl (pH 8.8) 200 mM (31.52 g/L), $MgSO_4$ 20 mM (4.93 g/L), 1% Triton® X-100, and 1 mg/mL nuclease-free BSA in 1 L pure H_2O.

2.3 Cell Transformation

1. Liquid LB (Luria-Bertani).
2. LB agar for plates: Dissolve *NaCl* (10 g/L), *Tryptone* (10 g/L), *Yeast extract* (5 g/L), and *agar* (15 g/L) in pure H_2O. Shake until the dissolution of solutes and autoclave the LB agar from 15 to 30 min at 15 psi (1.05 kg/cm^2) on liquid cycle. After cooling add *Ampicillin* (100 μg/mL) and mix the agar gently to avoid forming excess of bubbles (*see* **Note 4**).
3. Glycerol 30%:

   Dissolve 3 mL of absolute glycerol in 7 mL of pure H_2O and autoclave for 15 at 15 psi (1.05 kg/cm^2) on liquid cycle.
4. Recombinant, viral packaging, and viral envelope plasmids.
5. QIAGEN QIAfilter Plasmid Midi and Maxi Kits.
6. NanoDrop UV-Vis Spectrophotometer.
7. Polystyrene 100 mm cell culture dishes.
8. 1 L glass flasks.
9. 1 L Pyrex® round media storage bottles.
10. 1.5 mL microcentrifuge tubes.
11. Disposable L-shaped cell spreaders.
    SELECTIVE PLATES: Pour the agar in polystyrene 100 mm cell culture dishes (*see* **Note 5**) and then dry them in the laminar flow hood with the lid slightly off for 30 min.

2.4 Cell Transfection

Carry out all the procedures at room temperature unless otherwise specified.

1. Purified plasmids at known concentration.
2. Cell culture: T25 flasks with filter cap of HEK 293 cell line (*see* **Note 6**).
3. Lipofectamine transfection reagent.
4. OptiMEM-reduced serum medium.
5. HEK293T dedicated medium: DMEM high glucose + 10% FCS + 1% L-glutamine.

6. Polyethersulfone membrane syringe filters.
7. 1.5 mL microcentrifuge tubes.

2.5 Target Cell Line Killing Curve

1. Cell culture: 6-well tissue culture-treated plates of DU145 and PC3 cell lines (*see* **Note 7**).
2. DU145 and PC3 dedicated medium: EMEM high glucose + 10% FCS + 1% L-glutamine.
3. Puromycin dihydrochloride (*see* **Note 8**):

   Prepare stock at 1 mg/mL diluting 1 mL of Puromycin at 10 mg/mL concentration in 9 mL of pure H_2O and transferring 1 mL of diluted puromycin in 1.5 mL tubes.
4. 1.5 mL microcentrifuge tubes.

2.6 Target Cell Lines Infection (Transduction)

1. Cell culture: 6-well tissue culture-treated plates of DU145 and PC3 cell lines (*see* **Note 9**).
2. DU145 and PC3 dedicated medium: EMEM high glucose + 10% FCS + 1% L-glutamine.
3. Hexadimethrine bromide solution:
   Dissolve 1 mg/mL of HB in 0.9% NaCl and sterilizing by vacuum filtration in pre-rinsed Nalgene filter (0.45 μm pore size).

3 Methods

3.1 Primer Design Guidelines

Each mutagenic oligonucleotide primer must be designed individually per the desired mutation. In the design, the following considerations should be made:

1. The desired mutation must be present in both mutagenic primers and the primers should anneal to the same sequence on opposite strands of the plasmid.
2. Primers should be between 25 and 45 bases in length and the melting temperature (*Tm*) should exceed 78 °C.
3. The desired mutation should be in the middle of the primer with approximately 10–15 bases either side.
4. The primers should terminate in one or more C or G bases and should have a minimum GC content of 40%.
5. Primers must be purified either by FPLC or by PAGE. Mutation efficiency is decreased if primers are not purified.

3.2 Mutant Strand Synthesis Reaction

1. Complimentary primers containing the desired deletion of PML nuclear localization sequence (ΔNLS) and PML nuclear export sequence (ΔNES) are designed, synthesized, and purified:

   ΔNLS-sense
   5′-GCCCCAGGAAGGTCGGGAAGGAGGCAAG-3′

ΔNLS-antisense
5′-CTTGCCTCCTTCCCGACCTTCCTGGGGC-3′
ΔNES-sense
5′-ACATTAACAGGCTGTGGGAAGTGCCCGGGGC-3′
ΔNES-antisense
5′-GCCCCGGGCACTTCCCACAGCCTGTTAATGT-3′

2. ΔNLS and ΔNES reactions are set up on ice as outlined below in thin-walled PCR tubes:

   5 μL 10× reaction buffer, 50 ng pLKO/PMLI plasmid, 125 ng sense primer, 125 ng antisense primer, 1 μL dNTP mix, ddH_2O to a final volume of 50 μL. Mix the contents of the tube by gentle pipetting. Then add 1 μL *Pfu* Turbo DNA polymerase (2.5 U/μL).

3. Thermocycling parameters:
   Ensure that the heated lid is on the thermocycler. If no heated lid is available, then the reaction should be overlaid with mineral oil. The reaction is then cycled using the following PCR parameters: Hot start activation of the *Pfu* Turbo DNA polymerase at 95 °C, 30 s for 1 cycle, denaturation of the template at 95 °C, 30 s; annealing of the specific primers at 55 °C, 1 min; the denaturation, annealing and extension steps are repeated for 18 cycles. This is followed by a final extension step at 68 °C for 12 min. Place the reaction on ice for 2 min immediately following thermocycling to cool the reaction to less than 37 °C.

3.3 DPN I *Digestion of the Amplification Products*

1. 1 μL of *Dpn* I (10 U/μL) is added to each PCR reaction.
2. Each reaction mixture should be thoroughly and carefully mixed by gently pipetting the tube contents. The tubes are then spun down in a microcentrifuge for 1 min.
3. Immediately place the reaction tubes into a pre-warmed water bath at 37 °C and incubate the reactions for 1 h to digest the non-mutated pLKO/PMLI plasmid DNA.

3.4 Transformation of XL1-Blue Supercompetent Cells (XL1-B)

1. A vial of XL1-B cells should be gently thawed on ice. Fifty microliter of cells should be added to a prechilled round-bottom tube for each mutagenesis reaction to be transformed.
2. Carefully transfer 1 μL of the *Dpn* I-treated pLKO/PML1 plasmid reaction to separate aliquots of the XL1-B cells. DO NOT pipette up and down to mix. Gentle mix the transformation reactions by swirling and incubate the reactions on ice for 30 min.
3. The transformation reactions are then heat shocked at 42 °C for 45 s before being placed on ice for a further 2 min.
4. Five hundred microliter of preheated (42 °C) NZY+ broth is added to each of the transformation reactions and they are placed at 42 °C for 1 h with shaking at 225–250 rpm.

5. Each transformation reaction is plated in duplicate (250 μL/plate) onto pre-warmed agar plates containing 50 μg/mL ampicillin.
6. The transformation plates are incubated ay 37 °C for >16 h.
7. After incubation, the colony numbers are observed and up to ten selected clones are sequenced to verify that the selected clones contained the desired deletion.

3.5 Cell Transfection

Day 1—Late in the afternoon (*see* **Note 10**) [9]

1. For each sample premix in a polypropylene 1.5 mL tube 20 μL Lipofectamine 3000 and 500 μL Optimem medium (SOL. A). Incubate for 30 min.
2. For each sample premix in a polypropylene 1.5 mL tube 8 μg of target plasmid, 6 μg of viral packaging plasmid and 2 μg of viral envelope plasmid (SOL. B).
3. Mix SOL. A and SOL. B and add to each of T25 HEK 293T flasks.
4. Incubate HEK 293T cells at 37 °C, 5% CO_2, overnight.

Day 2—Early in the morning

1. Change media to HEK293T flasks with 5 mL/flask of normal dedicated medium.

Day 3

1. Collect spent medium from each HEK 293T flask to a fresh 15 mL tube, pour fresh dedicated medium in the flasks, and incubate them at 37 °C, 5% CO_2 until the following day.
2. Filter the collected medium through a 45 nm syringe filter (*see* **Note 11**).
3. Aliquot 1 mL of the filtered medium to 4 cryovials, label them as Fraction 1 (F1) and store at −20 °C.

Day 4

1. Collect spent medium from each HEK293T flask to a fresh 15 mL tube (*see* **Note 12**).
2. Filter the collected medium through a 45 nm syringe filter.
3. Aliquot 1 mL of the filtered medium to 4 cryovials, label them as Fraction 2 (F2) and store at −20 °C.

3.6 Target Cell Line Killing Curve

Day 1

1. Apply increasing amounts of puromycin to the DU145 and PC3 plates, maintaining one well without puromycin as a control (*see* **Note 13**).

Day 2

1. Check the viability of cells every day, searching for visual evidence of toxicity. Replace the medium containing the antibiotic every 2–3 days for up to a week (*see* **Note 14**).

3.7 Target Cell Line Infection (Transduction)

Day 1

1. Prepare the HB mix with 1 mL/well of EMEM and 8 μL/mL (final concentration 16 μL/well) of Hexadimethrine bromide (HB) solution.
2. Combine 1 mL of the HB mix and 1 mL of one of HEK-derived supernatants (Fraction 1) and add to one of each well of target cell lines 6-well plate and incubate overnight for about 24 h at 37 °C.

Day 2

1. Change media to target cell lines 6-well plate using normal dedicated medium.

Day 3

When cells reach about 80% confluence apply the optimum concentration of puromycin and keep them selected by regularly changing media plus puromycin.

3.8 Immuno-fluorescence

Day 1

1. Wash cells twice with PBS 1×.
2. Fix Cells in 4% paraformaldehyde for 30 min.
3. Wash cells three times with PBS 1×.
4. Add blocking buffer (10% Bovine Serum Albumin (BSA) in PBS 1×–0.1% Tween 20) and incubate at room temperature for 1 h.
5. Remove blocking solution and add primary antibodies (HA, E-Cadherin, and Vimentin) to fresh blocking solution and incubate on night at 4 °C [7].

Day 2

1. Remove the solution and wash three times 10 min with PBS 1×.
2. Incubate cells for 1 h in blocking solution containing fluorescent secondary antibodies [7].
3. Remove the solution and wash three times 10 min with PBS 1×.
4. Use a fluorescent microscope for imaging.

4 Notes

1. Use of high-quality DMSO should avoid the presence of oxidation products of DMSO, like dimethyl sulfone and dimethyl sulfide, that are inhibitors of transformation [10].
2. Chill to 0 °C before use.
3. It is possible to prepare LB agar directly in an autoclavable glass bottle, dissolving the weighed reagents in a small volume of water using a magnetic stir bar on a magnetic agitator. After the dissolution of the reagents take the solution to the final volume by adding water.
4. Since ampicillin degrades at temperatures higher than 55 °C, while agar starts solidifying from 50 °C it is recommended to put the medium cooling in a 55 °C bath before adding ampicillin to be sure that it will not degrade and that LB agar will not solidify until we are ready to pour the plates.
5. If the plates are for long-term storage 30 mL of LB-agar is a suitable amount, while if the plates are for quick use the volume of LB-agar can be decreased to 10–20 mL per plate.
6. Cells should not be too confluent so that they could survive for 3 days after transfection.
7. Seed cells in order to have the plate at a confluence of about 80% on the day of treatment with puromycin.
8. Puromycin is an antibiotic produced by *Streptomyces alboniger*. It works by inhibiting peptidyl transfer on prokaryotic and eukaryotic ribosomes.
9. Seed cells in order to have each well of the plate at 50–60% of confluence on the day of transduction.
10. It is more advisable to perform transfection late in the afternoon since cells should not remain in contact with transfection reagents for too long.
11. A membrane with 45 nm pore diameter blocks the passage of all cells and debris but allows the passage of viral particles through it.
12. From this point on, HEK 293T flasks will not be used anymore so they can be eliminated following the waste disposal procedures.
13. Test Puromycin for concentrations from 0 up to 1.5–2.0 μg/mL.
14. Ensure in this way that cells grow in a constant concentration of puromycin. The aim of the assay is to identify the optimum concentration, which is the lowest concentration of puromycin at which all cells are dead after 1 week of selection.

Acknowledgment

This work was supported by the John and Lucille van Geest Foundation, and the John van Geest Cancer Research Centre, Nottingham Trent University.

References

1. Lamouille S, Xu J, Derynck R (2014) Molecular mechanisms of epithelial–mesenchymal transition. Nat Rev Mol Cell Biol 15:178–196
2. de Thé H, Chomienne C, Lanotte M, Degos L, Dejean A (1990) The t (15; 17) translocation of acute promyelocytic leukaemia fuses the retinoic acid receptor α gene to a novel transcribed locus. Nature 347:558–561
3. Borrow J, Goddard AD, Sheer D, Solomon E (1990) Molecular analysis of acute promyelocytic leukemia breakpoint cluster region on chromosome 17. Science 249:1577–1580
4. Kakizuka A, Miller WH Jr, Umesono K, Warrell RP Jr, Frankel SR, Murty VV, Dmitrovsky E, Evans RM (1991) Chromosomal translocation t (15; 17) in human acute promyelocytic leukemia fuses RARα with a novel putative transcription factor, PML. Cell 66:663–674
5. Lallemand-Breitenbach V (2010) PML nuclear bodies. Cold Spring Harb Perspect Biol 2: a000661
6. Nisole S, Maroui MA, Mascle XH, Aubry M, Chelbi-Alix MK (2013) Differential roles of PML isoforms. Front Oncol 3:125
7. Buczek ME, Miles AK, Green W, Johnson C, Boocock DJ, Pockley AG, Rees RC, van Schalkwyk G, Parkinson R, Hulman J, Powe DG, Regad T (2015) Cytoplasmic PML promotes TGF-β-associated epithelial–mesenchymal transition and invasion in prostate cancer. Oncogene 35:3465–3475
8. Inoue H, Nojima H, Okayama H (1990) High efficiency transformation of *Escherichia coli with plasmids.* Gene 96:23–28
9. Merten OW, Hebben M, Bovolenta C (2016) Production of lentiviral vectors. Mol Ther Methods Clin Dev 3:16017. doi:10.1038/mtm.2016.17
10. Hanahan D (1985) Techniques for transformation of *E. coli.* In: Glover DM (ed) DNA cloning: a practical approach, vol vol. 1. IRL Press, Oxford, United Kingdom, pp 109–135

Chapter 13

Identification and Isolation of Cancer Stem Cells Using *NANOG-EGFP* Reporter System

Magdalena E. Buczek, Stephen P. Reeder, and Tarik Regad

Abstract

Cancer stem Cells or Cancer Stem-like Cells are thought to be associated with chemoresistance and recurrence in cancer patients following chemotherapy. Developing a method to study these malignant populations is the key to successful development of drug or immunotherapeutic assays. Here, we present a method of identification, isolation of Prostate Cancer Stem Cells (PCSCs) from the DU145 prostate cancer cell line using the *NANOG-GFP* expression system.

Key words Cancer stem cells (CSCs), Prostate cancer (PCa), NANOG, GFP reporter gene, Lentiviral expression system, Fluorescence-activated cell sorting, Sphere formation

1 Introduction

In the last decade, cancer stem cells (CSCs) have become a major topic in cancer research due to the role they play in cancer initiation, progression, and chemoresistance. Growing evidence suggests that a small population of CSCs residing within cancer tissues possess stem cells characteristics, which enable them to generate the bulk of tumors. These characteristics are associated with self-renewal and the capacity to generate differentiated progenies. Although advances have been made to develop methods capable of identifying and isolating CSCs, concerns remain about the specificity and accuracy of the used approaches for identification [1–6].

We have developed a new approach for identifying and isolating CSCs from prostate cancer cell lines. We used a lentiviral construct carrying the promoter of the stem cell marker *NANOG* to drive the expression of the reporter gene GFP (*NANOG-EGFP*) [7]. Nanog, together with other stem cell factors, is expressed during embryonic development where it plays an essential role in the maintenance of pluripotency and self-renewal of embryonic stem cells. This factor is re-expressed in cancer stem cells and contributes to cancer progression of several types of cancers [8–12]. In this study,

Gianpaolo Papaccio and Vincenzo Desiderio (eds.), *Cancer Stem Cells: Methods and Protocols*, Methods in Molecular Biology, vol. 1692, DOI 10.1007/978-1-4939-7401-6_13, © Springer Science+Business Media LLC 2018

lentiviruses that carry *NANOG-EFGP* were used to infect DU145 prostate cancer cells (Fig. 1a). GFP+ and GFP− cells were isolated using a class II MSC MoFlo cell sorter (Fig. 1b). To characterize their stem cell properties, sphere formation and differentiation assays were performed to investigate their capacity to self-renew and to generate differentiated progenies (Figs. 1c and 2). Thus, using this method, it is possible to isolate cancer stem cells or cancer stem-like cells from cell lines that could be used for further in vitro and in vivo investigations.

2 Materials

2.1 Lentiviral Plasmid Isolation

1. *Plasmids* (purchased from Addgene): *PL-SIN-Nanog-EGFP* (Cat no. 21321); *pMD2.G* (Cat no. 12259); *psPAX2* (Cat no. 12259).
2. QIAfilter Plasmid Midi Kit (25) (Qiagen, Cat no. 12243).
3. LB agar plates supplemented with Ampicillin (LB agar amp): 1% NaCl (Merk millipore, Cat no. 7760-5KG), 1% Tryptone (Oxoid, Cat no. LP0042), 0.5% Yeast Extract (Oxoid, Cat no. LP0021), 1.5% Agar Bacteriological (Oxoid, Cat no. LP0011), 100 μg/mL Ampicillin (Sigma, Cat no. A9518-5G).
4. LB (Luria-Betani) liquid medium supplemented with Ampicillin (Liquid LB amp) 1% NaCl, 1% Tryptone, 0.5% Yeast Extract, 100 μg/mL Ampicillin (Sigma, Cat no. A9518-5G).
5. Glycerol (Sigma, Cat no. G5516-1L).
6. TE buffer: 10 mM Tris, 1 mM EDTA (adjust pH up to 8.0 with HCl).
7. Kimwipes (Kimberly Clark Professional, Cat no. 3020).
8. 70% ethanol.
9. 50 mL centrifuge tubes (Sarstedt, Cat no. 62.547.254).
10. Sterile pipette tips.
11. Cryogenic vials (Star lab, Cat no. E30090-6212).
12. Shaking incubator at 37 °C.
13. Nanodrop 2000 Spectrophotometer (Thermo Fisher Scientific).

2.2 Plasmid Quantification

1. *TE buffer*: 10 mM Tris, 1 mM EDTA (adjust pH up to 8.0 with HCl).
2. Kimwipes (Kimberly Clark Professional, Cat no. 3020).
3. Nanodrop 2000 Spectrophotometer (Thermo Fisher Scientific).

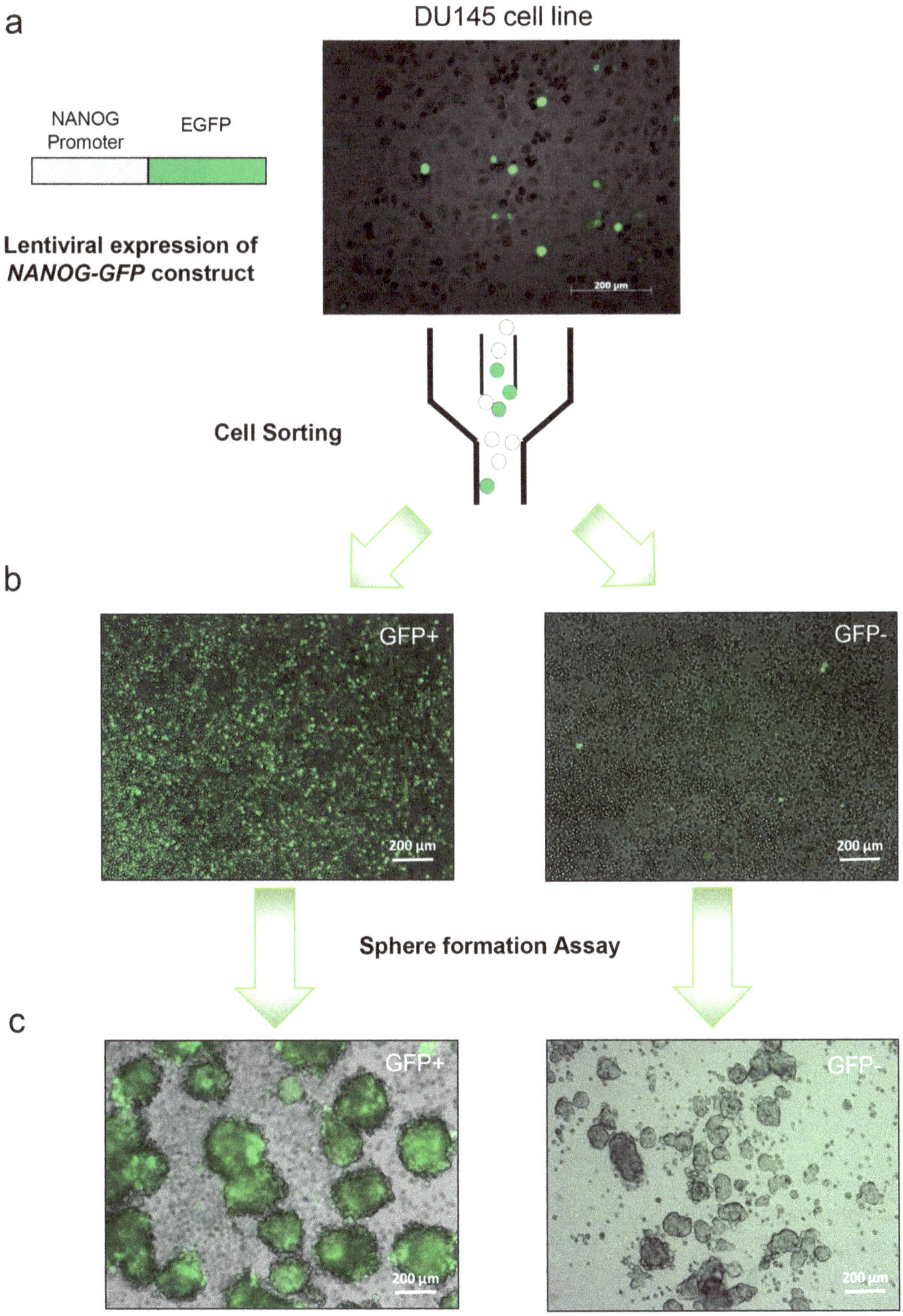

Fig. 1 Isolation and identification of PCSCs from the DU145 prostate cancer cell line. (**a**) Expression of *NANOG-GFP* construct in DU145 prostate cancer cell line. (**b**) Isolation of GFP *positive* and *negative* cells using MoFlow cell sorter. The percentage of GFP+ cells corresponds to 0.5–1% of total cells. (**c**) These cells are capable of cell renewal (sphere formation assay). GFP *positive* cells generate larger size spheres compared to GFP *negative* cells

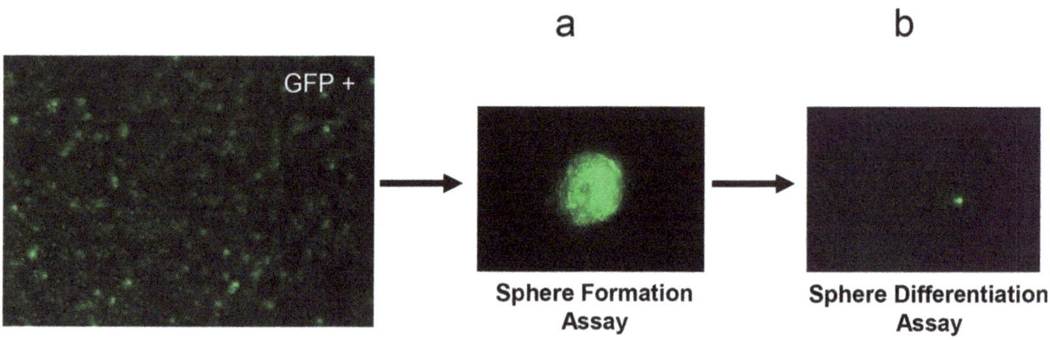

Fig. 2 Testing "stemness" properties of isolated GFP positive cells. (**a**) GFP *positive* spheres were cultured in DU145 media with serum. After 5 days in culture GFP *positive* spheres generated (b) GFP *positive* and GFP *negative* cells. Self-renewal (symmetric division) and the generation of differentiated progenies (asymmetric division) are characteristics of stem cells and cancer stem cells

2.3 HEK293T Transfection with Lentiviral Vectors

1. HEK293 T cell line (early passage).
2. HEK293T media: DMEM 4.5 g/L Glucose w/L-Gln, 500 mL (Lonza, Cat no BE12-604F), 10% FCS (HyClone, Cat no. SV30160.03), 1% L-glutamine (Lonza, Cat no. BE17-605E).
3. PBS-1X, w/o Ca^{++}, Mg^{++} 500 mL (Lonza, Cat no. BE17-516F).
4. Opti-MEM® I Reduced Serum Medium (ThermoFisher Scientific, Cat no. 31985047).
5. Lipofectamine 3000 Regent (ThermoFisher Scientific, Cat no. L3000015).
6. T25 flasks (Sarstedt, Cat no. 83.3910.002).
7. 50 mL centrifuge tubes (Sarstedt, Cat no. 62.547.254).
8. 5 mL plastic pipettes (Sarstedt, Cat no. 86.1253).
9. 1.5 mL polypropylene tubes (Sarstedt, Cat no. 72.690.001).
10. 10 mL Syringes (Medicina, Cat no. IVS10).
11. 0.45 μm syringe filters (Sartorius, Cat no. 16555).
12. Cryogenic vials (Star lab, Cat no. E30090-6212).

2.4 DU145 Infection with NANOG-GFP Lentiviral Vector

1. Fractions 1 and 2 of HEK293T-derived viral supernatant (*collected in the previous experiment*).
2. DU145 media: MEM Eagle-EBSS w/NEAA w/o L-Gln 500 mL (Lonza, Cat no. BE12-662F), 10% FCS (HyClone, Cat no. SV30160.03), 1% L-glutamine (Lonza, Cat no. BE17-605E).
3. Polybrene solution: Prepare 1 mg/mL Hexadimethrine bromide (Sigma, Cat no. H9268) in 0.9% NaCl solution and filter-

sterilize though 0.22 μm syringe filter (Sartorius, Cat no. 16534).

4. 6-well tissue culture plate (Sarstedt, Cat no. 83.3920).
5. 5 mL plastic pipettes (Sarstedt, Cat no. 86.1253).
6. Viral work-dedicated tissue culture cabinet and incubator adjusted to 37 °C, 5% CO_2.

2.5 Sorting DU145 NANOG+ (GFP+) and NANOG− (GFP−) Cells

1. DU145 *NANOG-GFP* cell line.
2. PBS (Lonza, Cat no. BE17-512F).
3. Trypsin 10× (Lonza, Cat no. BE02-00007E) diluted 1:10 with PBS, pre-warmed at 37 °C.
4. DU145 media (*see* above).
5. Trypan blue (Sigma, Cat no. T8154) diluted 1:3 with PBS.
6. Sorting media: 50 mL EMEM 2× (Lonza, Cat no. BEF17-512F) + 1% L-glutamine (Lonza, Cat no. BE17-605E) + 3 mM EDTA (Ambion, Cat no. AM9260G) + 25 mM HEPES (Lonza, Cat no. BE17-737M) + 0.05% Benzonase (Milipore, Cat no. 71205-25KUN) + 2% Penicillin/Streptomycin (Lonza, DE17-603E)—Filter-sterilized through a 0.22 μm pore filter.
7. Sphere media: Knock-out DMEM (Gibco, Cat no. 12660-012) + 10 mM $NaHCO_3$ (Thermo Fisher Scientific, Cat no. S/424053) + 20 mM D-(+)-Glucose (45%) (Sigma, Cat no. G8769) + 2% Stem Pro (Gibco, Cat no. A105008-01) + 20 ng/mL bFGF (Gibco, PHG0024) + EGF (Gibco, Cat no. PHG0314) + 1% L-glutamine (Lonza, Cat no. BE17-605E) + 2% Penicillin/Streptomycin (Lonza, DE17-603E)—Filter-sterilized through 0.22 μm pore filter.
8. Class II MSC MoFlo cell sorter (Beckman Coulter, Serial no. 2253).
9. 24-well plate (Sarstedt, Cat no. 83.3922).
10. Incubator at 37 °C, 5% CO_2.

3 Methods

3.1 Lentiviral Plasmid Isolation

Day 1

Perform following steps for each plasmid stab culture:

1. Using a sterile pipette tip touch the bacteria growing within the punctured area of the stab culture.
2. Gently spread the bacteria over a section of the LB agar plate supplemented with Ampicillin (LB agar + Amp) to create streak #1.

3. Using a fresh sterile pipette tip, drag through streak #1 and spread the bacteria over a second section of the same LB agar + Amp plate, to create streak #2.
4. Using a third sterile pipette tip, drag through streak #2 and spread the bacteria over the last section of the plate, to create streak #3.
5. Incubate the plate with newly plated bacteria overnight (12–18 h) at 37 °C (*see* **Note 1**).

Day 2

6. Using a sterile pipette tip touch the single bacterial colony growing on LB agar + amp plate and drop a tip into conical flask with 50 mL liquid LB amp.
7. Incubate bacterial culture overnight (12–18 h) at 37 °C in a shaking incubator (*see* **Note 2**).

Day 3

8. Following day collect bacterial culture into a 50 mL centrifuge tube.
9. Centrifuge at 1000 × *g* for 40 min at 4 °C.
10. Remove the supernatant.
11. Recover plasmid DNA from bacterial pellet using QIAfilter Plasmid Midi Kit (25) for plasmid isolation kit (*Follow manufacturer protocol*).
12. Resuspend the pellet in 20 μL TE buffer.
13. Determine DNA yield using Nanodrop Spectrometer and a suitable software (e.g., ND-8000 2.3.2.).

3.2 Plasmid Quantification

Perform these steps using Nanodrop 2000 equipment:

1. Clean the upper and lower optical surfaces (pedestals) of spectrophotometer with a Kimwipe soaked with 70% ethanol.
2. Pipet 1–2 μL of clean deionized water onto the lower optical surface. Close the lever arm gently. In DN-8000 programme select active pedestals and Press "Calibrate".
3. Wipe the pedestals with Kimwipe and pipet 1 μL of TE buffer onto the lower optical surface. Close the lever arm gently. In DN-8000 programme select active pedestals and Press "Blank".
4. Load 1 μL of each DNA sample onto lower optical surface. Close the lever arm gently. In DN-8000 programme select active pedestals and press "Measure".
5. Record the reading of DNA concentration and a purity (260/280 ratio and 260/230 ratio) (*see* **Notes 3** and **4**).
6. Store purified plasmid DNA at −80 °C.

3.3 HEK293T Transfection with Lentiviral Vectors

Day 1

1. Seed approximately 900,000 HEK293T cells into 1× T25 flask (with 4 mL of "HEK293T media"). Culture overnight at 37 °C, 5% CO_2 (*see* **Note 5**).

Day 2

2. For each transfection premix 20 μL Lipofectamine + 500 μL OPTIMEM media. Incubate for 30 min at RT (*see* **Note 6**).
3. For transfection premix 8 μg target plasmid *PL-SIN-Nanog-EGFP*) with 6 μg of packaging plasmid (*psPAX2*) + 2 μg envelope plasmid (*pMD2.G*).

NANOG transfection mix	20 μL Lipofectamine + 500 μL OPTIMEM	8 μg *PL-SIN-Nanog-EGFP* + 6 μg packaging plasmid + 2 μg envelope plasmid + 500 μL OPTIMEM

4. Combine the content of each of 4 L+O tubes with each of 4 PL+pack +env tubes (1 mL in total) and add to each of 4 T25 HEK 293 flasks.
5. Incubate transfected HEK293T at 37 °C overnight (in a viral cell culture-dedicated incubator to avoid cross contamination with other cell lines).

Day 2

6. Change media HEK293 media (5 mL per T25 flask). Incubate HEK293T at 37 °C overnight.

Day 3

7. Collect all the supernatants from each transfected HEK293T cell flask into fresh tube.
8. Filter through a 0.45 μm syringe filter into a fresh tube.
9. Aliquot 1 mL into cryogenic tubes (4 in total).
10. Label as Fraction 1 (F1) and store at −20 °C.

Day 4

11. Repeat steps for Day 3 and label supernatant aliquots as Fraction 2 (F2).

3.4 DU145 Infection with NANOG-GFP Lentiviral Vector

Day 1

1. Seed approximately 150,000 DU145 cells into each of 2× 6-well plates (with 3 mL of "DU145 media"). Culture overnight at 37 °C. They should reach approximately 60–70% of confluence for the following day (*see* **Note 7**).

Day 2

2. Prepare 10 mL DU145 media with 160 μL of 1 mg/mL Polybrene solution (final conc. 16 μg/mL).
3. Combine 1 mL DU145 media + Polybrene and 1 mL of one of HEK293-derived viral supernatants and add to one of each well of 6-well plate with DU145 cells (total of 2 mL/well). Incubate overnight at 37 °C in a viral-dedicated incubator (*see* **Note 8**).

Day 3

4. Change media for 4 mL of DU145 media.

3.5 Sorting of NANOG+ (GFP+) and NANOG− (GFP−) Cells

Day 1

1. Prepare 3 × 175 of DU145 NANOG-GFP cells (infected cell line) for sorting and DU145 cells (not infected) (*see* **Notes 9** and **10**).
2. Wash cells twice with 1× PBS.
3. Add pre-warmed Trypsin (5 mL/T175) and incubate for 10–20 min (until cells detach) at 37 °C, at 5% v/v CO2.
4. Stop trypsinization with adding an equal volume of DU145 medium (*see* above).
5. Centrifuge at 259 × *g* for 5 min.
6. Decant the supernatant and resuspend cells in Sorting medium.
7. Use the 40 μm cell strainer cap filter to obtain single-cell suspension.
8. Resuspend approximately 1 × 10^5 DU145 and 1 × 10^7 DU145 NANOG-GFP cells per 1 mL of Sorting media. Mix well.
9. Prepare a 24-well plate with 1 mL of Sphere medium.
10. Sort GFP+ and GFP− cells into a prepared 24-well plate from above, 10.000 cells/well. Perform sort on Beckman Coulter MoFlo cell sorter (see Materials) on Purify mode, Sort setup: 100 μm nozzle, sheath pressure 30 psi.
11. Assess whether sorted cells are evenly distributed across the well. Make sure cells are not clumping at this stage. Incubate cells under standard conditions in Spheres medium at 37 °C and 5% CO_2. Supplement every 2 days with bFGF (20 ng/mL) and EGF (20 ng/mL).

After 7 days

- Count numbers of emerging tumor spheres using a standard microscope with 4× or 10× magnification and a fluorescence microscope to detect fluorescence signal from the integrated reporter system.

- Count spheres with a diameter exceeding 100 μm as "large" spheres, and spheres with a diameter 50–100 μm as "small" spheres. Be sure that you count real spheres and not cell clusters.

4 Notes

1. In the morning, single colonies should be visible. A single colony should look like a white dot growing on the solid medium. This dot is composed of millions of genetically identical bacteria that arose from a single bacterium. If the bacterial growth is too dense and you do not see single colonies, re-streak onto a new agar plate to obtain single colonies.
2. It is recommended to use a 250 mL conical flask for 50 mL liquid LB media to allow a high rate of liquid movement during shaking incubation.
3. 260/280 ratio of sample absorbance at 260 nm and 280 nm. A ratio of approximately 1.8 is generally accepted as "pure" for DNA. 260/230 ratio of sample absorbance at 260 nm and 230 nm, a secondary measure of nucleic acid purity. The 260/230 values for "pure" nucleic acid are often higher than the respective 260/280 values. They are commonly in the range of 1.8–2.2.
4. Wiping the pedestals between measurements is usually sufficient to prevent sample carryover and avoid residue buildup. When loading anything on pedestals avoid bubbles. For more accurate reading it is recommended to load 2 μL volume per sample. Wipe thoroughly with Kimwipe and blank between each set of samples. For troubleshooting refer to *NanoDrop 8000 Spectrophotometer V2.0 User's Manual available on Thermo Scientific website.*
5. Seeding density may vary depending on the cell passage number (cells in earlier passage tend to grow slower than those of later passage). Perform the transfection in the late afternoon because the transfection mix should only be incubated with the cells for 12–15 h.
6. Make sure cells are approximately 80–90% confluent, as with lower confluency rate there might be a high rate of cell death.
7. Perform all the infection steps in a viral-dedicated cell culture cabinet.
8. The final concentration of Polybrene should be 8 μg/mL after it gets diluted with the viral supernatant.
9. GFP expression can be monitored by a fluorescent microscopy observation.

10. The number of cells needed for sorting depends on the proportion of GFP+ and GFP− cells and needs to be determined beforehand (based on the observation under the fluorescent microscope or flow cytometry). DU145 (not infected) would be used as a negative control for GFP fluorescence.

Acknowledgment

This work was supported by the John and Lucille van Geest Foundation, and the John van Geest Cancer Research Centre, Nottingham Trent University.

References

1. Visvader JE, Lindeman GJ (2008) Cancer stem cells in solid tumours: accumulating evidence and unresolved questions. Nat Rev Cancer 8 (10):755–768
2. Patrawala L, Calhoun T, Schneider-Broussard R, Li H, Bhatia B, Tang S, Reilly JG, Chandra D, Zhou J, Claypool K, Coghlan L, Tang DG (2006) Highly purified CD44+ prostate cancer cells from xenograft human tumors are enriched in tumorigenic and metastatic progenitor cells. Oncogene 25(12):1696–1708
3. Collins AT, Habib FK, Maitland NJ, Neal DE (2001) Identification and isolation of human prostate epithelial stem cells based on alpha (2) beta (1)-integrin expression. J Cell Sci 114 (21):3865–3872
4. Wei C, Guomin W, Yujun L, Ruizhe Q (2007) Cancer stem-like cells in human prostate carcinoma cells DU145: the seeds of the cell line? Cancer Biol Ther 6(5):763–768
5. Rybak AP, He L, Kapoor A, Cutz JC, Tang D (2011) Characterization of sphere-propagating cells with stem-like properties from DU145 prostate cancer cells. Biochim Biophys Acta 13(5):683–694
6. Regad T (2017) Tissue-specific cancer stem cells: reality or a mirage? Transl Med Rep 1 (1):6535
7. Hotta A, Cheung AY, Farra N, Vijayaragavan K, Séguin CA, Draper JS, Pasceri P, Maksakova IA, Mager DL, Rossant J, Bhatia M (2009) Isolation of human iPS cells using EOS lentiviral vectors to select for pluripotency. Nat Methods 6(5):370–376
8. Zhang K, Zhou S, Wang L, Wang J, Zou Q, Zhao W, Fu Q, Fang X (2016) Current stem cell biomarkers and their functional mechanisms in prostate cancer. Int J Mol Sci 17(7): E1163
9. Zbinden M, Duquet A, Lorente-Trigos A, Ngwabyt SN, Borges I, Ruiz I, Altaba A (2010) NANOG regulates glioma stem cells and is essential in vivo acting in a cross-functional network with GLI1 and p53. EMBO J 29:2659–2674
10. Golestaneh AF, Atashi A, Langroudi L, Shafiee A, Ghaemi N, Soleimani M (2012) miRNAs expressed differently in cancer stem cells and cancer cells of human gastric cancer cell line MKN-45. Cell Biochem Funct 30:411–418
11. Liu J, Ma L, Xu J, Liu C, Zhang J, Chen R, Zhou Y (2013) Spheroid body-forming cells in the human gastric cancer cell line MKN-45 possess cancer stem cell properties. Int J Oncol 42:453–459
12. Zhang J, Espinoza LA, Kinders RJ, Lawrence SM, Pfister TD, Zhou M, Veenstra TD, Thorgeirsson SS, Jessup JM (2013) NANOG modulates stemness in human colorectal cancer. Oncogene 32:4397–4405

Chapter 14

Determination of miRNAs from Cancer Stem Cells Using a Low Density Array Platform

Hiromichi Kawasaki, Angela Lombardi, and Michele Caraglia

Abstract

A microarray approach has been extensively used for global gene expression profiles in many biological research fields such as understanding of pathological mechanism in malignancies and defining of molecular biomarkers to monitor disease status. The most attractive advantage of microarray technology is its application to simultaneous analysis of miRNA expression pattern with a large amount of assessments. In this chapter, we provide a facile and universal protocol for divergent miRNA expression profiles in prostate cancer stem cells with a low density array-based microarray analysis.

Key words Microarray, MicroRNA, Total RNA extraction, Reverse transcription, Pre-amplification

1 Introduction

MicroRNAs (miRNAs) are a category of short, endogenous non-coding RNAs that have a crucial role in the control of gene expression through promoting mRNA destabilization or inhibiting translation machinery. Recently, over 2000 miRNA sequences have been identified in human genome. In silico prediction tool has estimated that more than 30% of the genome is controlled by miRNAs [1, 2]. Each miRNA targets several mRNAs, through the hybridization with the perfect or nearly perfect complementary site in the 3′-untranslated regions (3′-UTR) of mRNA [3, 4]. To date, it is widely known that miRNAs are closely associated with cell proliferation, differentiation, apoptosis, and metastasis of malignancies [2, 5, 6]. A number of studies have demonstrated that miRNAs are aberrantly expressed in various tumors, including prostate cancer [7, 8]. Therefore, miRNAs are highlighted as intriguing tools for understanding biological mechanism in tumors and developing predictive biomarkers for disease occurrence and progression.

Several methods, including quantitative real-time PCR, low density array, and next-generation sequencing, are currently available to determine a profile of gene expression levels in both

Gianpaolo Papaccio and Vincenzo Desiderio (eds.), *Cancer Stem Cells: Methods and Protocols*, Methods in Molecular Biology, vol. 1692, DOI 10.1007/978-1-4939-7401-6_14,

physiological and pathological specimens [9–11]. Although relatively large amount of initial samples are required to perform an assay, the microarray-based technique is a very useful and powerful tool for discovery as well as for exploring biological function of genes, owing to its effective and attractive utilities. One of the major advantages of microarray technology applied to miRNA expression profiles is that it is extremely suitable for a large-scale identification and can simultaneously determine the divergent miRNA expression pattern in a single experiment. Recently, several platforms have been developed and used for the profiling [12–14]. To elucidate molecular biology and general pathology in clinical samples such as tissue, blood, and saliva, comprehensive microarray screening is currently used for comparison studies of miRNA expression levels between cancerous and noncancerous specimens [15–18]. In addition, this high-throughput identification can also assess gene alternations between treated and untreated cells with therapeutic compounds or radiation [19, 20]. For the evaluation of miRNA expression in prostate cancer obtained from cancer stem cells, we applied TaqMan Array cards, which is based on a low density array platform and can identify mature miRNA expressions with high specificity and sensitivity [21, 22]. For example, a method using this array card for the evaluation of salivary miRNAs was reported [23]. Here, we describe a simple and widely available technique regarding total RNA isolation from cells and miRNA expression profile for defining pathological status in prostate tumor stem cells. RNA preparation was carried out with a conventional acid-phenol:chloroform extraction and an effective column-based purification step. Conversion of total RNA into cDNA was conducted by a reverses transcription procedure with a stem-loop primer system. A pre-amplification process was performed in order to obtain a sufficient amount of products for microarray analysis [24]. This promising approach can also be available for predictive and prognostic biomarker studies of cancers in many other types of cells and clinical samples.

2 Materials

2.1 Total RNA Extraction

Crushed ice, 2-mercaptoethanol, 100% ethanol (ACS grade or better), miRVana PARIS kit (Ambion), Heat block, Centrifugal separator, Nanodrop ND-1000 (Thermo Scientific), Nuclease-free 1.5 mL tube.

2.2 Reverse Transcription

Crushed ice, nuclease-free water, TaqMan® MicroRNA Reverse Transcription Kit (Applied Biosystems), Megaplex RT Primers Human Pool A v2,1 (Applied Biosystems), Thermal cycler, Microcentrifuge, Nuclease-free PCR tube.

2.3 Pre-amplification

Crushed ice, nuclease-free water, Megaplex TaqMan® PreAmp Primers Human Pool A v2.1 (Applied Biosystems), Megaplex TaqMan® PreAmp Master Mix (Applied Biosystems), Thermal cycler, Microcentrifuge, Nuclease-free PCR tube.

2.4 Low Density Array

Nuclease-free water, 0.1× TE buffer at pH 8.0, TaqMan® Array Human MicroRNA A Cards v2.0 (Applied Biosystems), TaqMan® Universal PCR Master Mix No AmpErase® UNG, (Applied Biosystems), ViiA 7 real-time PCR system (Applied Biosystems), Centrifugal separator with special card holder (Applied Biosystems), Nuclease-free 1.5 mL tube.

3 Methods

3.1 Total RNA Extraction from Cell Pellet

1. Prepare a prostate cancer cell pellet in a nuclease-free 1.5 mL tube and the reagents supplied with miRVana PARIS kit according to the manufacturer's manuals (*see* **Notes 1** and **2**).
2. Add 300 μL of ice-cold Cell Disruption buffer to the cell pellet and mix thoroughly, and then mix with 300 μL of 2× Denaturing Solution. Warm 2× Denaturing Solution at 37 °C if it appears a crystal before starting the experiment.
3. After incubation on ice for 5 min, add 600 μL of Acid-Phenol: Chloroform to the mixture and mix gently by pipetting (*see* **Note 3**).
4. Centrifuge at 10,000 × *g* for 5 min at room temperature to distinguish the mixture into aqueous (upper) and organic phases. If the interphase is not compact, repeat the centrifugation (*see* **Note 4**).
5. Transfer carefully the aqueous phase into a new fresh 1.5 mL tube without disturbing the interphase or the lowest phase.
6. Add 1.25 volumes of 100% ethanol into the collected solution and mix thoroughly.
7. Place a Filter Cartridge in a Collection Tube.
8. Put 700 μL of the mixture onto the Filter Cartridge (*see* **Note 5**).
9. Centrifuge at 10,000 × *g* for 20 s. Discard flow-through from the Collection Tube.
10. Repeat **steps 8** and **9** using the same filter, if the mixture remains.
11. Apply 700 μL of miRNA Wash Solution 1 to the filter and centrifuge at 10,000 × *g* for 15 s. Discard flow-through (*see* **Note 6**).
12. Apply 500 μL of Wash Solution 2/3 to the filter and centrifuge at 10,000 × *g* for 15 s. Discard flow-through (*see* **Notes 7** and **8**).

13. Repeat **step 12**.
14. Centrifuge the Filter Cartridge in the same Collection Tube at 10,000 × *g* for 1 min to get rid of any residual fluids from the filter.
15. Transfer the Filter Cartridge into a new Collection Tube.
16. Add 50 μL of Elution Solution preheated at 95 °C into the center of the filter, and then centrifuge at 10,000 × *g* for 30 s. This eluate contains total RNA (*see* **Note 9**).
17. Measure the quantity and quality of total RNA in the eluate using a NanoDrop instrument (*see* **Note 10**).
18. Proceed to the Megaplex reverse transcription experiment immediately or store the eluate at −80 °C until use.

3.2 Megaplex Reverse Transcription (RT)

1. Thaw the reagents on ice, mix gently, and then spin down briefly. Do not vortex RT reagents.
2. Prepare a mixture for revers transcription in a nuclease-free tube as shown in the below list.

Components	RT reaction volume (μL)
Nuclease-free water	0.20
RT buffer (10×)	0.80
$MgCl_2$ (25 mM)	0.90
dNTPs with dTTP (100 mM)	0.20
RNase inhibitor (20 U/μL)	0.10
Megaplex RT primers (10×)	0.80
MultiScribe reverse transcriptase (50 U/μL)	1.50
Total	4.50

3. After mixing, transfer 4.5 μL of the mixture for RT reaction into each PCR tube.
4. Add 3 μL of a solution including 200 ng of total RNA into each PCR tube containing RT reaction mixture, mix gently by pipetting, and then spin down briefly (*see* **Note 11**).
5. Incubate the mixture on ice for 5 min.
6. Set up the RT run method as follows: 2 min at 16 °C and 1 min at 42 °C and 1 s at 50 °C × 40 cycles, 5 min at 85 °C and then holding at 4 °C.
7. Start the RT run.
8. Proceed to the Megaplex pre-amplification experiment immediately or store the product at −20 °C until use for up to 1 week.

3.3 Megaplex Pre-amplification

1. Thaw the reagents on ice, mix gently, and then spin down briefly. Do not vortex all reagents.
2. Prepare a mixture for pre-amplification in a nuclease-free tube as shown in the below list.

Components	Pre-amplification reaction volume (μL)
Nuclease-free water	7.5
Megaplex PreAmp primers (10×)	2.5
TaqMan® PreAmp master mix (2×)	12.5
Total	22.5

3. After mixing, transfer 22.5 μL of the mixture for pre-amplification into each PCR tube.
4. Add 2.5 μL of the RT product into each PCR tube containing the mixture, mix gently by pipetting, and then spin down briefly.
5. Incubate the mixture on ice for 5 min.
6. Set up the run method as follows: 10 min at 95 °C, 2 min at 55 °C, 2 min at 72 °C, 15 s at 95 °C and 4 min at 60 °C × 12 cycles, 10 min at 99.9 °C, and then holding at 4 °C.
7. Start the pre-amplification run.
8. Dilute the pre-amplified product with 75 μL of 0.1× TE buffer at pH 8.0 (*see* **Note 12**).
9. Proceed to microarray assay immediately or store the pre-amplified product at −20 °C until use for up to 1 week.

3.4 Microarray Assay

1. Prepare a reaction solution in a nuclease-free 1.5 mL tube as shown in the below table

Components	Microarray reaction volume (μL)
Diluted pre-amplified product	9
Nuclease-free water	441
TaqMan® master mix, no UNG (2×)	450
Total	900

2. Dispense 100 μL of the reaction solution into each port in the MicroRNA Array Card.
3. Centrifuge at 1200 × *g* for 1 min for two times (*see* **Note 13**).

4. Set up the run method: as follows: 2 min at 50 °C, 10 min at 95 °C, 15 s at 95 °C and 1 min at 60 °C × 40 cycles.
5. Load the card into the instrument and run the microarray assay.

3.5 Calculation of Fold Change

1. Determine the most appropriate endogenous control in your samples for normalization.
2. Determine the reference sample, which is usually untreated or non-pathological sample.
3. Calculate the relative miRNA expression with the ΔΔCt method the following formula:

   $Ct_{Target}—Ct_{Target, endogenous} = \Delta Ct_{Target}$
   $Ct_{Reference}—Ct_{References,endogenous} = \Delta Ct_{Normal}$
   $\Delta Ct_{Target} - \Delta Ct_{Normal} = \Delta\Delta Ct$

   In this formula, Ct_{Target} and $Ct_{Target,endogenous}$ are the expression level of miRNA or endogenous control, respectively, in your target sample. $Ct_{Reference}$ and $Ct_{Reference,endogenous}$ are also the level of miRNA or endogenous control, respectively, in your reference sample.
4. Calculate the fold change with the equation $2^{-\Delta\Delta Ct}$ method in the following formula: Fold change $= 2^{-\Delta\Delta Ct}$.

4 Notes

If you need more detailed information on how to use the reagents, you can refer to the manufacturer's instructions.

1. Use 10^2–10^7 cells for extraction experiment. More than 10^6 cells are recommended.
2. Add 375 μL of 2-mercaptoethanol into the bottle of 2× Denaturing Solution before first use.
3. Do not use the upper layer of Acid-Phenol:Chloroform that is the aqueous buffer.
4. The interphase should be much compact than other phases or nothing.
5. Up to 700 μL can be applied to the Filter Cartridge at a time.
6. Add 21 mL of 100% ethanol into the bottle of miRNA Wash Solution 1 before first use.
7. Add 40 mL of 100% ethanol into the bottle of Wash Solution 2/3 before first use.
8. If a crystal is precipitated in Wash Solution 2/3 the bottle, do not use a crystal from the bottle when washing step.
9. Nuclease-free water can be applied to collect an eluate instead of Elution Solution.

10. Measure a 260/280 ratio of total RNA sample on a spectrophotometer. Purified total RNA is allowed a ratio of 1.8–2.2.
11. The total amount of RNA is acceptable from 1 to 350 ng.
12. Nuclease-free water can be applied to dilute a pre-amplified product instead of 0.1× TE buffer at pH 8.0.
13. Do not centrifuge the array card more than three times.

References

1. Pasquinelli AE, Reinhart BJ, Slack F, Martindale MQ, Kuroda MI, Maller B, Hayward DC, Ball EE, Degnan B, Müller P, Spring J, Srinivasan A, Fishman M, Finnerty J, Corbo J, Levine M, Leahy P, Davidson E, Ruvkun G (2000) Nature 408:86–89
2. Lewis BP, Burge CB, Bartel DP (2005) Conserved seed pairing, often flanked by adenosines, indicates that thousands of human genes are MicroRNA targets. Cell 120 (1):15–20
3. Zamore PD, Haley B (2005) Ribo-gnome: the big world of small RNAs. Science 309:1519–1524
4. Bartel DP (2004) MicroRNAs: genomics, biogenesis, mechanism, and function. Cell 116 (2):281–297
5. Ambros V (2004) The functions of animal microRNAs. Nature 431:350–355
6. Zhang Y, Yang P, Wang X-F (2014) Microenvironmental regulation of cancer metastasis by miRNAs. Trends Cell Biol 24(3):153–160
7. Kimura S, Naganuma S, Susuki D, Hirono Y, Yamaguchi A, Fujieda S, Sano K, Itoh H (2010) Expression of microRNAs in squamous cell carcinoma of human head and neck and the esophagus: miR-205 and miR-21 are specific markers for HNSCC and ESCC. Oncol Rep 23:1625–1633
8. Kojima S, Chiyomaru T, Kawakami K, Yoshino H, Enokida H, Nohata N, Fuse M, Ichikawa T, Naya Y, Nakagawa M, Seki N (2012) Tumour suppressors miR-1 and miR-133a target the oncogenic function of purine nucleoside phosphorylase (PNP) in prostate cancer. Br J Cancer 106:405–413
9. Toiyama Y, Takahashi M, Hur K, Nagasaka T, Tanaka K, Inoue Y, Masato K, Richard Boland C, Goel A (2013) Serum miR-21 as a diagnostic and prognostic biomarker in colorectal cancer. J Natl Cancer Inst 05(12):849–859
10. Git A, Dvinge H, Salmon-Divon M, Osborne M, Kutter C, Hadfield J, Bertone P, Caldas C (2010) Systematic comparison of microarray profiling, real-time PCR, and next-generation sequencing technologies for measuring differential microRNA expression. RNA 16:991–1006
11. Pritchard CC, Cheng HH, Tewari M (2012) MicroRNA profiling: approaches and considerations. Nat Rev Genet 13(5):358–369
12. Callari M, Dugo M, Musella V, Marchesi E, Chiorino G, Grand MM, Pierotti MA, Daidone MG, Canevari S, De Cecco L (2012) Comparison of microarray platforms for measuring differential MicroRNA expression in paired normal/cancer colon tissues. PLoS One 7(9):e45105
13. Ozen M, Creighton CJ, Ozdemir M, Ittmann M (2008) Widespread deregulation of microRNA expression in human prostate cancer. Oncogene 27:1788–1793. (or ref7)
14. Hsieh I-S, Chang K-C, Tsai Y-T, Ke J-Y, Lu P-J, Lee K-H, Yeh S-D, Hong T-M, Chen Y-L (2013) MicroRNA-320 suppresses the stem cell-like characteristics of prostate cancer cells by downregulating the Wnt/beta-catenin signaling pathway. Carcinogenesis 34 (3):530–538
15. Abrahamsson A, Dabrosin C (2015) Tissue specific expression of extracellular microRNA in human breast cancers and normal human breast tissue in vivo. Oncotarget 6 (26):22959–22969
16. Lerner C, Wemmert S, Bochen F, Kulas P, Linxweiler M, Hasenfus A, Heinzelmann J, Leidinger P, Backes C, Meese E, Urbschat S, Schick B (2016) Characterization of miR-146a and miR-155 in blood, tissue and cell lines of head and neck squamous cell carcinoma patients and their impact on cell proliferation and migration. J Cancer Res Clin Oncol 142:757–766
17. Momen-Heravi F, Trachtenberg AJ, Kuo WP, Cheng YS (2014) Genomewide study of salivary MicroRNAs for detection of oral cancer. J Dent Res 93(7):86S–93S
18. Iborra M, Bernuzzi F, Correale C, Vetrano S, Fiorino G, Beltrán B, Marabita F, Locati M, Spinelli A, Nos P, Invernizzi P, Danese S

(2013) Identification of serum and tissue micro-RNA expression profiles in different stages of inflammatory bowel disease. Clin Exp Immunol 173(2):250–258

19. Singh S, Chitkara D, Mehrazin R, Behrman SW, Wake RW, Mahato RI (2012) Chemoresistance in prostate cancer cells is regulated by miRNAs and hedgehog pathway. PLoS One 7 (6):e40021
20. Li B, Shi X-B, Nori D, Chao CKS, Chen AM, Valicenti R, de Vere White R (2011) Down-regulation of microRNA106b is involved in p21-mediated cell cycle arrest in response to radiation in prostate cancer cells. Prostate 71:567–574
21. Chen C, Ridzon DA, Broomer AJ, Zhou Z, Lee DH, Nguyen JT, Barbisin M, Xhu NL, Mahuvakar VR, Andersen MR, Lao KQ, Livak KJ, Guegler KJ (2005) Real-time quantification of microRNAs by stem-loop RT-PCR. Nucleic Acids Res 33:e179
22. Mestdagh P, Feys T, Bernard N, Guenther S, Chen C, Spelemann F, Vandesompele J (2008) High-throughput stem-loop RT-qPCR miRNA expression profiling using minute amounts of input RNA. Nucleic Acids Res 36: e143
23. Yoshizawa JM, Wong DTW (2013) Salivary microRNAs and oral cancer detection. Methods Mol Biol 936:313–324
24. Mengual L, Burset M, Marín-Aguilera M, Ribal MJ, Alcaraz A (2008) Multiplex preamplification of specific cDNA targets prior to gene expression analysis by TaqMan arrays. BMC Res Notes 1:21–28

Chapter 15

Assessing DNA Methylation in Cancer Stem Cells

Sudipto Das, Bruce Moran, and Antoinette S. Perry

Abstract

Many cancer-associated epigenetic signatures are also commonly observed in stem cells, just as epigenetic stem cell patterns are in cancer cells. DNA methylation is recognized as a hallmark of cancer development and progression. Herein, we describe two approaches to analyze DNA methylation, which can be applied to study or discover DNA methylation aberrations throughout the genome, as well as a more targeted investigation of regions of interest in cancer stem cells.

Key words DNA methylation, PCR, Methylomic, Regions of interest, Differentially methylated regions, Methyl capture, 5mC

1 Introduction

Epigenetic modifications are centrally involved in stem cell identity, and play an especially important role in pluripotent embryonic stem cells (ESCs) [1–3]. Epigenetic modifications include cytosine methylation in DNA, posttranslational modifications of histone tails, nucleosome remodeling, and the activity of noncoding RNAs, which act in a concerted manner to regulate gene expression without directly changing the genetic code. For example, the polycomb group (PcG) proteins act as key epigenetic regulators in ESCs, by impeding transcription of developmental genes through creating repressive histone marks [4]. In addition, alterations in DNA methylation patterns are known to play essential roles in reprogramming during induced pluripotent stem cells (iPSC) generation [5].

Alterations in DNA methylation patterns were first described in cancer cells more than 30 years ago [6]. Today, DNA promoter hypermethylation is recognized as a bone-fide mechanism of epigenetic gene inactivation in cancer, targeting tumor suppressor genes and genes with important regulatory functions. Cancer cells

Sudipto Das and Bruce Moran contributed equally to this work.

Gianpaolo Papaccio and Vincenzo Desiderio (eds.), *Cancer Stem Cells: Methods and Protocols*, Methods in Molecular Biology, vol. 1692, DOI 10.1007/978-1-4939-7401-6_15, © Springer Science+Business Media LLC 2018

demonstrate gene methylation patterns in which some genes are shared and other genes are methylated in a tumor type-specific manner [7]. Notably, many genes that become de novo hypermethylated in cancer are also targets of the PcG repressor complex in ESCs. ESCs rely on PcG proteins to reversibly repress genes encoding transcription factors required for differentiation [8]. It has been shown that stem cell PcG group targets are up to 12 times more likely to display cancer-specific promoter DNA hypermethylation than non-PcG target genes, lending support to the theory of a "stem cell origin of cancer" [9]. In this model reversible gene repression is replaced by permanent silencing by de novo methylation, thus locking the cell into a perpetual state of self-renewal, and thereby predisposing to subsequent malignant transformation. Interestingly, certain cancer-associated hypermethylation signatures are also observed in histologically normal stem cells. A contributing factor to the de novo methylation could be age, which is considered to be one of the most important demographic risk factors for cancer; PcG target genes are significantly more likely to become methylated with age than non-PcG targets [10]. Furthermore, an age-dependent PcG target gene methylation signature has been detected in pre-neoplastic conditions, suggesting that it may drive gene expression alterations associated with carcinogenesis and that age may in fact predispose to malignant transformation by irreversibly stabilizing stem cell features.

Many methods have been developed to study DNA methylation. The most widely used techniques employ bisulfite modification of DNA. In this reaction, treatment of genomic DNA with sodium bisulfite followed by an alkali deaminates cytosine residues thus converting them to uracil, while 5-methylcytosine (5mC) is protected from this modification [11, 12]. The DNA sequence under investigation is then PCR amplified with primers designed to anneal specifically with bisulfite-converted DNA. This combination of bisulfite treatment and PCR introduces an artificial SNP at every CpG dinucleotide, which can then be exploited to discriminate methylation status based on the presence of a cytosine (5mC) or uracil (unmethylated cytosine). Bisulfite-based approaches are used for large-scale analysis (e.g., MeDipSeq, methylation beadchip arrays, among many others) [13, 14], as well as more targeted studies (e.g., quantitative methylation-specific PCR, bisulfite sequencing, pyrosequencing) [12, 15]. The choice in approach is largely dependent on the type(s) of question being asked and the degree of previous knowledge. For example, methylomic approaches are often suitable for discovery-type experiments, which can be subsequently followed up and validated with more targeted approaches, once regions of interest (RoI) have been identified. In other instances, RoI are already well defined, and so, one can proceed straight to a targeted analysis of these. Other important considerations are the type, quality, and abundance of

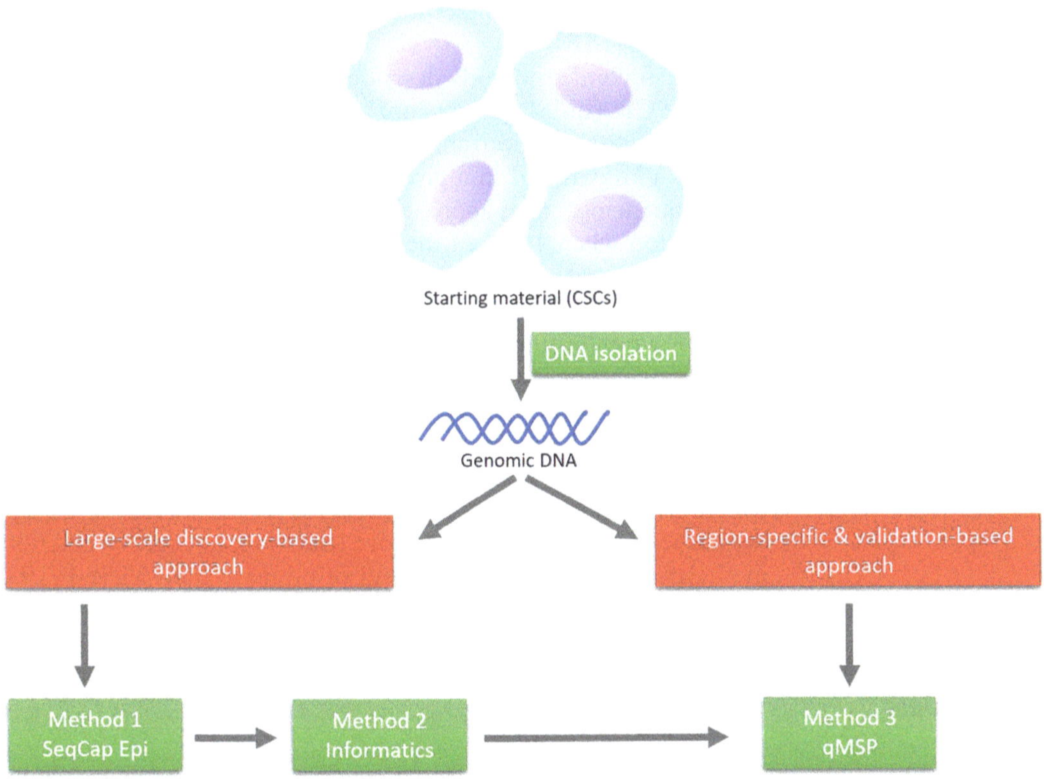

Fig. 1 Experimental strategy to study DNA methylation of cancer stem cells (CSCs). Techniques/methods are indicated in *green*. The two approaches can be carried out independently or sequentially together as in the strategy indicated

starting material, the size of the study (e.g., the number of samples) and budgetary constraints.

Herein, we describe methods to enable both approaches, as well as a bioinformatic pipeline to support their analysis (Fig. 1). For genome-wide approaches, the complexity of the samples can first be reduced by enriching the genomic regions of interest with enzymatic treatment (e.g., reduced representation bisulfite sequencing), or enriching for DNA sequences containing 5mC, by antibody-based or methyl-binding-domain-based immunoprecipitation [16]. Next-generation sequencing platforms allow genome-wide characterization of methylomic profiles with a high resolution. SeqCap Epi (Roche Nimblegen) is a relatively new probe-based enrichment approach that allows capture and subsequent sequencing of a substantially large proportion of the epigenome (>50 Mb) across different species. It effectively allows assessment of DNA methylation status of over 5.5 million CpG sites interspersed across the genome. One of the most important features of this method is the ability to design custom-based capture to encompass various RoI specific to the study, thus circumventing issues arising through a much wider global discovery approach [17, 18].

The second method described, quantitative methylation-specific PCR (qMSP, methylight), is a technique that delivers a semi-quantitative indication of the proportion of fully methylated DNA at a known RoI in a given sample. In contrast to the large-scale sequencing-based approach, qMSP will only reliably quantify methylation when 100% of the CpG sites being interrogated by a primer/probe set are methylated. This is achieved by incorporating CpG dinucleotides into the primer and probe-binding sites. Thus, the PCR amplification will only take place when all of the CpGs in the hybridization sites are represented by 5mC and not uracil. Therefore, if anything, this technique can underestimate the degree of methylation at a given locus. qMSP is especially useful for high-throughput analysis because it is inexpensive and quick to perform, which means that it can be easily applied to the analysis of a large sample set. It is also highly sensitive (down to 1/10,000–100,000 methylated alleles in a background of unmethylated alleles) [19], making it suitable for small amounts of starting material.

2 Materials

All chemicals and reagents, required in these experiments should be of analytical grade quality and stored in accordance with the manufacturer's instructions. Prepare buffers and solutions using distilled water and store at room temperature (unless stated otherwise). Adhere to local regulations in regard the handling and disposal of reagents and chemicals.

2.1 General Materials

1. Molecular biology grade DNase-free, RNase-free water.
2. Microcentrifuge tubes (1.5 mL).
3. 96-well PCR plates.
4. Microseal ® "B" PCR plates sealing film, adhesive, optical #msb1001 (Bio-rad).

2.2 Targeted Methyl Capture Approach Using SeqCap Epi

1. DNA quantification Quant-iT® dsDNA assay kit (cat. P7589, Invitrogen).
2. Covaris ultrasonicator M220.
3. microTUBE AFA pre slit snap cap (cat. E7023-500 mL, Covaris).
4. Agencourt AMPure XP beads (cat: A63800, Beckam Coulter).
5. DNA vacuum concentrator (Eppendorf or similar).
6. DynaMag 96 side magnet (Cat no: 12321D, Life Technologies).
7. KAPA HTP DNA library preparation kit (cat. 07138008001, Roche NimbleGen).

8. SeqCap Epi CpGiant enrichment kit (cat. 07138881001, Roche NimbleGen)—This is the standard off the shelf assay for 4 reactions—1 sample per reaction. For custom design assays use choice or developer enrichment kit.
9. NimbleGen SeqCap Adapter kit A and B (cat: 07141530001, 07141548001, Roche NimbleGen).
10. Agilent high sensitivity DNA bioanalyzer kit (cat. 5067-4626, Agilent Technologies).
11. EZ DNA methylation-lightening kit, Zymo Research cat. no. D5030).
12. MiSeq Reagent kit v3.0—150 cycles (MS-102-3001, Illumina Ltd.).
13. HiSeq 2000 v4.0 PE cluster kit (cat. PE-401-4001).

2.3 SeqCap Epi Data Analysis

1. General tools required for analysis: SAMtools [20], BWA [21, 22], Java.
2. Quality control and preprocessing of sequence data: fastQC [23]; BBDuk from the BBTools package [24]; markDuplicates from the PicardTools package (http://broadinstitute.github.io/picard).
3. Alignment of sequence data and postprocessing: BWA-meth [25], markDuplicates.
4. Methylation event calling: PileOMeth (https://github.com/dpryan79/PileOMeth), bisSNP [26].
5. Differential methylation analysis: methylKit [27].

2.4 Quantitative Methylation-Specific PCR (qMSP)

1. Commercially available bisulfite modification kit (e.g., EpiTect Fast Bisulfite Conversion kit, Qiagen cat. no. 59824, EZ DNA methylation-lightening kit, Zymo Research cat. no. D5030).
2. qPCR mastermix without AmpErase® Uracil N-Glycosylase (e.g., TaqMan® Universal PCR Master Mix, No AmpErase® UNG, Life Technologies cat. no. 4364341).
3. Appropriate qPCR plates (either 48-well, 96-well of 384-well) for intended instrument (e.g., ABgene FAST 96-well PCR plate, Thermo Scientific cat. no. AB-1900, MicroAmp^R Fast optical 96-well reaction plates, Life Technologies cat. no. 4366932).
4. Optical adhesive covers (e.g., Thermo Scientific cat. no. AB-0558, MicroAmp^R Optical adhesive covers, Life Technologies, cat. no. 431171).
5. DNA primers (standard desalting purified) and fluorescently labeled probe (e.g., Zen-double quenched probes, Integrated DNA Technologies, MGB-quenched probes, Life Technologies).

6. gBlocks Gene Fragments for constructing standard curves and interplate calibration (e.g., Integrated DNA Technologies).
7. Control Human methylated DNA for relative quantification of methylation (e.g., EpiTect Control methylated DNA, Qiagen cat. no. 59655).

3 Methods

3.1 SeqCap Epi-Based Target Enrichment Approach for Discovery of Differentially Methylated Loci

3.1.1 DNA Quantification

Day 1

1. Successful generation of high-quality DNA libraries largely depends on the concentration of the dsDNA sample. The Quant-iT® dsDNA Picogreen assay is used to measure the precise concentration of dsDNA in a given sample. Make 25 μL aliquots of Picogreen dye and store, protected from light, at −20°C. Prepare "DNA standards" from a stock DNA solution (provided; 100 μg/mL) as outlined in Table 1, and store at 4°C.
2. Prepare a 96-well PCR plate with the DNA standards and sample/test DNAs to be quantified, as follows: Add 150 μL of each DNA standard to the 8 wells in the first column of the plate. Use the remaining 11 columns, as required, to add sample DNA, diluting each 100× (1.5 μL DNA + 148.5 μL 1× TE buffer) (*see* **Note 1**).
3. Thaw an aliquot of Picogreen to room temperature and add 4975 μL 1× TE. Add 50 μL of diluted Picogreen to each standard/sample DNA, thus bringing the total volume of

Table 1
Preparation of DNA standards for Picogreen dsDNA quantification

	1× TE volume (mL)	Stock DNA (100 μg/mL) volume (μL)	Standard concentration (ng/mL)
Standard 1	10	100	1000
Standard 2	10	70	700
Standard 3	10	50	500
Standard 4	10	30	300
Standard 5	10	10	100
Standard 6	10	5	50
Standard 7	10	2.5	25
Blank	10	0	0

each well up to 200 μL. Shield the plate from light and shake gently.

4. Measure the absorbance on a UV spectrophotometer or plate-reader, with the appropriate software (e.g., Softmax Gemini) using the following settings: automix 5 s before measurement, excitation at 485 nm (T_x), Emission at 520 nm (E_m).
5. Calculate the concentration of dsDNA by plotting the absorbance of the standards against their concentrations, and extrapolating the concentrations of the sample DNAs using the slope calculated from the standard curve.

3.1.2 DNA Sonication

Day 2

1. The amount of input dsDNA required for sonication is between 500 and 1000 ng. Bring each DNA sample to a final volume of 52.5 μL, by diluting in 1× TE as required, and transfer to a Covaris microTUBE for sonicating.
2. Fragment DNA samples to an average size of 180–220 bp using the following parameters on the M220 Covaris: duty cycle: 20%, intensity: 5, cycles per burst: 200, time: 120 sec, and temperature: 15–22 °C (*see* **Note 2**).
3. Following sonication, transfer the entire sample (≥50 μL) to a fresh 1.5 mL microcentrifuge tube.
4. Take 1 μL of the sonicated sample to assess the fragment size using the Bioanalyzer high-sensitivity DNA kit (Agilent). Upon confirming the correct fragment size (180–220 bp), the remainder of the sonicated DNA sample (≥50 μL) may be used for library generation.

3.1.3 DNA Library Preparation and Bisulfite Conversion

Day 2 (continued)

1. Ideally, library preparation should be carried out on the same day or within 24 h of DNA sonication (*see* **Notes 3** and **4**).
2. The first steps of DNA end-repair and A-tailing are carried out using the buffer and enzyme provided with the KAPA HTP DNA library preparation kit, and in accordance with the manufacturer's instructions (*see* **Note 5**).
3. Dilute the adaptors (provided, 10 μM) to 0.2 μM, before proceeding to the ligation step, using only 2.2 μL diluted adapter and 2.8 μL of water per ligation reaction.
4. Perform two clean-up reactions using the PEG/SPRI solution at a 1:1 ratio (DNA:PEG/SPRI). Elute the cleaned-up ligation reaction into 26 μL water (*see* **Note 6**).
5. Use 25 μL of the DNA library for bisulfite conversion, as per the manufacturer's instructions (*see* **Note 7**).

Day 3

6. Complete bisulfite conversion, eluting the modified DNA into 20 μL water.
7. Proceed to the ligation-mediated (LM) PCR reaction using the Kapa HiFi HotStart Uracil + ready mix (provided). We recommend only 12 PCR cycles.
8. Clean the LM-PCR reactions using Ampure beads (1:8 ratio, DNA:beads), resuspending in 20 μL water.
9. Assess the library quality and quantity using the Bioanalyzer high-sensitivity DNA kit. Store the library at –20 °C (*see* **Notes 8** and **9**).

3.1.4 Estimating Bisulfite Conversion Efficiency of the DNA Library

Day 4

1. Differential methylation calls are dependent on the bisulfite conversion rate. Therefore, it is critical to estimate the bisulfite conversion efficiency of each DNA library. This can be done using the Kapa DNA library qPCR quantification kit (or alternative appropriate for qPCR instrument of choice). Based on the library concentration (determined using the bioanalyzer), a 1:100–1:1000 dilution should be made, to enable subsequent serial dilutions in the range of 1:8000–1:32,000, depending on the initial concentration of the library.
2. The final dilution (e.g., the most dilute) is used as input for the qPCR, along with the standards (provided). Include a melt curve step with the amplification reaction.
3. Estimate the molarity of the library by extrapolating from the standard curve generated from the standards.

Day 5

4. Denature exactly 4 nm of each library using NaOH. If working with >1 library, libraries may be pooled together, taking care to avoid repeated use of unique adapters (*see* **Note 10**).
5. Sequence the library (or pool thereof) on a MiSeq, in either a 1× 50 or 2 × 75 bp fashion.

Day 6–7

6. Retrieve the fastq sequencing files from the system, and carry out some standard QC analysis by generating mapped/aligned and basic metrics for each sample. This is a good basis for estimating the bisulfite conversion efficiency (*see* **Note 11**).

3.1.5 Sequence Capture and Sequencing

Day 8–10

1. Once the QC is complete, and the bisulfite conversion efficiency has been confirmed, the library is ready for hybridization.

2. Prepare the hybridization reaction using 1 μg of the library along with hybridization buffer, blocking oligonucleotides (specific to the adapter being used), universal oligonucleotides, and bisulfite capture enhancer. Mix thoroughly before transferring to a 96-well plate and sealing. Carefully pierce the adhesive microfilm (using a $\leq$ 18–20 gauge needle) above the sample-containing wells, to enable evaporation of liquid.
3. Dehydrate the hybridization reaction using a DNA vacuum concentrator at 60 °C for 1–1.5 h. Ensure that all of the liquid in each well has evaporated before removing the plate.
4. Add hybridization buffer and hybridization component A to each lyophilized sample and mix thoroughly. Denature the samples at 95 °C for 10 min and then store at room temperature (*see* **Note 12**).
5. Add 4.5 μL of SeqCap Epi probes to each sample and seal the plate, before incubating at 47 °C for 72 h. in a thermal cycler. It is important to ensure that the lid of the thermal cycler is heated to 57 °C to prevent evaporation.
6. Meanwhile, prepare the capture beads by thoroughly cleaning them in bead wash buffer in a fresh 96-well plate, taking care to ensure that the wells containing the beads correspond to the wells containing samples in the hybridization reaction plate.

Day 11

7. Carefully, but quickly, transfer the hybridization reactions to the plate containing the washed beads and mix thoroughly using a multichannel micropipette, before incubating at 47 °C for 45 min in a thermal cycler. As the beads start to settle at the bottom of the well during the incubation, it is important to mix the sample (by pipetting) every 15 min (*see* **Note 13**).
8. Following incubation, clean the capture-bound beads thoroughly to ensure removal of any unbound probes (*see* **Note 14**). First carry out the temperature-dependent washes: the prepared "stringent wash buffer" and "wash buffer I" are heated to 47 °C and aliquoted in a 96-well plate in the required volumes for each wash, such that the wells correspond to the reaction plate. This will enable efficient addition of the two buffers to each reaction with minimal reduction in set temperature.
9. Next, carry out three washes using wash buffers I, II, and III respectively, all at room temperature.
10. Resuspend the beads in 50 μL water (molecular biology grade) and split the reaction into two aliquots, as per the manufacturer's guidelines.

11. To each reaction, add 25 μL of Kapa HiFi HotStart ready mix and 5 μL post-LM PCR oligonucleotides, yielding a final reaction volume of 50 μL (in duplicate).
12. Perform the PCR reaction for a total of 16 cycles.
13. Upon completion of PCR, combine the duplicate reactions and subject to a post-PCR cleanup using a 1:1.8 ratio (DNA: Ampure beads), followed by two 80% ethanol washes and finally eluting into 50 μL water.
14. Assess the quality of the eluted captured sample using the bioanalyzer and quantify by Picogreen (*see* Subheading 3.1.1, *DNA quantification*).
15. Take 4 nm of the captured sample for denaturing and clustering on the c-bot, and thereafter sequencing on a HiSeq 2000 v4 (Illumina sequencing platform or similar high-throughput NGS platforms) in a 2 × 150 bp approach, by multiplexing four samples per lane (to yield an average coverage of 30× per sample).
16. Following sequencing and de-multiplexing, retrieve the fastq files for processing using an established bioinformatic pipeline (*see* Subheading 3.2, Fig. 2).

3.2 Bioinformatic Analysis of SeqCap Epi Data

This method assumes a single-end sequence dataset. Paired-end data can be used with minimal revision. Variables are capitalized and preceded with a dollar sign ($) as is the format for "bash" script. Variable names should make the subject obvious. A backslash indicates a continuation from the previous line.

3.2.1 Quality Control (QC) and Preprocessing

1. It is important to determine sequence quality prior to analysis; the fastQC tool allows visualization of multiple metrics for assessment:

```
fastqc $FASTQ -outdir=$OUTDIR
```

2. Poor quality sequence is more likely to contain errors. This is indicated by the Phred score. It is also possible that adapters were sequenced. Therefore, sequence data should be trimmed using a Phred score (here $q = 20$), giving as input a file containing known adapter sequence (supplied with the tool). Parameters "k" (kmer size) and "mink" (minimum kmer size) are left as defaults, but can be adjusted to maximum and minimum at the cost of increased runtime (*see* **Note 15**):

```
bbduk.sh in=$FASTQ out=$OUTDIR/$SAMPLE".trim.fastq.gz" \
trimq=20 qtrim=rl ref=$BBDUK_REF stats=$OUTDIR"/metrics"
```

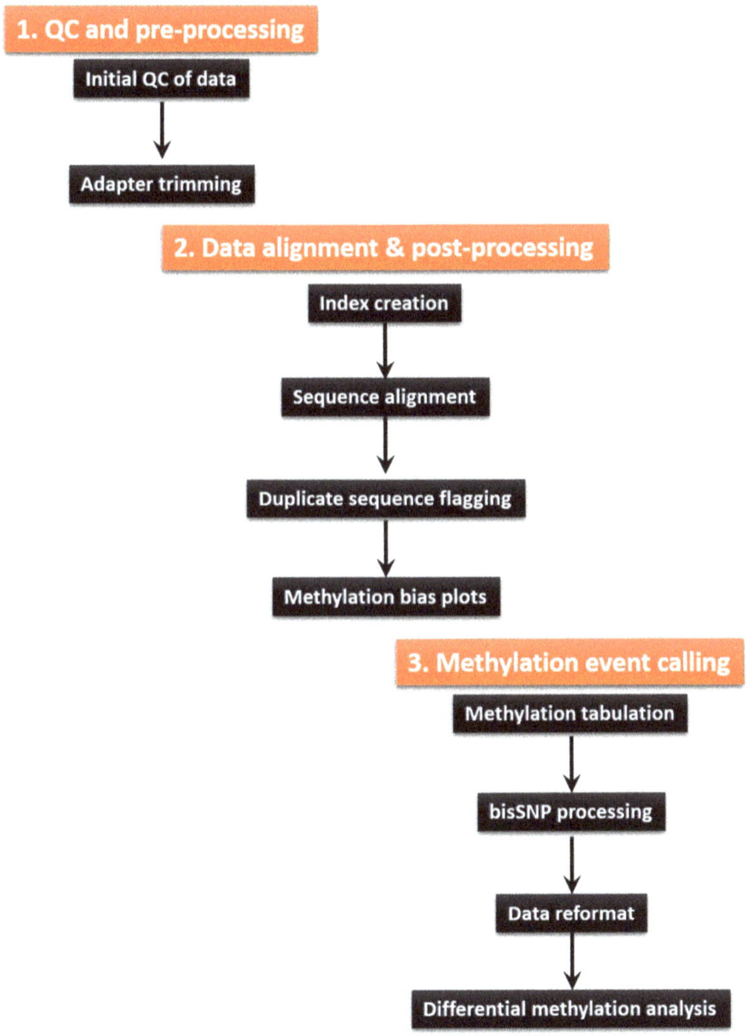

Fig. 2 Bioinformatic analysis pipeline of methylomic sequencing data (e.g., SeqCapEpi dataset). Abbreviations: *QC* quality control, *bis* bisulfite

3.2.2 Alignment and Postprocessing

1. Once the sequence data are trimmed and quality is checked and approved, the data can be aligned to a reference genome. First create an index (*see* **Note 16**):

```
bwameth.py index $REFERENCE
```

2. Next, align the data. The BWA-meth aligner is a fast and efficient tool, which is based on the BWA-mem algorithm [20, 25]. BWA-meth outputs SAM format. Catch this output as a file, then postprocess (it is also possible to "pipe" into SAMtools for further processing):

```
  bwameth.py -reference $REFERENCE \
  $OUTDIR/$SAMPLE".trim.fastq.gz" >
$OUTDIR/$SAMPLE".trim.sam"
```

3. Sequence data require removal of duplicate sequence. To do this, mark (rather than remove) the duplicates, which will be subsequently disregarded based on their flags attached at this stage. PicardTools MarkDuplicates outputs a metrics file specifying the level of duplication, which is also a good indication of data quality.

```
java -jar $PICARD_JAR MarkDuplicates \
INPUT$OUTDIR/$SAMPLE".trim.sam" \
OUTPUT=$OUTDIR/$SAMPLE".trim.markdup.bam" \
METRICS_FILE=$OUTDIR"/metrics/markdup.metrics" \
REMOVE_DUPLICATES=FALSE \
ASSUME_SORTED=TRUE \
VALIDATION_STRINGENCY=LENIENT
```

4. Use SAMtools to Index the BAM File Output for Further use:

```
samtools index $OUTDIR/$SAMPLE".trim.markdup.bam"
```

3.2.3 Methylation Event Calling

1. Use the PileOMeth tool to "extract" methylation calls. This requires a reference genome as used previously (*see* Subheading 3.2.2, step 1). This step by default tabulates methylation in a "bedGraph" format.

```
 PileOMeth              extract         $REFERENCE
$OUTDIR/$SAMPLE".trim.markdup.bam"
```

2. Produce a "methylation bias-plot," indicating the level of CpG methylation per base across the aligned sequence reads. This gives a good visualization of sequence quality and is an important determination of sample utility.

```
 PileOMeth              mbias           $REFERENCE
$OUTDIR/$SAMPLE".trim.markdup.bam" \
 $OUTDIR/$SAMPLE".mbias_plot"
```

3. Filter for SNPs using the bisSNP tool suite, which is modeled on the GATK method for genome/exome DNA sequence data. It uses known indels to realign data and uses known SNPs to recalibrate mapping scores, following which the data are genotyped to allow filtering of SNPs. Prior to running bisSNP, sequence data must have "readgroup" information attached using PicardTools.

```
java -jar $PICARD_JAR AddOrReplaceReadGroups \
INPUT=$OUTDIR/$SAMPLE".trim.markdup.bam" \
OUTPUT=$OUTDIR/$SAMPLE".trim.markdup.rg.bam" \
RGID=$SAMPLE RGLB="libraryX" RGPL="Illumina" \
RGPU="UnitX" RGSM=$SAMPLE \
CREATE_INDEX=TRUE VALIDATION_STRINGENCY=SILENT

java -jar $BISSNP_JAR \
-R $REFERENCE \
-T BisulfiteRealignerTargetCreator \
-I $OUTDIR/$SAMPLE".trim.markdup.rg.bam" \
-o $OUTDIR/$BS/indel_realign_target.intervals"
-known $KNOWN_INDELS \

java -jar $BISSNP_JAR \
-R $REFERENCE \
-T BisulfiteIndelRealigner \
-I $OUTDIR/$SAMPLE".trim.markdup.rg.bam" \
-o $OUTDIR/$SAMPLE".trim.markdup.rg.realign.bam"
-targetIntervals $OUTDIR/$BS/"indel_realign_target.intervals" \
-known $KNOWN_INDELS \

java -jar $BISSNP_JAR \
-R $REFERENCE \
-T BisulfiteCountCovariates \
-I $OUTDIR/$SAMPLE".trim.markdup.rg.realign.bam" \
-knownSites $COSMIC \
-knownSites $DBSNP \
-cov ReadGroupCovariate \
-cov QualityScoreCovariate \
-cov CycleCovariate \
-recalFile $OUTDIR/$BS/"recalFile_before.csv"

java -jar $BISSNP_JAR \
-R $REFERENCE \
-T BisulfiteTableRecalibration \
-I $OUTDIR/$SAMPLE".trim.markdup.rg.realign.bam" \
-o $OUTDIR/$SAMPLE".trim.markdup.rg.realign.recal.bam" \
-maxQ 40 \
-recalFile $OUTDIR/$BS/"recalFile_before.csv"

java -jar $BISSNP_JAR \
-R $REFERENCE \
-T BisulfiteCountCovariates \
-I $OUTDIR/$SAMPLE".trim.markdup.rg.realign.recal.bam" \
-knownSites $COSMIC \
-knownSites $DBSNP \
```

```
-cov ReadGroupCovariate \
-cov QualityScoreCovariate \
-cov CycleCovariate \
-recalFile $OUTDIR/$BS/"recalFile_after.csv"

java -jar $BISULFITEANALYZECOVARIATES_JAR \
-recalFile $OUTDIR/$BS/"recalFile_after.csv" \
-outputDir $OUTDIR/$BS \
-ignoreQ 5 \
-max_quality_score 40

java -jar $BISSNP_JAR \
-R $REFERENCE \
-T BisulfiteGenotyper \
-I $OUTDIR/$SAMPLE".trim.markdup.rg.realign.recal.bam" \
-trim5 5 -trim3 5 -mmq 30 \
-vfn1 $OUTDIR/$SAMPLE".trim.markdup.rg.realign.recal.cpg.vcf" \
-vfn2 $OUTDIR/$SAMPLE".trim.markdup.rg.realign.recal.snp.vcf" \
-C CG,1 \
-intervals $CAPTURE_INTERVALS

java -jar $BISSNP \
-R $REFERENCE \
-T VCFpostprocess \
-oldVcf
$OUTDIR/$SAMPLE".trim.markdup.rg.realign.recal.cpg.vcf" \
-newVcf
$OUTDIR/$SAMPLE".trim.markdup.rg.realign.recal.cpg.filter.vcf" \
-snpVcf
$OUTDIR/$SAMPLE".trim.markdup.rg.realign.recal.snp.vcf" \
-o $OUTDIR/"metrics/bisSNP.cpg_filter.summary.txt"
```

4. Finally, process the data for methylKit input. Data from bisSNP are not correctly formatted for methylKit, and must be reformatted. An example Perl script to convert from VCF is given at www.github/bruce.moran/perl-scripts/vcf2methylKit.sh. This can be used to generate a *.methylKit.input file.

3.2.4 Differential Methylation Analysis with Methylkit

1. We recommend carrying out differential methylation analysis using MethylKit, a Bioconductor package used in the R statistical environment (R core team). R-script for methylKit Analysis:

```
library(methylKit)
wd<-c("/path/to/input")
setwd(wd)
filesIn<-dir(pattern="methylKit.input")
```

```
##Given some condition 0,1 and samples a,b,c,d
condition<-c(0,0,1,1)
samples<-c("a","b","c","d")

##Read in data
myObj<-mread(location=as.list(filesIn),
sample.id=as.list(samples),
     assembly="hg19", header=F,
     treatment=condition)
meth<-unite(myObj)
getCorrelation(meth, plot = T)
PCASamples(meth)
myDiff<-calculateDiffMeth(meth,slim=F)
myDiff25p=get.methylDiff(myDiff,difference=25,qvalue=0.01)
```

3.3 Quantitative MSP to Study Region-Specific DNA Methylation and/or to Validate Findings from Discovery/–Omic-Based Approach (Subheading 3.1)

3.3.1 Primer Design for qMSP

1. The genomic DNA sequence of a "region of interest" (RoI), e.g., CpG island, promoter, 5′ untranslated region, enhancer etc., can be freely viewed and downloaded using the UCSC Human Genome Browser: http://genome.ucsc.edu/.
2. Copy and paste the DNA code for the RoI into a word document and transform it into a virtual bisulfite-modified, fully methylated sequence (*see* **Note 17**). Do this by first making sure that all of the sequence is in lower case (the font-type and size is unimportant). Use the "Find and Replace" function to replace all of the "cg" doublets with uppercase "CG." Next, replace all "c" with "t," taking care to ensure that "match case" option is selected. Save this sequence and use it to design the oligonucleotides for qMSP.
3. When considering where to position oligonucleotides within the RoI (*see* **Notes 18** and **19**), comply with these rules to avoid spurious results (Fig. 3a):
   - Oligonucleotides should *each* contain ≥2 CpG sites, preferably toward the 3′ end of their sequence (e.g., a minimum of 6 per assay), to bias amplification in favor of bisulfite-converted methylated DNA only.
   - Oligonucleotides should *each* contain several non-CpG cytosine residues (which appear as thymine in the in silico modified sequence), to ensure amplification of bisulfite-modified DNA only (and not of any residual unconverted genomic DNA).
4. In parallel with PCR amplification of a RoI, or multiples of, a control reaction should *always* be performed using oligonucleotides that will *only* amplify bisulfite-modified DNA, regardless of DNA methylation. This "housekeeping" reaction serves to normalize for varying amounts of bisulfite-modified DNA between test samples. Therefore, control oligonucleotides

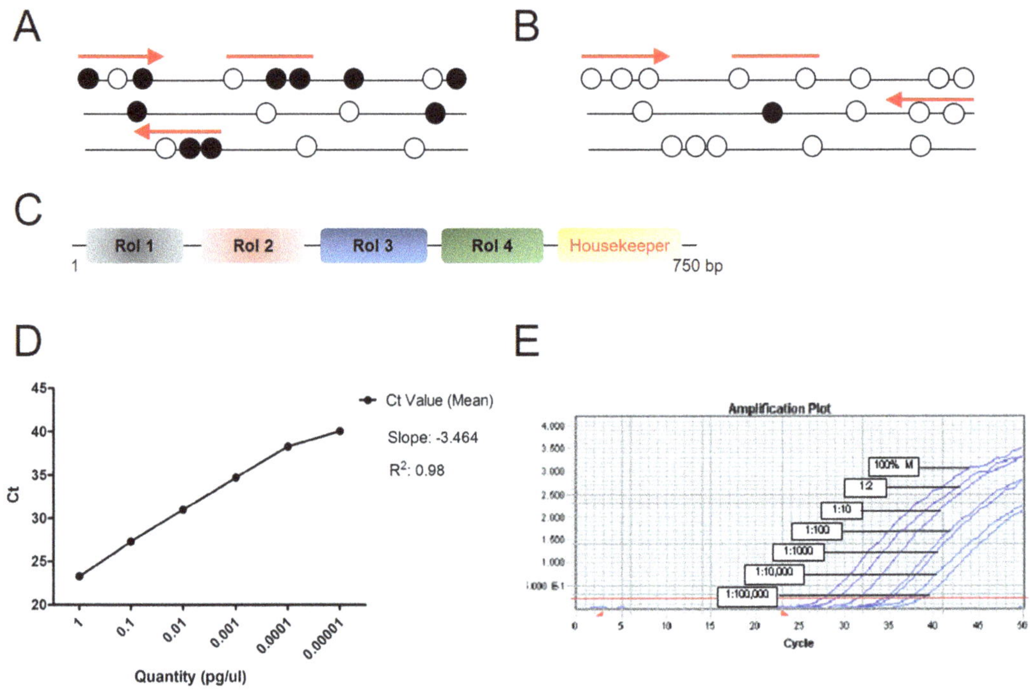

Fig. 3 The principles of qMSP for DNA methylation analysis. (**a**) Primers and fluorescently labeled probe (depicted in red) amplify bisulfite-converted fully-methylated DNA. (**b**) A control PCR reaction that does not discriminate between methylated and unmethylated templates is used to normalize the amount of input bisulfite-modified DNA. Filled circles indicate 5-methylcytosine, white circles represent cytosine. (**c**) Depiction of gBlock design, encompassing multiple regions of interest (RoI) and a control for normalization. (**d**) Standard curve results from a qMSP performed on serial dilutions of a gBlock gene fragment. (**e**) Sensitivity of detection of DNA methylation (1/10,000–1/100,000) and quantitative accuracy of qMSP. Amplification plot of fluorescence intensity (*y axis*) against PCR cycle (*x axis*). Each curve represents a different input quantity of in vitro methylated DNA into unmethylated DNA

should avoid CpG sites but must contain several non-CpG cytosines (Fig. 3b). The same housekeeping region can be used in multiple experiments.

5. In addition, oligonucleotides should also meet standard parameters for primer design, e.g., avoid secondary structures, self-dimers, and hetero-dimers. Ensure that the melting temperature of the primers is matched, preferably within 1 °C and typically between 58 and 60 °C. The amplicon length should be <150 bp and the melting temperature of the probe should be approximately 10 °C greater than that of the primers, to comply with standard real-time PCR parameters. We recommend using the freely available Oligo Analyzer from Integrated DNA technologies (http://eu.idtdna.com/analyzer/Applications/OligoAnalyzer/), or the UCSC In-Silico PCR platform (http://www.genome.ucsc.edu/), to ensure these parameters are met.

Table 2
Confirming the specificity of a new qMSP assay

	Unmodified genomic DNA	Modified unmethylated genomic DNA	Modified methylated genomic DNA	NTC
Amplification	No	No	Yes	No

3.3.2 Optimizing qMSP Assays

When testing the performance of new qMSP assay, several factors need to be taken into consideration.

1. The specificity of the assay for bisulfite-modified methylated DNA should first be confirmed using a set of controls: unmodified genomic DNA, modified methylated DNA, and modified unmethylated DNA. Such controls are readily commercially available (e.g., Qiagen EpiTect® Control DNA set, Zymo Research Human Control Methylated, and Non-Methylated DNA Set). A suitable cell line can also be used, if the methylation status of the RoI has already been determined.
2. Prepare qMSP reactions as follows: qPCR mastermix without AmpErase® Uracil N-Glycosylase, 900 nM final concentration of both forward and reverse primers, 300 nM final concentration of fluorescently labeled probe, 10 ng of bisulfite-modified DNA and H_2O to bring total reaction volume to 20 μL. Perform all reactions in triplicate (this should be factored in when calculating volumes for a PCR master-mix) for 50 cycles of amplification under standard real-time PCR thermal cycling conditions.
3. Once specificity is confirmed (Table 2), the primer and probe concentrations should be optimized across a range, typically 300, 600, and 900 nM for primers and 100, 200,and 300 nM for the probe, using a modified methylated control sample.
4. Amplification curves should be visualized to assess the cycle number of amplification (Ct) and the height of the change in fluorescence emitted (ΔRn). Choose the concentrations that deliver the lowest Ct and highest ΔRn (*see* **Note 20**).
5. Once assays have been optimized for specificity and performance, serially diluted standards can be prepared, which are used to construct a standard curve for quantifying methylation levels. For constructing standard curves for qMSP, we recommend using synthetic ds DNA fragments such as gBlocks™ (Integrated DNA Technologies), which can be in silico designed as described in Subheading 3.3.1. gBlocks™ gene fragments have capacity up to 3 kb and can thus be designed to house multiple RoI and a housekeeper region for normalizing input amounts of bisulfite-modified DNA between test samples (Fig. 3b). Alternatively, commercially available bisulfite-modified methylated DNA can be used.

Table 3
Preparation of serially diluted methylation standards for qMSP

Standard	Copy number	Volume of gBlock™ (μL)	Volume of molecular grade H_2O (μL)
1	1000,000	10 (WS[a])	173.8
2	100,000	10 (S1)	90
3	10,000	10 (S2)	90
4	1000	10 (S3)	90
5	100	10 (S4)	90
6	10	10 (S5)	90

[a] We suggest preparing a working solution (WS) of the gBlock™ at a concentration of 10 pg/μL

6. Prepare a working solution of the gBlocks™ (or alternative) at a concentration of 10 pg/μL and use this to prepare tenfold serial dilutions, which will be used to construct a standard curve for Absolute Quantification (AQ) (Table 3, *see* **Note 21**). Examine the slope and R^2, which should ideally be −3.3 (+/− 0.2) and >0.997, respectively. It is essential that the concentrations of the standards are such that their amplification range spans that of the unknowns (e.g., test DNAs) to be measured.

3.3.3 Quantitative Methylation-Specific PCR on CSCs

Day 1

1. Isolate and quantify DNA from CSCs using a method of choice (*see* **Note 22**).

Day 2

2. Carry out bisulfite conversion of DNA. Many commercially available kits are optimized to modify as little as 100 pg up to 2 μg DNA. In our hands, this technique performs best using 100–500 ng of input genomic DNA. Take care at the final elution step to avoid over-concentrating the bisulfite-converted sample. We recommend eluting into a final volume that yields a concentration in the region of 10 ng/μL, e.g., 500 ng of input genomic DNA eluted into a final volume of 50 μL, thus providing sufficient volume of converted DNA for multiple PCR reactions, as required. There are no methods to specifically quantify bisulfite-modified DNA. Therefore, calculations of concentration are based on the assumption of >98% conversion rate of the reaction.
3. Perform qMSP reactions as described in Subheading 3.3.2.
4. For each test DNA and standard, a housekeeping qMSP reaction should be carried out in parallel with RoI, using oligonucleotides targeted to a control gene (e.g., *ACTB),* to normalize for the amount of input bisulfite-modified DNA between samples.

5. Each RoI being quantified (for methylation levels) must be amplified in the test samples, a positive control (fully methylated human DNA) and a negative template control and at least two of the methylation standards (*see* **Note 21**). For studies involving large numbers of test samples, we recommend using the same positive control across all reactions (e.g., plates).
6. Perform qMSP under standard AQ real-time settings, adjusting to 50 cycles of amplification.
7. Examine the amplification of the controls and standards first. Adjust the threshold and baseline, if required, so that the Ct of the standards is the same as that of the reference standards.
8. Extrapolate from the reference standard curve to yield quantities (ng) of methylation for each unknown/sample.
9. Analyze qMSP data by calculating a normalized index of methylation (NIM) for each sample, as previously described [15, 28]. This will determine the ratio of the normalized amount of methylated RoI to the normalized amount of control, by applying the formula:

   $$[(\mathrm{TARGET}_{\mathrm{sample}}/\mathrm{TARGET}_{\mathrm{MC}})/(\mathrm{CONTROL}_{\mathrm{sample}}/\mathrm{CONTROL}_{\mathrm{MC}})] \times 1000.$$

   where $\mathrm{TARGET}_{\mathrm{sample}}$ is the quantity of fully methylated copies of a RoI in any individual sample, $\mathrm{TARGET}_{\mathrm{MC}}$ is the quantity of fully methylated copies of a RoI in the methylated control DNA, $\mathrm{CONTROL}_{\mathrm{sample}}$ is the quantity of bisulfite-modified templates in any individual sample, and $\mathrm{CONTROL}_{\mathrm{MC}}$ is the quantity of bisulfite-modified templates in the universally methylated control DNA.

4 Notes

1. Space permitting on the 96-well plate, we recommend performing the Picogreen quantification assay in technical duplicates for both DNA standards and samples to be quantified, to increase the precision of the final result.
2. It is important to pause the sonication procedure at increments of 25% during the process and flick the tube, as constant sonication leads to formation of droplets, which adhere to the walls of the tube preventing even sonication of the entire sample. Flicking the tube will allow collection of the droplets at the bottom of the tube hence facilitating homogenous sonication of the sample.
3. If not proceeding directly to library preparation, sonicated DNA may be stored at −20 °C.
4. To streamline pipetting and washing steps, we recommend using a 96-well plate when preparing >3 libraries at a time.

However, no more than 16 libraries should be prepared at one time.

5. It is important to remember that during the clean-up procedure (which is performed multiple times: (1) between the end-repair and A-tailing, (2) between A-tailing and ligation and (3) before and after LM-PCR), the ethanol washes are carried out for 30 s each and after the second ethanol wash, the tubes/plate are/is centrifuged at full speed for 10–15 s. This allows sedimentation of any residual ethanol left in the sample and prevents any carry-over. The beads are allowed dry for 2–3 min and then resuspended in TE/water, before cracks begin to appear.
6. Given that the efficiency of the fragmentation and ligation reactions is usually high, there is essentially no need to carry out a dual size-selection, as this is a source of DNA loss, which needs to be minimized in lieu of the fact that bisulfite conversion is an unavoidable source of DNA loss when performing methyl capture.
7. There are several commercially available "fast" bisulfite modification kits, with incubation times <4 h. However, to facilitate the protracted nature of the library preparation, we recommend setting up this reaction and leaving at 4 °C overnight, to complete cleanup and wash steps the following day.
8. In case an adapter dimer is present following the PCR amplification of the bisulfite-converted library (evident by a sharp peak between 120 and 130 bp on the Bioanalyzer), the library should be further cleaned using a 1:0.8 ratio of DNA:beads.
9. There are several safe stopping points throughout the library preparation, refer to the manufacturer's instructions. However, the LM-PCR needs to be carried out within 1–2 days of bisulfite conversion because modified DNA is highly unstable and will be readily degraded thus potentially drastically reducing efficiency of LM-PCR.
10. It is important to ensure that each library has a unique adaptor in order to successfully de-multiplex the libraries after sequencing.
11. These metrics estimate the ratio of CpG vs. non-CpG (CHH, CHG) methylation which provides basic information on the bisulfite conversion efficiency. A high ratio (>98%) is regarded as good bisulfite conversion efficiency. However, if the efficiency is estimated as <98%, the library preparation should be repeated. This is thus a very appropriate internal QC measure that can also be used as a "GO NO-GO" indication.
12. We recommend briefly incubating hybridization reactions on ice for 2 min.
13. Regular mixing of samples and beads is important during the incubation step in order to maintain homogeneity of the

reaction and also ensure effective binding of captured sample to the probes.

14. It is critically important to thoroughly clean the hybridization reactions to remove any unbound probes, as inefficient cleanup will lead to a high off-target percentage.
15. The fastQC tool supplies a "stats" output, which indicates the percentage of each adapter sequence detected, given total adapters detected. Output to the screen also shows the total and percentage of both bases and reads that were trimmed, an efficient metric for determining data quality.
16. An index can be used for multiple samples as long as the genome used is appropriate.
17. For optimal qMSP results, amplicons should be $\leq$150 bp in length. Therefore, depending on the size of the RoI, multiple qMSP assays may need to be designed to ensure adequate coverage of the region and permit methylation interrogation at CpGs throughout the region.
18. The output from qMSP will give information on the CpG sites only within the oligonucleotide hybridization sequence. It is thus important to carefully consider which CpG sites are of primary interest, and design assays with these in mind.
19. In some instances, due to high GC content, it is practically impossible to successfully design oligonucleotides while adhering to the design rules. Because DNA methylation is palindromic, a viable alternative strategy is to take the reverse complement strand and design assays.
20. Often, there is no discriminable difference in Ct or ΔRn between different primer and probe concentrations. In this instance, choose the combination with the lowest probe concentration, as this is typically the most costly reagent in this method. Primer concentrations are best matched within a pair and are typically higher than probe concentration used.
21. When constructing standard curves for qMSP, we recommend performing the qMSP reaction five times, independently, each with three technical replicates. This will enable the construction of a "reference standard curve," which can be used time after time to extrapolate sample DNAs, by simply including two of the six standards on each qMSP plate. In other words, it eliminates the need to repeatedly construct standard curves, once the standards on a given plate amplify in accordance with the reference standards. We set a cut-off value of coefficient of variation <30% between the reference standard curve and the standards performed on individual plates.
22. A nanodrop spectrophotometer can be used to quantify DNA. However, for low yields, Picogreen or qubit fluorescence can perform more accurate levels of detection.

References

1. Spivakov M, Fisher AG (2007) Epigenetic signatures of stem-cell identity. Nat Rev Genet 8 (4):263–271
2. Li M, Liu GH, Izpisua Belmonte JC (2012) Navigating the epigenetic landscape of pluripotent stem cells. Nat Rev Mol Cell Biol 13 (8):524–535
3. Tung PY, Knoepfler PS (2015) Epigenetic mechanisms of tumorigenicity manifesting in stem cells. Oncogene 34(18):2288–2296
4. Fisher CL, Fisher AG (2011) Chromatin states in pluripotent, differentiated, and reprogrammed cells. Curr Opin Genet Dev 21 (2):140–146
5. Lund RJ, Narva E, Lahesmaa R (2012) Genetic and epigenetic stability of human pluripotent stem cells. Nat Rev Genet 13(10):732–744
6. Bird AP (1986) CpG-rich islands and the function of DNA methylation. Nature 321:209–213
7. Esteller M, Corn PG, Baylin SB, Herman JG (2001) A gene hypermethylation profile of human cancer. Cancer Res 61(8):3225–3229
8. Ringrose L, Paro R (2004) Epigenetic regulation of cellular memory by the polycomb and trithorax group proteins. Annu Rev Genet 38:413–443
9. Widschwendter M et al (2007) Epigenetic stem cell signature in cancer. Nat Genet 39 (2):157–158
10. Teschendorff AE et al (2010) Age-dependent DNA methylation of genes that are suppressed in stem cells is a hallmark of cancer. Genome Res 20(4):440–446
11. Wang RY, Gehrke CW, Ehrlich M (1980) Comparison of bisulfite modification of 5-methyldeoxycytidine and deoxycytidine residues. Nucleic Acids Res 8(20):4777–4790
12. Frommer M, McDonald LE, Millar DS, Collis CM, Watt F, Grigg GW, Molloy PL, Paul CL (1992) A genomic sequencing protocol that yields a positive display of 5-methylcytosine residues in individual DNA strands. Proc Natl Acad Sci U S A 89(5):1827–1831
13. Bibikova M et al (2011) High density DNA methylation array with single CpG site resolution. Genomics 98(4):288–295
14. Bock C et al (2010) Quantitative comparison of genome-wide DNA methylation mapping technologies. Nat Biotechnol 28 (10):1106–1114
15. Eads CA, Danenberg KD, Kawakami K, Saltz LB, Blake C, Shibata D, Danenberg PV, Laird PW (2000) MethyLight: a high-throughput assay to measure DNA methylation. Nucleic Acids Res 28(8):E32
16. Harris RA et al (2010) Comparison of sequencing-based methods to profile DNA methylation and identification of monoallelic epigenetic modifications. Nat Biotechnol 28 (10):1097–1105
17. Duhaime-Ross A (2014) Revved-up epigenetic sequencing may foster new diagnostics. Nat Med 20(1):2
18. Li Q et al (2015) Post-conversion targeted capture of modified cytosines in mammalian and plant genomes. Nucleic Acids Res 43(12): e81
19. Perry AS et al (2007) In silico mining identifies IGFBP3 as a novel target of methylation in prostate cancer. Br J Cancer 96 (10):1587–1594
20. Li H et al (2009) The sequence alignment/map format and SAMtools. Bioinformatics 25 (16):2078–2079
21. Li H, Durbin R (2009) Fast and accurate short read alignment with burrows-wheeler transform. Bioinformatics 25(14):1754–1760
22. Li H (2013) Aligning sequence reads, clone sequences and assembly contigs with BWA-MEM. arXiv. 1303.3997(v1[q-bio.GN])
23. Andrews, S. FastQC A quality control tool for high throughput sequence data Available from: http://www.bioinformatics.babraham.ac.uk/projects/fastqc/
24. Bushnell, B. *BBMap*. 2015.; Available from: http://sourceforge.net/projects/bbmap/
25. Pedersen BS, Eyring K, De S, Yang IV, Schwartz DA (2014) Fast and accurate alignment of long bisulfite-seq reads. arXiv. 1401.1129v2([q-bio.GN])
26. Liu Y et al (2012) Bis-SNP: combined DNA methylation and SNP calling for Bisulfite-seq data. Genome Biol 13(7):R61
27. Akalin A et al (2012) MethylKit: a comprehensive R package for the analysis of genome-wide DNA methylation profiles. Genome Biol 13 (10):R87
28. Yegnasubramanian S, Kowalski J, Gonzalgo ML, Zahurak M, Piantadosi S, Walsh PC, Bova GS, De Marzo AM, Isaacs WB, Nelson WG (2004) Hypermethylation of CpG islands in primary and metastatic human prostate cancer. Cancer Res 64(6):1975–1986

Chapter 16

Histones Acetylation and Cancer Stem Cells (CSCs)

Vivian Petersen Wagner, Manoela Domingues Martins, and Rogerio Moraes Castilho

Abstract

Chromatin decondensation is a key mechanism that guarantees gene transcription and repair of the genome, regulated mainly by the acetylation of histones. Emerging evidence has pointed out to histones as a new controlling mechanism of stem cell maintenance and fate. In this chapter, we will focus on the methods used to enrich tumor cell lines for cancer stem cells, and in the methods to identify the status of the histone acetylation in cancer cells and stem cells using immunofluorescence, invasion, and adhesion assays and identification of nuclear size.

Key words Histones acetylation, HDACs, Chromatin, Cytospin, BMI-1, EMT

1 Introduction

Posttranslational modification of histones dynamically influences gene expression independent of alterations in the DNA sequence. These mechanisms are often mediated by histone linkers and by the recruitment of DNA-binding proteins. HDAC I and II interacting proteins along with transcriptional activators, coactivators, or corepressors are also associated with posttranslational events. Histones are molecular markers of epigenetic changes [1]. We found that histological sections of human head and neck squamous cell carcinoma (HNSCC) present a mix expression of histone acetylation throughout the tumor mass. Tumors of epithelial origin like the HNSCC are comprised of malignant cells presenting a plethora of cellular morphologies ranging from small cells displaying a compacted nucleus, to tumor cells showing enlarged nucleus. Neoplastic cells found at the invasive front of tumors often display a fusiform shape containing elongated nucleus. Nuclear sizes reflect the heterogeneity of transcriptional activity found in solid cancers being associated with the status of histone acetylation. While enlarged nuclear size is prone to transcriptional factors binding due to histone acetylation, the smaller nucleus is overall associated

Gianpaolo Papaccio and Vincenzo Desiderio (eds.), *Cancer Stem Cells: Methods and Protocols*, Methods in Molecular Biology, vol. 1692, DOI 10.1007/978-1-4939-7401-6_16, © Springer Science+Business Media LLC 2018

with the deacetylation of histones and silent chromatin (reviewed in [2]). In general, an invasive tumor cell requires high transcription levels of genes driving tumor behavior like increased cellular motility, enhanced invasiveness, and resistance to apoptosis among other tumor characteristics. Histone acetylation is often observed in tumor cells presenting an aggressive behavior, like cells undergoing an epithelial- mesenchyme transition (EMT) [3]. On the contrary, tumor cells presenting reduced levels of histone acetylation are characterized by slow cycling cells and the maintenance of tumor quiescence.

Changes in histone acetylation also impact the "stemness" of cancer stem cells, a subpopulation of tumors cells characterized by slow cycling and retention of the ability to self-renewal. Stem cells and its malignant counterparts are characterized by the expression of high levels of aldehyde dehydrogenase (ALDH). Cancer stem cells account for about 0.5–3% of the total number of tumor cells growing in monolayers. Interestingly, changes in the culture techniques allowing tumor cells to grow under ultra-low adhesion conditions generate tumorspheres that are enriched for CSCs [4]. Differences in the clonogenic potential and aggressiveness between the distinct populations of HNSCC spheres (named holoclones, meroclones, and paraclones) are likely to play a critical role in tumor behavior and resistance to therapy. Tumor cells undergoing sphere-forming assays are reprogramed to express low levels of histone acetylation when compared to high levels of histone acetylation observed on same tumor cells growing in monolayer. Pharmacological induction of histone acetylation also enhances the expression of BMI-1, a major component of the polycomb group complex 1. BMI-1 functions as a vital epigenetic repressor involved in embryonic development and self-renewal of somatic stem cells. BMI-1 overexpression is often upregulated in a variety of cancers and associated with tumor aggressiveness and poor survival [3], (reviewed in [1]). Along BMI-1 expression, histone deacetylase inhibitors also result in increased tumor invasion and the acquisition of EMT phenotype, along with the expression of the mesenchyme marker vimentin [3].

Thus, our studies have set up a series of technical conditions to explore the role of histone modifications in the maintenance of cancer stem cells. Much of our effort is focus on solid tumors from the head and neck anatomical that includes squamous cell carcinomas, mucoepidermoid carcinomas, and adenoid cystic carcinomas. We have described many of these techniques in this chapter hoping to facilitate the development of new research focusing on cancer biology of solid tumors.

2 Materials

As the basis for the experiments described herein, all the solutions were prepared using ultrapure water (purified deionized water to achieve a sensitivity of 18 MΩ-cm at 25 °C) and analytical grade reagents. Buffers and reagents were stored at room temperature, at 4 °C, or at −20 °C as indicated. Waste disposal follows Occupational Safety and Health Administration (OSHA) and institutional safety regulations.

2.1 Cell Lines

We have used a series of solid tumor cell lines derived from the head and neck anatomical area. Below are the most common cell lines we use along with its origin. A similar protocol applies to cell lines of different origin.

1. Head and neck squamous cell carcinoma cell lines generated at the Wayne State University [5].
2. Head and neck squamous cell carcinoma cell lines generated at the University of Michigan School of Medicine [6, 7].
3. Mucoepidermoid carcinoma cell lines generated at the University of Michigan School of Dentistry [8].
4. Adenoid cystic carcinoma primary human cell lines generated at the University of Michigan School of Dentistry [9].
5. Normal oral keratinocyte cell line generated at the National Institute of Dental and Craniofacial Research [10].

2.2 Spheres Assay

Stem cells possess anchorage independence growth abilities. Therefore, these cells have the capacity to survive and proliferate under adherent-free culture conditions. Sphere assays represent a cost-effective method for drug screening in which CSCs are the target population.

1. Costar® 6 Well Clear Flat Bottom Ultra-Low Attachment Multiple Well Plates, Individually Wrapped and Sterile.
2. Medium (*see* **Note 1**).
   (a) DMEM1, for the oral squamous cell carcinoma and oral keratinocyte cell lines: 500 mL of DMEM/High glucose with L-glutamine; without sodium pyruvate. Add 10% of Fetal Bovine Serum and 1% of antibiotic/antimycotic cocktail.
   (b) DMEM2, for the oral squamous cell carcinoma UMSCC22A and UMSCC22B cells line: 500 mL of DMEM/High glucose with L-glutamine; without sodium pyruvate. Add 10% of Fetal Bovine Serum; 1% L-glutamine, 1% amino acids, and 0.1% of gentamicin.
   (c) RPMI, for mucoepidermoid carcinoma cell lines and adenoid cystic carcinoma primary cells: 500 mL of RPMI

1640 supplement with 10% of Fetal Bovine Serum, 1% antibiotic, 1% L-glutamine, 1 mL of 10 μg/mL epidermal growth factor, 4 mL of 50 μg/mL hydrocortisone, and 250 μL of 10 μg/mL insulin.

3. Histone acetyltransferase inhibitor: Curcumin, Curcuma longa L.
4. Histone deacetylase inhibitor: SAHA/Varinostat.

2.3 Cytospin

1. Fisherbrand™ Superfrost™ Plus Microscope Slides.
2. Cytospin tank (*see* **Note 2**).
3. Gel Blot Paper (*see* **Note 3**).
4. Drive Punch (*see* **Note 4**).
5. PBS.
6. Centrifuge.
7. Ethanol.
8. Hematoxylin.
9. Eosin.
10. Safeclear (Nonhazardous alternative to Xylene).
11. Paraformaldehyde.
12. PBS.
13. Coverslip (60 × 24 mm).
14. Slide mounting medium (e.g., Permount).

2.4 Immunofluorescence

1. PBS.
2. Tween-20.
3. BSA.
4. Primary antibodies:
   (a) Acetyl- histone H3.
   (b) Phospho-p65.
   (c) DNMT1.
   (d) Acetyl-CBP/p300.
   (e) NF-kappa-B p65.
   (f) BMI-1.
5. Secondary antibodies of appropriate source/fluorochrome for double staining.
6. Hoechst 33342.
7. Fluoroshield® aqueous histology mounting medium (Sigma-Aldrich) or similar.

2.5 Tumorsphere Isolation According to Morphology

1. Inverted phase contrast microscope.

2.6 Adhesion Assay

1. Culture dish for adherent cells, 60 mm Polystyrene dish.

2.7 Nuclear Size Assay

1. Trypsin-EDTA (0.025%).
2. PBS.
3. Methanol.
4. Cytospin materials.

2.8 Invasion Assay

1. Fibronectin.
2. Millicell Cell Culture Inserts® containing polycarbonate filter membrane with 8 μm-diameter pores in 24-well plates (Millipore, Billerica, MA, USA) or similar.
3. Medium supplemented with 20% of fetal bovine serum (*see* **Note 5**) according to cell lines.
4. Hematoxylin.
5. Eosin.

3 Methods

Carry out all the procedures at room temperature unless otherwise specified.

3.1 Spheres Assay

1. Add Trypsin/EDTA to detach your cells.
2. Seed between 2.5×10^3 and 5×10^3 cells in each well of the Ultra-Low Attachment plates (6-well plate). The final volume should be 2 mL per well.
3. Leave cells growing for 5 days in a 5% CO_2-humidified incubator at 37 °C. Avoid disturbing cells during this period. Some cell lines may require more days to form spheres. We suggest performing an initial assay to establish the correct time of culturing for each cell line.
4. After 5 days of culture, tumorspheres are formed. At this period, analysis on the number of spheres, the proportion between holoclones, meroclones and paraclones, adhesion assay, and invasion assay can proceed. Single-cell suspension following flow cytometry and the evaluation of nuclear size can also be conducted.

   Here is an example of drugs used in our laboratory to study the behavior of CSCs upon changes in chromatin organization. It is critical to take in consideration when the chosen drug should be administered to the spheres.

Drugs intent to therapy of solid tumors should be administered 5 days after seeding of tumor cells under low adhesion conditions. Administration of drugs designed to enrich the population or CSC or SC should initiate the treatment at day 2. By the second day, the primordial sphere is already formed and composed of few cells. At this time, administration of pro-stem cells factors/small molecules has the potential to enrich the population of stem cells/CSCs. In each case, the timing of drug administration is the key for the outcome.

(a) Inducing stem cell differentiation using histone deacetylase inhibitors on tumor spheres: In this assay, the goal is to study the ability of HDAC inhibitors in reducing the population of CSCs. Toward this aim, tumor cells are seeded for 5 days until tumorspheres are formed. Tumorspheres are exposed to SAHA (HDACi) for 24 h at the specific concentration (IC_{50}) determined for each tumor cell line (*see* **Note 6**). Follow-up of tumor sphere shape, form, and the number should be recorded every hour. Typically, morphological changes of sphere will be evident within the first 5 h.

(b) Accumulation of CSCs driven by histone acetyltransferase inhibition: This essay challenges the potential ability of HATi in maintaining the "stemness" of tumor cells. We expect to observe the maintenance of tumorspheres for a longer period compared to control spheres. Curcumin is a HAT inhibitor (*see* **Note 7**). Tumor cells are seeded in ultra- low adhesion culture plates and left to grow for 2 days. Once small spheres are observed under a microscope, Curcumin is administered to the culture media and tumorspheres are closely monitored for changes in number, growth rate, size, and potential selective outgrowth of holoclones, meroclones, or paraclones.

Upon completion of the sphere forming assay, all tumorspheres can be analyzed either by transferring all spheres to a glass slide (Cytospin), or by challenging tumorsphere properties using adhesion, or invasion assays. Spheres can also be disrupted into single-cell suspension using a gentle mechanical pipetting in combination with trypsin/EDTA to be further processed for cell sorting and nuclear sizing (Scheme 1).

3.2 Cytospin

1. Preferentially use refrigerated centrifuge (4 °C) during Cytospin.
2. Prepare Gel Blot papers to be used with a Cytospin tank. Dip the chamber stamp on a stain solution (ex: crystal violet; trypan blue) and print it on the Gel Blot Paper. Cut the paper according to the stamp format (Fig. 1).

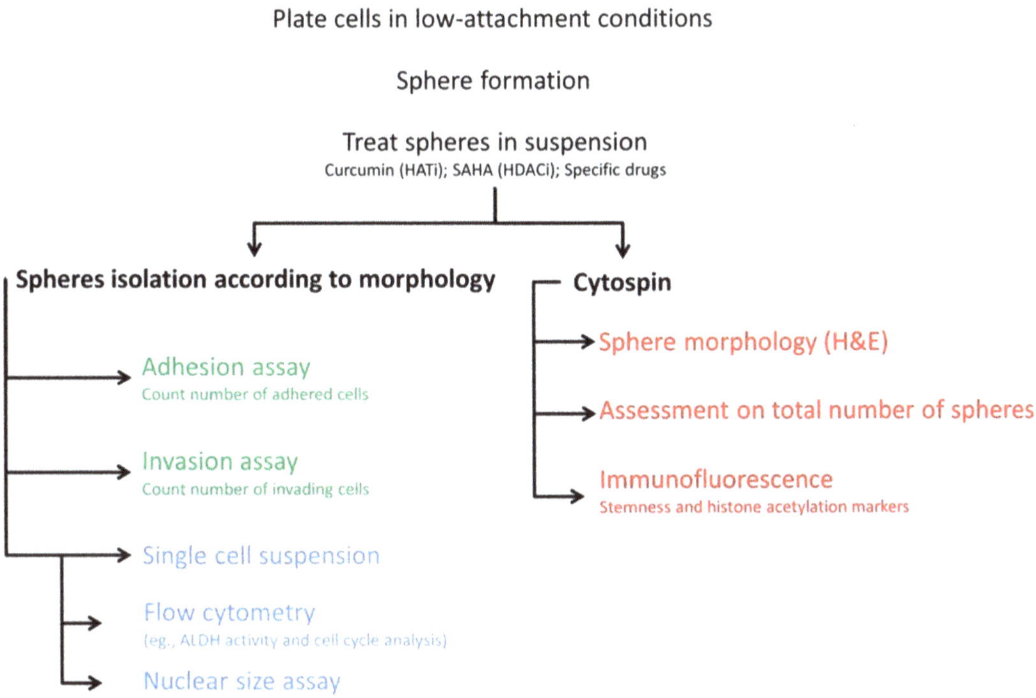

Scheme 1 Examples of potential assays using tumorspheres. Spheres can be isolated by its morphology (Holo, mero, and paraclones) (*green* and *blue*), or can be transferred to glass slides using Cytospin (*red*)

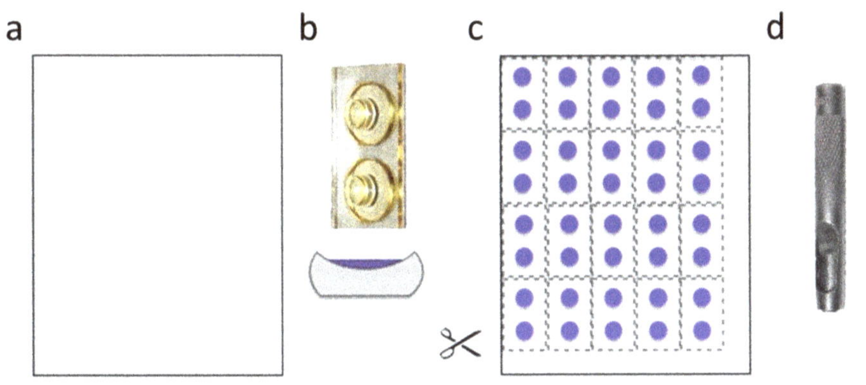

Fig. 1 Gel Blot paper preparation. (**a**) Gel Blot Paper. (**b**) Cytos pin chamber stamp and staining solution. (**c**) Gel Blot Paper appearance after stain with Cytos pin chamber stamp. Once dry, cut according to the chamber size and remove the round stained part with a drive punch (**d**). The punch diameter must match the Cytos pin chamber diameter; an 8 mm drive punch is represented

3. Identify superfrost slides. Use one slide for each well according to the assay.
4. Assemble the Cytospin tank according to Fig. 2.
5. For each culture dish well, carefully collect the medium (2 mL) containing the spheres in suspension and pippet 1 mL of the medium in each cylinder of the chamber.

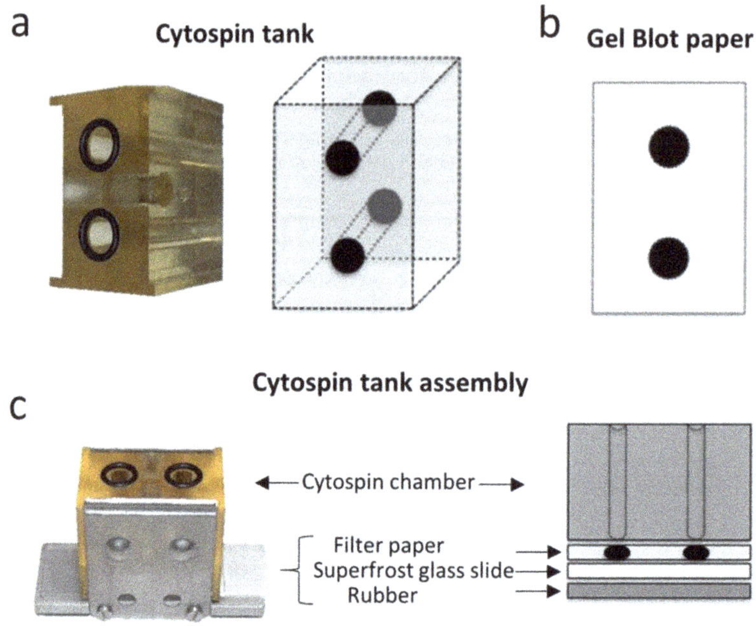

Fig. 2 Cytos pin tank preparation. (**a**) Cytospin chamber containing two hollow cylinders. (**b**) Gel Blot paper cut in the same size of the chamber and containing two holes that match the hollow areas of the cytos pin tank. (**c**) In the Cytos pin tank place 1—the rubber (offers protection to the slide); 2—the superfrost identified slide; 3—the filter paper; 4—the Cytos pin chamber (observe that holes of chamber and paper must coincide)

6. Further, remove any sphere leftover in the culture wells by washing with 2 mL of PBS. Pippet 1 mL of PBS containing spheres in each cylinder of the tank.
7. Place the Cytospin tank into the centrifuge. Ensure that the centrifuge is correctly balanced.
8. Centrifuge at 300 × *g* 4 °C for 10 min.
9. After finished, slides may be fixed and further processed for immunofluorescence or stained with eosin & hematoxylin.
10. Fixation:
    (a) Fixate slides with paraformaldehyde 4% in PBS for 20 min at room temperature (*see* **Note 8**).
11. Staining:
    (a) Eosin staining—1 min.
    (b) Water bath.
    (c) Hematoxylin staining—30 s.
    (d) Water bath.
    (e) Alcohol 70%—5 min.
    (f) Alcohol 95%—5 min.
    (g) Alcohol 100%—5 min.

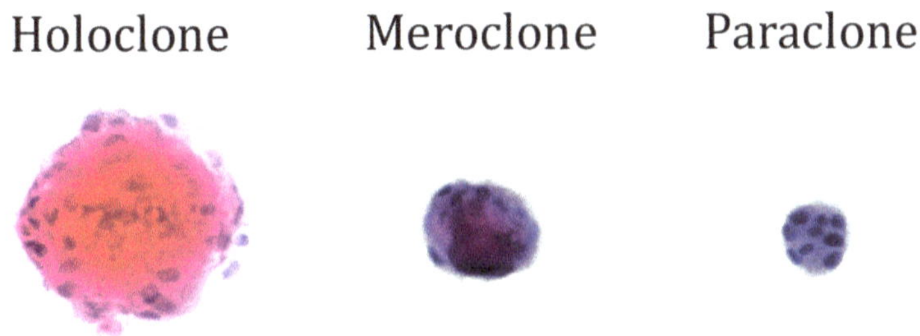

Fig. 3 Representative images of holoclone, meroclone, and paraclone stained with H&E. Its size and shape define the type of sphere

(h) Mount coverslips with permount without any pressure on the spheres. For optimal results use coverslips with high edges (e.g., Arrayit Corporation, Arrayit LifterSlip™ coverslips (Cat. CST1).

3.3 Spheres Analysis (H&E Stained Slides)

1. Using a conventional light microscope count the number of spheres according to each subtype in each slide (Fig. 3).

3.4 Immunofluorescence

1. After spheres are fixed with paraformaldehyde, Wash slides with PBS 3 × 5′ each.
2. Incubate slides with PBS-T + BSA 3% (*see* **Note 9**) for 60 min at room temperature.
3. Incubate primary antibody diluted in PBS-T + BSA 3% overnight in a humid chamber at 4 °C (*see* **Note 10**)—ensure that all slide is covered with the antibody once that spheres can be spread throughout the slide after cytospin. The antibodies and dilutions suggested are the following (*see* **Note 11**):
   (a) Acetyl-H3 (lys9)—1:200.
   (b) CBP/p300—1:100.
   (c) DNMT1—1:40.
   (d) p65—1:50.
   (e) BMI—1:50.
4. Wash each slide with PBS 3 × 5 min.
5. Incubate secondary antibody for 90 min in a humid chamber at room temperature in the dark (*see* **Note 12**) 1:200 diluted in PBS-T + BSA 3%.
6. Wash slides with PBS 3 × 5 min each.
7. DNA staining—Hoechst 33342 (stored at 4 °C) diluted 1:500 in water for 5 min.
8. Wash slides with PBS 3 × 5 min each.
9. Wash slides with water 2 × 5 min each.
10. Mount coverslips with fluoroshield.

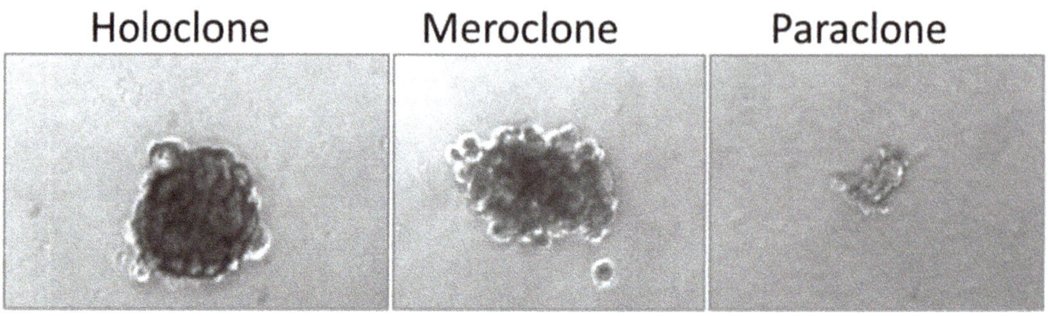

Fig. 4 Images obtained from the inverted microscope (Nikon Eclipse TS100) coupled to an external camera (Qimaging Publisher 5). No coloration is used to identify tumorspheres subtype

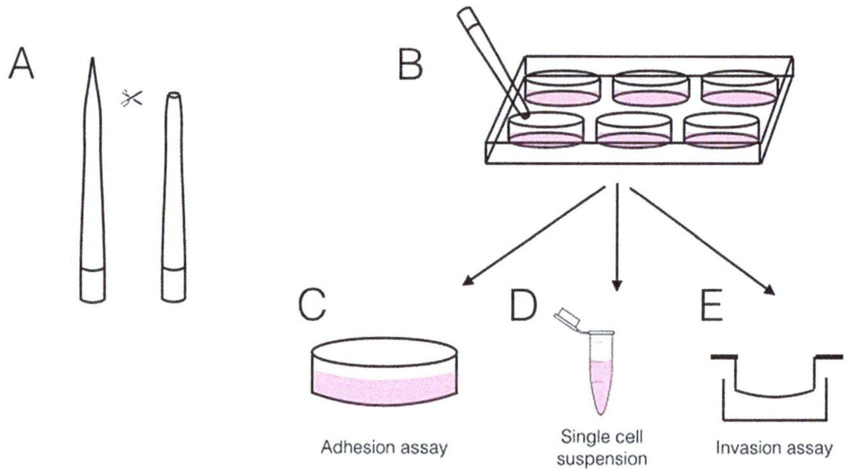

Fig. 5 (**a**) P1000 pipette tips must be cut at the tip before tumorspheres collection. (**b**) Collect each subtype of tumorspheres (holoclones, meroclones, and paraclones) under an inverted microscope. (**c**) Seed each subtype of tumorspheres ($n = 10$) in a new regular cell culture dish for adhesion assay or (**d**) place tumorspheres in 1.5 mL test tubes to disrupt spheres into single-cell suspension or (**e**) seed tumorspheres in a Millicell Cell Culture Inserts containing a fibronectin layer for invasion assay

3.5 Tumorsphere Isolation According to Morphology

1. Observe spheres under ultra-low adhesion conditions and identify each tumorsphere subtype (holoclone, meroclone, and paraclone) under an inverted phase contrast microscope (Fig. 4).
2. Cut the tip of a P1000 pipette tip to reduce stress over tumor spheres during pipetting.
3. Under an inverted microscope, collect the tumorspheres of a particular subtype (Fig. 5b) and:
   (a) Seed 10 tumorspheres in a conventional culture dish to perform an adhesion assay (Fig. 5c).
   (b) Place tumorspheres in a test tube to process for cytospin (Fig. 5b).

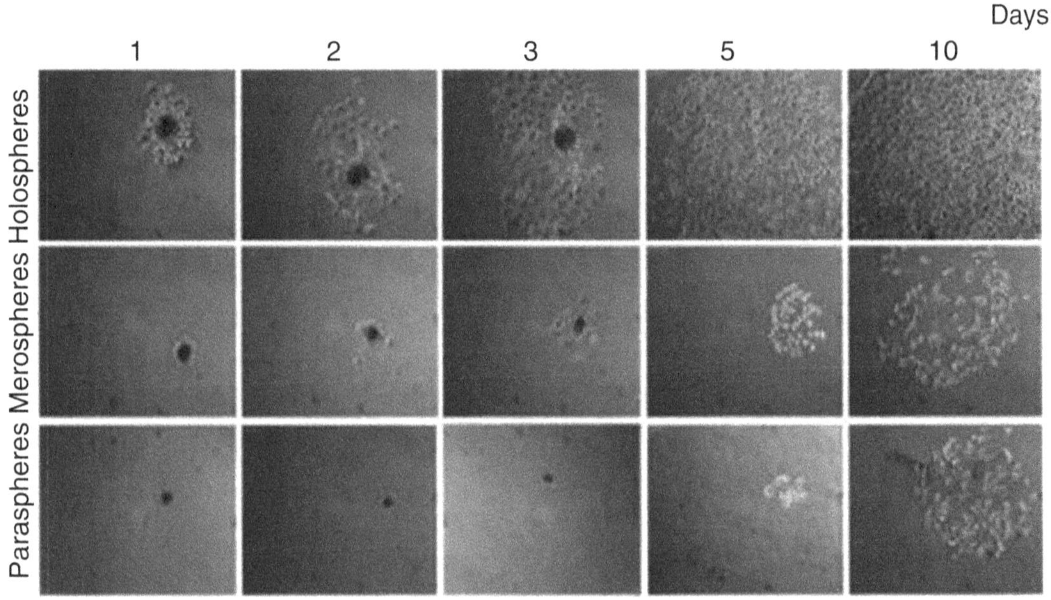

Fig. 6 Representative examples of holospheres, merospheres, and paraspheres attachment potential during a 10-day follow-up period. (*Source*: Almeida et al. Cancers 2016, 8(1):7; doi:10.3390/cancers8010007 [4]).

(c) Seed tumorspheres in a Millicell Cell Culture Inserts containing a fibronectin layer previously prepared for an invasion assay (Fig. 5c).

3.6 Adhesion Assay

1. Seed ten tumorspheres of each subtype (holoclones, meroclones, and paraclones) in a conventional culture dish.
2. Observe under an inverted microscope each sphere for 10 days and note the day of attachment of each sphere to obtain the adhesion efficiency of each subtype of tumorspheres.
3. Images should be taken at each day during the follow-up period (Fig. 6).

3.7 Nuclear Size

1. Place tumorspheres in 1.5 mL test tubes containing 1 mL of trypsin/EDTA. Incubate for 5 min at 37 °C following by gently pipetting tumorspheres up and down to detach spheres and create a single cell suspension.
2. Centrifuge cells at 300 rpm for 5 min at room temperature.
3. Aspirate the supernatant containing trypsin/EDTA.
4. Add 1 mL of PBS and centrifuge cells for 300 rpm for 5 min at room temperature.
5. Aspirate the supernatant containing PBS.
6. Fix cells by adding 1 mL of precooled methanol 100% (*see* **Note 13**) and incubate for 5 min at −20 °C.

7. Centrifuge cells at 300 rpm for 5 min at room temperature.
8. Remove methanol and wash cells with PBS.
9. Proceed to Cytospin assay following staining with hematoxylin & eosin.
10. Using a microscope, capture representative images of cells dispersed throughout the slide.
11. Quantification of number of cells and nuclear size can be performed using ImageJ (Open source NIH software https://ima gej. nih. go v/ij/inde x. html) following the next steps:
    (a) Open the image on ImageJ.
    (b) Using the "freehand selections" option underline the edges of cell nuclei and then click on analyze > measure and note the area (in pixels).
    (c) All cells nuclei can be underlined before asking for the areas.

3.8 Invasion Assay

1. Preparation of Millicell Cell Culture Inserts should be conducted inside a cell culture laminar flow. One day before the experiment, add 250 μL of fibronectin 10 μg/mL to each chamber of the Millicell Cell Culture Inserts.
2. Leave the Millicell Cell Culture Inserts containing fibronectin for 1 h until fibronectin is dry, wash twice with dH_2O.
3. Store the Millicell Cell Culture Inserts containing fibronectin at 4 °C until tumorspheres are ready for seeding.
4. Seed tumorspheres on the Millicell Cell Culture Inserts coated with fibronectin. The number of spheres seeded in each invasion chamber reflected a total of 1×10^3 cells; therefore, the total number of spheres varied among holospheres, merospheres, and paraspheres.
5. Add 400 μL of medium supplemented with 10% FBS inside the Millicell Cell Culture Inserts. To create a gradient between the upper and the lower part of the invasion chamber, add 700 μL of medium supplemented with 20% FBS in the lower compartment (Fig. 7).
6. Incubate chambers for 24 h inside a cell culture incubator at 37 °C, and 5% CO_2 atmosphere.
7. Fix the membrane with precooled Methanol 100% (*see* **Note 13**) and incubate for 5 min at −20 °C.
8. Wash the membrane with PBS.
9. Stain with Hematoxylin for 10 min.
10. Wash with H_2O 2 × 5 min.
11. Stain with eosin for 5 min.

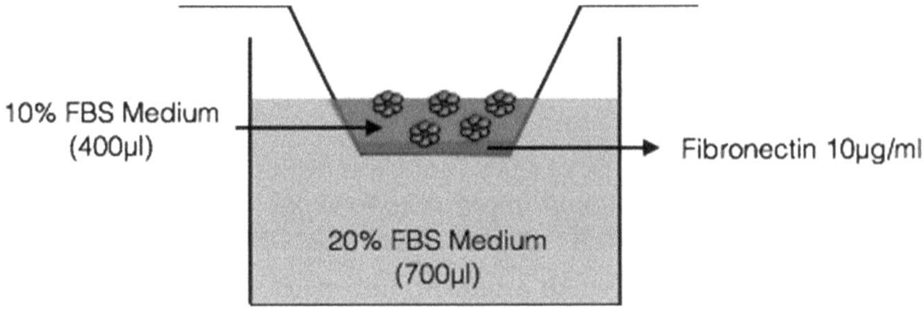

Fig. 7 Representative image of Millicell Cell Culture Inserts. The spheres are seeded on the upper part containing 10% FBS medium with a bottom of fibronectin layer. The cells invade during 24 h through the membrane to the lower part containing 20% FBS medium

12. Wash with H_2O 2 × 5 min.
13. Using a swab, clean the upper portion of the Millicell Cell Culture Inserts containing cells that did not invade, and also removing the fibronectin coat. Only cells located underneath and outside of the insert are considered invasive.
14. Using a surgical blade, carefully cut the bottom of the inserts (membrane portion) containing the invasive cells and mount onto a glass slide (facing up) using water base mounting media (e.g., Fluoroshield).
15. Photograph at least four representative areas for each insert and count the number of invading cells.

3.9 Reproducibility and Rigor

The maintenance of reproducibility and rigor in research are essential to better understanding the biological process. Toward this goal, the incorporation of blinding and randomization to reduce bias, clear laboratory practices for data collection and analyses, and transparency in reporting results and feasibility assays are essential. A quality system of operation in the laboratories should be emphasized through the development of Standard Operating Procedures (SOP). Blind administration of drugs and small molecules should be carried out as a routine, as well as the data collection and analyses of the results. The selection of a control group should be specified for each experiment and taking into consideration all the variables regarding population, drug, and conditions. Experiments should be repeated independently and in triplicates for each condition.

4 Notes

1. Use the appropriate medium that your cells grow under normal conditions.
2. The Cytospin tank is composed of a tank that fits in the centrifuge with an internal space for the chamber to adapt; the

Cytospin chamber containing two hollow cylinders; a rubber to protect the slide. Cytospin technique can also be performed using a variety of products (e.g., Biomedical Polymers Cytology Funnels, and Cytospin starter kit from ThermoFisher).

3. The use of a Gel Blot paper with the appropriate thickness is of paramount importance to avoid loss of spheres during centrifugation (e.g., Whatman® Gel Blot GB003).
4. The punch diameter must match the diameter of the Cytospin chamber cylinders. We use an 8 mm drive punch. Note: several Cytospin systems offer precut filters that dispense the use of the punch.
5. Use the appropriate medium for each cell line supplemented with 20% fetal bovine serum instead of 10%.
6. SAHA IC50 must be determined for each cell type. In our experience, these concentrations ranged from 15 to 50 μM/mL.
7. Curcumin concentrations must be determined for each cell type. In our experience, concentrations ranging from 25 to 50 μM/mL were effective in inhibiting HAT activity.
8. Prepare the solution immediately before using.
9. Prepare the solution using 1.5 g of BSA and 125 μL of Tween in 50 mL of PSB. After use store the solution on 4 °C.
10. The humid chamber is of paramount importance to avoid spheres to dry.
11. Some antibodies might need new standardization in different cell lines.
12. All the steps from now must be performed in the dark.
13. Cool methanol on −20 °C for at least 24 h before use.

References

1. Martins MD, Castilho RM (2013) Histones: controlling tumor signaling circuitry. J Carcinog Mutagen 1(Suppl 5):1–12
2. Struhl K (1998) Histone acetylation and transcriptional regulatory mechanisms. Genes Dev 12(5):599–606
3. Giudice FS, Pinto DS Jr, Nor JE, Squarize CH, Castilho RM (2013) Inhibition of histone deacetylase impacts cancer stem cells and induces epithelial- mesenchyme transition of head and neck cancer. PLoS One 8(3):e58672
4. Almeida LO, Guimaraes DM, Squarize CH, Castilho RM (2016) Profiling the behavior of distinct populations of head and neck cancer stem cells. Cancers (Basel) 8(1):E7
5. Cardinali M, Pietraszkiewicz H, Ensley JF, Robbins KC (1995) Tyrosine phosphorylation as a marker for aberrantly regulated growth-promoting pathways in cell lines derived from head and neck malignancies. Int J Cancer 61(1):98–103
6. Carey TE, Van Dyke DL, Worsham MJ et al (1989) Characterization of human laryngeal primary and metastatic squamous cell carcinoma cell lines UM- SCC-17A and UM-SCC-17B. Cancer Res 49(21):6098–6107
7. Bradford CR, Zhu S, Ogawa H et al (2003) P53 mutation correlates with cisplatin sensitivity in head and neck squamous cell carcinoma lines. Head Neck 25(8):654–661

8. Warner KA, Adams A, Bernardi L et al (2013) Characterization of tumorigenic cell lines from the recurrence and lymph node metastasis of a human salivary mucoepidermoid carcinoma. Oral Oncol 49(11):1059–1066
9. Acasigua GA, Warner KA, Nor F et al (2015) BH3-mimetic small molecule inhibits the growth and recurrence of adenoid cystic carcinoma. Oral Oncol 51(9):839–847
10. Castilho RM, Squarize CH, Leelahavanichkul K, Zheng Y, Bugge T, Gutkind JS (2010) Rac1 is required for epithelial stem cell function during dermal and oral mucosal wound healing but not for tissue homeostasis in mice. PLoS One 5(5):e10503

Chapter 17

Immunohistochemistry for Cancer Stem Cells Detection: Principles and Methods

Martina Intartaglia, Rosalaura Sabetta, Monica Gargiulo, Giovanna Roncador, Federica Zito Marino, and Renato Franco

Abstract

Cancer stem cells (CSCs) are rare immortal cells within a tumor that can self-renew and drive tumorigenesis. CSCs play a pivotal role in the tumor development, progression and relapse, as well as in the resistance of anticancer therapy. Different tools could help in the analysis of CSCs, especially Immunohistochemistry (IHC) represents a useful technique able to identify several specific CSC markers. The main aims of this chapter are the description of the explain immunohistochemical methods used in the characterization of CSCs. Furthermore, focus on the most common troubleshooting in CSCs IHC is provided, especially the pitfalls of the CSCs markers IHC on tissue microarrays.

Key words Cancer stem cells (CSCs), Antigen retrieval, Detection methods, Fixation, Immunohistochemistry, Standardization, Troubleshooting

1 Introduction

Cancer stem cells (CSCs) comprise a rare subpopulation of tumor cells quiescent and self-renewing that play a key role in the tumor development, progression, and relapse. CSCs have an unlimited potential cell division leading to possible metastasis and relapse of the disease [1]. Several findings reported that CSCs have been identified in many tumor types, including colorectal, breast, ovary, pancreas, prostate, melanoma, head, and neck cancer [2, 3].

Since CSCs survive to radio and chemotherapies treatments, they give rise to recurrence or new primary tumors. Therefore, CSCs are frequently associated with the resistance to the treatment providing the requirements to optimize cancer therapy.

CSC could be identified through the cell surface marker expression by using staining techniques in tumor sections or by gene expression arrays [4, 5].

Several CSC markers have been identified for many cancer types, their expression is often evaluated by IHC that ensures an

Gianpaolo Papaccio and Vincenzo Desiderio (eds.), *Cancer Stem Cells: Methods and Protocols*, Methods in Molecular Biology, vol. 1692, DOI 10.1007/978-1-4939-7401-6_17, © Springer Science+Business Media LLC 2018

easy clinical applicability. Each different cancer type could express specific markers, as shown in Table 1.

The main aims of this chapter are to explain materials and methods, as well as the standardization and troubleshooting in immunohistochemistry assay. Finally, we describe the pitfalls of the IHC on tissue microarrays (TMA) to detect cancer stem cells.

Immunohistochemistry (IHC) is a technique that allows the visualization of an antigen and its location in tissue sections using a specific antigen-antibody reaction.

Over time, many improvements have been made in the standardization of IHC methods in order to use this assay in various fields including immunology, histology, and chemistry. To date, being a high sensitive and specific method, IHC represents an essential tool for routine diagnosis and research. The application of IHC has been widely expanded in pathology field, for example it is used for the differential diagnosis, the identification of the site of the primary tumor in metastatic patients.

Two different IHC approaches could be used: indirect and direct methods. The indirect method involves an unlabeled primary antibody that binds the specific antigen, a labeled secondary antibody that reacts with primary antibody. In particular, the secondary antibody is conjugated to an enzyme, most often horseradish peroxidase (HRP) or alkaline phosphatase (AP), that reacts with substrate yielding a chromogenic development. Conversely, the direct method uses a primary antibody directly conjugated to an enzyme, which is then activated by adding a substrate producing a detectable product. The direct detection not requires the use of a secondary antibody. (Fig. 1).

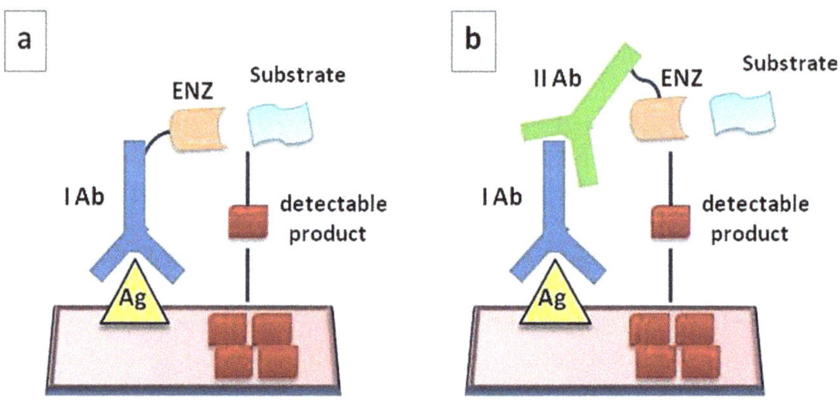

Fig. 1 Immunohistochemistry methods: direct (**a**) and indirect (**b**). *Ag* Antigen of interest; *I Ab* Primary Antibody; *II Ab* Secondary Antibody; *ENZ* Enzyme

Table 1
The main cancer stem cells markers [6].

Cancer types	Cancer stem cells markers
BLADDER	Aldehyde dehydrogenase, 1-A1/ALDH1A1, CD44, CD47, CEACAM-6/CD66c
BREAST	Aldehyde dehydrogenase, 1-A1/ALDH1A1, BMI-1, CD24, CD44, CD133, Connexin 43/GJA1, CXCR4, DLL4, EpCAM/TROP1, ErbB2/Her2, GLI-1, GLI-2, IL-1 alpha/IL-1F1, IL-6 R alpha, CXCR1/IL-8 RA, integrin alpha 6/CD49f, PON1, PTEN
COLON	ALCAM/CD166, aldehyde dehydrogenase, 1-A1/ALDH1A1, CD44, CD133, DPPIV/CD26, EpCAM/TROP1, GLI-1, Lgr5/GPR49, Musashi-1
GASTRIC	CD44, DLL4, Lgr5/GPR49
GLIOMA/ MEDULLOBLASTOMA	A20/TNFAIP3, ABCG2, aldehyde dehydrogenase, 1-A1/ALDH1A1, BMI-1, CD15/Lewis X, CD44, CD133, CX3CL1/Fractalkine, CX3CR1, CXCR4, HIF-2 alpha/EPAS1, IL-6 R alpha, integrin alpha 6/CD49f, L1CAM, c-Maf, Musashi-1, c-Myc, nestin, Podoplanin, SOX2
HEAD and NECK	ABCG2, aldehyde dehydrogenase, 1-A1/ALDH1A1, BMI-1, CD44, HGF R/c-MET, Lgr5/GPR49
LEUKEMIA	BMI-1, CD34, CD38, CD44, CD47, CD96, CD117/c-kit, GLI-1, GLI-2, IL-3 R alpha/CD123, MICL/CLEC12A, Musashi-2, TIM-3
LIVER	Alpha-fetoprotein/AFP, Aminopeptidase N/CD13, CD45, CD45.1, CD45.2, CD90/Thy1CD90, NF2/Merlin
LUNG	ABCG2, aldehyde dehydrogenase, 1-A1/ALDH1A1, CD90/Thy1, CD117/c-kit, EpCAM/TROP1
MELANOMA	ABCB5, ABCG2, ALCAM/CD166, CD133, MS4A1/CD20, nestin, NGF R/TNFRSF16
MYELOMA	ABCB5, CD19, CD27/TNFRSF7, CD38, MS4A1/CD20, Syndecan-1/CD138
OSTEOSARCOMA	ABCG2, CD44, Endoglin/CD105, nestin, STRO-1
OVARIAN	Alpha-Methylacyl-CoA, Racemase/AMACR, CD44, CD117/c-kit, Endoglin/CD105, Ovastacin
PANCREATIC	Aldehyde dehydrogenase, 1-A1/ALDH1A1, BMI-1, CD24, CD44, CXCR4, EpCAM/TROP1, PON1
PROSTATE	ABCG2, ALCAM/CD166, aldehyde dehydrogenase, 1-A1/ALDH1A1, alpha-Methylacyl-CoA, Racemase/AMACR, BMI-1, CD44, CD151, c-Maf, c-Myc, TRA-1-60(R)

2 Materials

2.1 Buffers, Diluents, and Antigen Retrieval Solutions

1. Wash buffer: It corresponds to tris buffer normal saline (TBS) (0.05 M Tris, 0.15 M NaCl, 0.05% Tween 20, pH 7.6). It employs TBS 10× and dilutes with distilled water to obtain a working solution (*see* **Notes 1** and **2**).
2. Antibody diluent, background reducing (e.g., Dako #S2022).
3. Target retrieval solution citrate, pH 6 (e.g., Dako #S2031). Add 900 mL of distilled water to 100 mL of target retrieval solution to prepare a working dilution.
4. Target retrieval solution EDTA, pH 9.0 (e.g., Dako #S2367). To prepare a working dilution, add 900 mL of distilled water to 100 mL target retrieval solution.
5. Target retrieval solution, high pH Tris, pH 10.0 from Dako. To prepare a working dilution, add 900 mL of distilled water to 100 mL target retrieval solution (*see* **Note 3**).
6. Proteinase K.

2.2 Substrates, Chromogens, and Counterstain Solutions

1. Hydrogen peroxide-DAB Solution (e.g., Dako #K3467), used for peroxidase-based immunohistochemical methods (*see* **Notes 4** and **5**).
2. Permanent red substrate-chromogen (e.g., Dako #K064).
3. Mayer's hematoxylin (*see* **Note 6**).

2.3 Endogenous Activities Blocking Solutions

1. Peroxidase and alkaline phosphatase blocking reagent (e.g., Dako S2003) (*see* **Notes 7** and **8**).
2. Protein block, serum free (e.g., Dako #X0909) (*see* **Note 9**).
3. Biotin blocking system from (e.g., Dako #X0590) (*see* **Note 10**).

3 Methods

In order to maintain cell morphology, tissue architecture, and the antigenicity of target epitopes, the complete preparation of the sample is very important, while, for signal visualization, the use of the right antibodies to target the correct antigens is critical.

3.1 Tissue Fixation and Processing

There are several critical points in procedures of IHC, including the correct handling of the sample from the appropriate fixation to adequate paraffin block preparation.

Fixation chemically is critical because it crosslinks proteins or reduces protein solubility, which can mask target antigens during prolonged or improper fixation. The gold standard fixative for routine histology and immunohistochemistry is formaldehyde, which is a semi-reversible, covalent crosslinking reagent that can be used for perfusion or immersion fixation for any length of time, depending on the level of fixation required. Minimal fixation of 1–2 days is recommended (*see* **Note 11**).

After fixation, tissue samples are embedded in paraffin to maintain the natural shape and architecture of the sample during long-term storage and sectioning for IHC.

Paraffin-embedded tissue samples are sectioned into slices as thin as 4–5 μm with a microtome. Then these sections are mounted on glass slides. These glass slides are particular because they are coated with an adhesive, which is added by surface-treating glass slides with 3- aminopropyltriethoxysilane (APTS) or poly-L-lysine, which both leave amino groups on the surface of the glass to which the tissue directly couples.

After mounting, the sections are dried in an oven or microwave in preparation for deparaffinization.

Before proceeding with the staining protocol, the slides must be deparaffinized and rehydrated.

The paraffin from sections must be completely removed for the antibodies to reach the target antigens with xylene, which is a flammable, toxic, and volatile organic solvent. So, the samples are heated to 55 °C for 10 min to melt the paraffin and then washed two times with xylene for 7 min each. Then the sample is rehydrated through graded washes of ethanol in water, ending in pure water (Fig. 2). From this point until final mounting, the slides must remain wet to prevent nonspecific antibody binding and high background staining.

Formalin-fixed, paraffin-embedded tissue sections always need a treatment to unmask the antibody epitopes, either by heat (heat-induced epitope retrieval; HIER) or enzymatic degradation (proteolytic-induced epitope retrieval; PIER). These steps represent a critical phase because, if the antibodies will not have complete access to the tissue, they will be unable to bind to the correct epitopes.

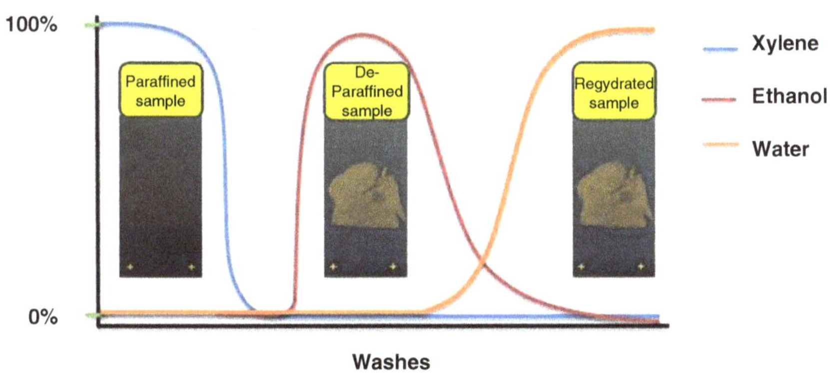

Fig. 2 The optimal washes used to deparaffinize and rehydrate formalin fixed paraffin embedded tissue samples (FFPE). Two consecutive washes with xylene are used to deparaffinize the tissues. Xylene is then removed by an ethanol decreasing scale (from 100 to 70%) and finally the sample is hydrated by graded washes of ethanol to water

In order to avoid false positive and high background detection, endogenous biotin, peroxidase, phosphatases, or other enzyme activity must be blocked; to reach this aim, physically or chemically blocking strategies are employed.

Antibodies bind with avidity to specific epitopes, but they may partially or weakly bind to reactive sites that are sites on nonspecific proteins and these sites are similar to the cognate-binding sites on the target antigen. This nonspecific binding causes high background staining that can mask the detection of the target antigen.

In order to decrease background staining in IHC, tissue samples are incubated with a buffer that blocks the reactive sites to which the primary or secondary antibodies may bind. Among common blocking buffers there are normal serum, nonfat dry milk, BSA, or gelatin, and commercial blocking buffers.

Process:

1. Samples must be <4 mm thick.
2. Immerse directly the sample to be fixed in 10% neutral buffered formalin for 12–24 h.
3. Trim samples.
4. Embed samples in paraffin.
5. Cut 3–5 mm-thick slices with a microtome.
6. Place sections on glass slides for IHC (*see* **Note 12**).
7. Dry sections in a 55–60 °C oven for about an hour (*see* **Note 13**).
8. Stain the sections after deparaffinizing.

3.2 Antigen Retrieval Methods

The tertiary and quaternary structures of many antigens are modified by fixation with cross-linking agents, and this makes antigens undetectable by antibodies. In order to retrieve the loss of antigenicity, antigen retrieval (AR) methods are used and proteins return to their pre-fixation conformation. About 85% of antigens fixed in formalin need some type of AR to optimize the immunoreactions [7]. The request of AR depends on both the antigen examined and the antibody used.

Epitope recognition by the primary antibodies can be hampered by methylene bridges between proteins due to formaldehyde. To remove these bridges there are two methods, heat-induced epitope retrieval (HIER) and proteolytic-induced epitope retrieval (PIER).

3.2.1 Detergents in Antigen Retrieval

Detergents solubilize membrane proteins by mimicking the lipid bilayer environment, giving life mixed micelles consisting of lipids and detergents and detergent micelles containing proteins (usually one protein molecule per micelle). In IHC the more common detergents used are of nonionic type (e.g., Triton R-X 100, Tween 20, saponin, BRIJR, and Nonidet P40). These are generally added to wash buffers (e.g., 0.05% for Tween 20).

3.2.2 Enzymatic Antigen Retrieval

Protease-induced epitope retrieval (PIER) was the most commonly used antigen retrieval method before the invention of heat-based antigen retrieval methods. The PIER approach uses the enzymatic activity of pronase, pepsin, ficin, trypsin, or proteinase K to partially digest proteins to unmask the antibody epitopes, and the efficacy of using PIER depends on enzyme concentration and incubation time. In this chapter, we support the utilization of proteinase K because it is active at room temperature. The method of PIER is a digestion of protein cross-linkages introduced during formalin fixation, but this cleavage is nonspecific and so some antigens may be negatively poked by this treatment. The effect of PIER is related to the concentration and type of enzyme, incubation parameters (time, temperature, and pH), as well as to the duration of fixation.

3.2.3 Heat-Induced Epitope Retrieval

Heat-Induced Epitope Retrieval (HIER) is based on the concept that the chemical reactions between proteins and formalin may be reversed by high temperature or strong alkaline hydrolysis [8]. HIER is the most common approach to antigen retrieval, and temperature, pH, and time of incubation are very important factors that must be optimized for proper antigen unmasking without causing morphological damage. Sodium citrate (pH 6) and Tris/EDTA (pH 9) buffers are commonly used with HIER in conjunction with the heat source (microwave oven, pressure cooker, or steamer).

The grade of fixation can drastically change the response of antigens to antigen retrieval. Normally, unfixed proteins are denatured at temperatures of 70–90 °C, while such proteins do not suffer denaturation at the same temperatures when they have been fixed in formaldehyde. According to the HIER method and after dewaxing and rehydration, do not let the slides dry out at any time.

HIER in a Microwave Oven

1. Using a microwave, heat 500 mL of target retrieval solution (either citrate pH 6.0 or EDTA pH 9.0 or Tris pH 10.0) in a plastic jar that will hold the slides and a plastic beaker with 200 mL of water for 2 min at 750 W. After, remove the beaker of water.
2. Place slides in the heat buffer and cover the container loosely with its lid.
3. The solution needs to boil and so put the microwave at 750 W for 5 min.
4. Add warm water to the solution in order to obtain the original volume.

5. Repeat **steps 3** and **4** for 15–20 min.
6. After removing the container from the microwave oven, put it for 15 min in col. tap water.
7. Wash the slides in distilled water and transfer to wash buffer.

HIER in a Pressure Cooker

1. Connect the unit and place the pan into the decloaker's body.
2. Grout the pan of the decloaker (Biocare Medical) with 500 mL of deionized water and turn the unit on.
3. Put the slides into Tissue TekTM containers filled with 250 mL of target retrieval solution (either citrate pH 6.0 or EDTA pH 9.0 or Tris pH 10.0).
4. Put the containers with slides into center of pan.
5. Put the heat shield in the center of the pan.
6. Collocate the monitor steam strip on the top of the staining dish, put the lid on and secure.
7. Put the weight on the vent nozzle.
8. Push the display set and verify each of the displayed parameters.
9. Depending on the antigen, set the SP1 function (heating time) between 30 s and 5 min,
10. Push the display set button to SP1 and push start.
11. Push the start/stop button when the timer goes off.
12. The timer will sound off again when the temperature gets to 90 °C.
13. Push the start/stop button to end the program. The pressure should be 0.
14. Open the lid and let the slides to become cold for several minutes.
15. Remove the slide container and slowly wash the slides in running tap water.
16. Transfer slides to wash buffer.

HIER in a Steamer

1. Grout the bottom of steam container with water.
2. Place into a steamer basket the Tissue TekTM containers filled with 250 mL of retrieval buffer.
3. Turn steamer on and preheat the AR buffer in the Tissue TekTM containers/Coplin jars, bringing the buffer up to 95 °C.
4. When the temperature get to 95 °C, quickly place the slides in the AR buffer (get attention and do not touch it with bare hands), and increase the buffer temperature back to 95 °C.
5. After the temperature reaches 95 °C, steam for 20 min or the required time for antigen retrieval.

6. Remove the beaker with the slides from the steamer and let it cool for 20 min at room temperature.
7. Wash in tap water for 10 min.
8. Put the slides in wash buffer and continue with immunohistochemical staining.

3.3 Immunoenzyme Techniques

The final intent of any immunohistochemical method is to identify the maximum quantity of antigen with the minimal possible background. The option of method will depend on the quantity of antigen present, the level of sensitivity required, and the technical capabilities of the laboratory. The methods included in this chapter use commercial kits in an automatic stainer but it is possible to do the same procedure in manual staining.

3.3.1 Direct Methods

The manual staining follows these procedures:

1. Dewax sections in three changes of xylene or substitute, 7 min each.
2. Hydrate sections using 100% ethanol (3 min), 95% ethanol (3 min), and 70% ethanol (3 min). Rinse slides in water to adequately remove alcohol (3 min).
3. HIER or PIER at 37 °C, if needed (*see* **Note 3**).
4. Place the slides in rinse buffer for 5 min and transfer to the autostainer.
5. Block endogenous peroxidase with peroxidase and alkaline phosphatase-blocking reagent and block endogenous biotin with biotin-blocking system.
6. Rinse in wash buffer for 5 min.
7. Antigen retrieval with proteinase K at RT (if needed), 5 min.
8. Wash in rinsing buffer for 5 min.
9. Incubate sections with a serum-free nonspecific binding blocking solution for 20 min.
10. WITHOUT washing, take (blot if done manually) the fluid off the slide.
11. Incubate with primary labeled antibody for 30 min (*see* **Note 14**).
12. Wash with rinsing buffer for 5 min.
13. Incubate sections in the DAB solution for 5–10 min.
14. Rinse sections in distilled water for 5 min.
15. Counterstain with Mayer's hematoxylin for 30 s.
16. Rinse sections in distilled water. Blue sections using diluted ammonium hydroxide solution.

17. Dehydrate using water (3 min), 70% ethanol (3 min), 95% ethanol (3 min), 100% ethanol (3 min), and xylene or substitute (two changes, 7 min).
18. Mount in a synthetic mounting medium.

3.3.2 Indirect Methods

Two-Step Method

1. Follow **steps 1–12** as in Subheading 3.3.1.
2. Incubate with labeled secondary antibody for 30 min.
3. Follow **steps 11–17** as in Subheading 3.3.1.

Polymer-Based Immunoenzyme Method

In this method, an inert backbone of polymer (e.g., dextran), which bounds molecules of immunoglobulin (e.g., goat anti-rabbit immunoglobulins) recognizing the primary antibody (in this case, rabbit immunoglobulins), is labeled with many molecules (e.g., peroxidase). The advantages of this method are that it is more sensitive than the indirect method and also the presence of the lack of avidin or biotin molecules involved in the reaction and therefore the lack of endogenous avidin–biotin activity (EABA) background. There is also a second generation of polymer-based immunoenzyme methods which uses a second (link) unlabeled antibody between the primary and the polymer incubations. This method is more sensitive than the one-step polymer-based method.

1. Follow **steps 1–12** as in Subheading 3.3.1.
2. Incubate with polymer–immunoglobulin–enzyme complex for 30 min.
3. Follow **steps 12–18** as in Subheading 3.3.1.

3.3.3 Multiple-Step Methods

This method is based on the high affinity of avidin (glycoprotein found in egg white) or streptavidin (glycoprotein from *Streptomyces avidinii*) for biotin (glycoprotein present in egg yolk). Furthermore, thanks to its lack of oligosaccharide residues and its neutral isoelectric point, streptavidin produces less background. Multiple-step methods are more sensitive but also more laborious than indirect methods; moreover, avidin–biotin methods are currently the most widely used IHC methods.

Streptavidin–Biotin Complex (ABC) Method

1. Follow **steps 1–11** as in Subheading 3.3.1.
2. Incubate for 30 min with biotinylated secondary antibody.
3. Wash with wash buffer three times.
4. Incubate for 30 min with tertiary reagent (preformed avidin/streptavidinperoxidase complex).
5. Follow **steps 11–17** as in Subheading 3.3.1.

Tyramide-Based Methods

Compared with a conventional ABC method, tyramide-based methods amplify the immune reaction 100–1000 fold;

furthermore, also the dilution of the primary antibody can be enhanced several hundredfold.

In these methods, there is the deposition of molecules of labeled (biotin, fluorescein) tyramide followed by a secondary reaction with peroxidase conjugated to streptavidin- or peroxidase-conjugated anti-fluorescein.

1. Follow **steps 1–11** as in Subheading 3.3.1.
2. Incubate with F(ab′)2 biotinylated secondary antibody (avidin–biotin method) or peroxidase–IgG secondary antibody (fluorescein method) for 15 min.
3. Wash with wash buffer three times.
4. Incubate with primary peroxidase–streptavidin–biotin complex (avidin–biotin method) or fluorescyl-tyramide amplification reagent (fluorescein method), 15 min.
5. Wash with wash buffer three times.
6. Incubate with biotinyl–tyramide amplification reagent (avidin–biotin method), 15 min or anti-fluorescein-peroxidase (fluorescein method), 15 min.
7. Wash with wash buffer three times.
8. Incubate with peroxidase–streptavidin complex (avidin–biotin method), 15 min.
9. Follow **steps 11–17** as in Subheading 3.3.1. For the fluorescein method, follow **steps 12–17** as in Subheading 3.3.1.

3.4 Immunohistochemical Detection of Multiple Antigens

In commerce there are detection kits that allow the detection of at two or more antigens using two different enzymes as labels (e.g., peroxidase and alkaline phosphatase). These detection kits are highly effective but also very expensive. The quality of the detection of antigens depends on their location (different or same tissues, cells, or cellular compartments). A accurate selection of the chromogen for each antigen is also necessary to achieve the best distinction between antigens. The possibility of good visualization of both antigens is reduced if they are anatomically close to each other (e.g., both antigens are within the nucleus or the cytoplasm of the same cell type). Double immunodetection is complicated by the variety of AR methods used for different antigens, in other words, an AR necessary for one antigen might have deleterious effects for the second antigen to be detected. For a comprehensive review of multiple immunostaining, read van der Loos' monograph [9] on multiple immunoenzymatic staining. The method included can be used for primary antibodies from same or different species.

3.4.1 Sequential Double Immunoenzymatic Staining Using Primary Antibodies from Same or Different Species (Modified from Van der Loos) [9] (See **Note 15**)

1. Refer to **steps 1–11** as in Subheading 3.3.1.
2. Incubate with ENVISION™/peroxidase reagent for 30 min.
3. Rinse with wash buffer three times.
4. Incubate sections in the DAB solution for 5 min.
5. Elution step with DAKO double staining block or alternatively for 5 min boiling in citrate pH 6.0.
6. Rinse with wash buffer three times.
7. Incubate samples with the nonspecific binding blocking solution for 10 min.
8. WITHOUT rinsing, blow (blot if done manually) the fluid of the slide.
9. Incubate with second unlabeled antibody for 30 or 90 min in based to type of antibody in use.
10. Rinse with wash buffer three times.
11. Incubate with ENVISION™/alkaline phosphatase reagent for 30 min.
12. Rinse with wash buffer three times.
13. Develop alkaline phosphatase activity with Fast Red, 5–30 min.
14. Rinse with distilled water.
15. Counterstain with Mayer's hematoxylin.
16. Mount in aqueous mounting medium.

3.4.2 Standardization of a New Immunohistochemical Test

Many factors influence the result of a new IHC testing, therefore, its standardization is a laborious process. Usually, commercial antibodies are tested in human tissues and rarely in other species. In order to determine the suitability of antibody for a particular species, as well as the IHC detection of a particular antigen in frozen sections and/or western blot, it is essential to have information from the manufacturer of the antibody. However, often the researcher is forced to develop a standard protocol for testing new antibodies, because this information is not available.

The following protocol considers that the tissues were fixed in formalin and embedded in paraffin.

1. Select the fabric that can be used as a positive control. Theoretically, it should have areas known to lack the antigen of interest.
2. Processing (for example, fixation, embedding) of the control and the test tissues must be done in the same way. Furthermore, the control tissue should be of the same species as the test tissues, and, if present, we can take an additional control tissue from a species known to react with the antibody.
3. Prepare dilutions of the primary antibody.

4. Put on three sets of slides: one without AR; another with enzymatic AR (e.g., proteinase K); the third set of slides with heat-induced epitope retrieval (HIER) with citrate buffer at pH 6.0.
5. Follow a standard procedure for the IHC test. Incubation of the primary antibody (time, temperature) will depend on the antigen in question, generally 1 h.
6. After the IHC test is done, examine the slides to determine staining quality and the test result (*see* **Note 16**).

3.4.3 Troubleshooting

Excessive Background Staining

1. Pre-staining problems.
   (a) Insufficient fixation, necrosis, and autolysis.
   (b) Tissue sections allowed to dry out. Then, reduce incubation time and/or incubate in a humidified chamber.
   (c) If sections are not completely deparaffinized, use fresh dewaxing solutions.
   (d) Slide adhesive inappropriate or too thick. Make use of adhesives specific for IHC or positive charged slides.
   (e) Tissue section too thick, then prepare thinner sections.
   (f) Inappropriate antigen retrieval used, then upgrade antigen retrieval conditions.
   (g) Incubation temperature too elevated, then reduce temperature.
2. Blocking problems
   (a) If endogenous enzyme activity is not suppressed, increase concentration of blocking agent.
   (b) Inappropriate protein blocking. Change blocking agent.
   (c) Inappropriate blocking of endogenous avidin-binding activity. Employ an avidin–biotin blocking step or use a nonavidin-biotin detection method.
   (d) Inappropriate blocking of endogenous biotin. Employ an avidin– biotin blocking step or a nonavidin–biotin detection method.
   (e) Blocking serum not from same species. Employ blocking serum from same species as the link (secondary) antibody.
3. Primary antibody problems
   (a) Primary antibody too concentrated, then dilute the primary antibody.
   (b) Primary antibody incubation time too long, then decrease incubation time.
   (c) If primary antibody is from a similar or identical species as the test tissue (mouse on mouse, rat on mouse, etc.), use specific protocols or additional blocking steps.

   (d) Insufficient buffer washes (inappropriate buffer ion concentration), then change ionic strength of the buffer solution.
4. Secondary antibody problems
   (a) Secondary antibody and label concentration too high.
   (b) Secondary antibody and label incubation time too long.
   (c) Buffer washes inadequate.
   (d) Secondary antibody identifies endogenous (tissue) immunoglobulins.
5. Chromogen and counterstains problems
   (a) Chromogen concentration too elevated. Decrease concentration of chromogen.
   (b) Chromogen allowed to react too long, then decrease incubation time with chromogen.
   (c) Buffer washes are inadequate. Extend buffer washes.
   (d) Counterstain hides the IHC reaction. Use another type of counterstain that does not interfere with the immunohistochemical staining.

Inadequate or No Staining of the Test Slide and Adequate Staining of the Positive Control Slide

1. The test tissue does not present the antigen in question.
2. The antigen is present in the test tissue in a very low concentration. Use an amplification procedure, or increase the primary antibody concentration, incubation time or temperature, or a combination thereof.
3. There is an over- or under-fixation of the test tissue. Change antigen retrieval protocol.
4. If the test tissue is from a different species than the control tissue, it has different reactivity with the primary antibody. Then, validate the IHC test with same species control and test tissues.

Weak or No Staining of Positive Control and Weak or No Staining of Test Slides

1. If all slides from some of the primary antibodies used in the run are affected, control inadequacy of the primary antibody, method incompatibility, primary and link antibody incompatibility, or inadequate antigen retrieval.
2. If the whole run has a negative result, control assay log, adequacy of reagent volumes, and sequence of reagent delivery to the slide. Assess whether the reagents have been passed on all slides (e.g., buffer, chromogen).
3. If it is hit-and-miss throughout the run, there are technical problems or problems with the tissues. Control inadequate sequence of reagents, unbalanced autostainer, and inadequate drop zone.

No Staining of Positive Control Slide and Adequate Staining of the Test Slide

1. Review the checklist if there is a technical error in the staining or handling of the positive control slide, and repeat the assay if everything is in order.
2. Tissue photo-oxidation and dehydration during prolonged storage of tissue control sections can lead to tissue section aging [10–13]. Use a known positive case to test the tissue control section by IHC.

4 Notes

1. TBS working solution at room temperature survives 4 days and at 4 °C it is 7 days.
2. Sodium azide inhibits enzyme activity of the enzyme-labeled reagents. Then, do not mix.
3. When using heat-induced epitope retrieval (antigen retrieval), employ the target retrieval solution more appropriate to detect that particular antigen of the three included in Materials.
4. The incubation time is related to the amount of antigen; in fact, background increases with longer incubation time.
5. Disposal of DAB. DAB (3,3′-diaminobenzidine) is a commonly used chromogen for immunohistochemical staining. In the presence of a peroxidase enzyme, DAB, in correspondence of the antigen-antibody complex, will produce a brown precipitate that is insoluble in alcohol. The working solution should be prepared before use: add 2 μL of DAB in 100 μL of DAB substrate. The main drawback of DAB is that it is irritating and considered potential carcinogen. Handle with care and add several drops of sodium hypochlorite to inactivate it. As it is photosensitive, handle and store in the dark. The solution will turn black (due to oxidation of DAB) and can be washed down.
6. In order to highlight the precipitates of the DAB-peroxidase reaction, we use Mayer's hematoxylin as a counterstain.
7. Pretreatment of the sections for antigen retrieval can follow or anticipate the endogenous peroxidase blocking step.
8. This treatment can damage same antigens, in particular those in the cytoplasmic membrane, and for this reason it should be done after the incubation with the primary antibody.
9. A solution of bovine serum albumin (BSA) or normal serum can be used too.
10. Add this solution before the incubation with the biotinylated antibody [14].
11. Other fixatives. Many of the formalin substitutes are coagulating fixatives that precipitate proteins by breaking hydrogen

bonds in the absence of protein crosslinking, and the typical non-crosslinking fixative is ethanol. Other fixatives employed in IHC are glyoxal (dialdehyde), a mixture of glyoxal and alcohol, 4% paraformaldehyde (PFA), and zinc formalin.

12. Other slide adhesives can be used (e.g., poly-l-lysine).
13. Do not use temperatures above 60 °C, because this may destroy antigenity [15].
14. As necessary, incubation duration and incubation temperature (e.g., 37 °C, 4 °C) can be modified.
15. In this method an elution or blocking step between the primary and second immune reactions is needed. There are kits based on polymer-based technology (e.g., ENVISION™). The concentrations of the primary antibodies should be at least double concentrated to those used in separate IHC methods. For sequential double immunostaining, peroxidase activity using DAB as chromogen must be developed first [16]. It is very important to choose the right color combination, which will depend greatly on the amount of antigen and its location in the tissue section, because the counterstain should not mask the color of the immune reaction.
16. At the end of this procedure and depending on the results achieved, you need to obtain the best signal-to-noise ratio or to modify the experimental conditions (such as the concentration of the primary antibody, incubation and temperature time and antigen retrieval procedures).

5 Pitfalls in TMA Use to Detect CSCs by IHC

IHC is often used to study markers expression on TMA sections. TMA is a paraffin block in which several tissue cores are assembled in an array fashion with the aim of putting in place multiplex histological analysis. Cantile et al. [17] performed IHC analysis on breast and lung cancer TMAs in order to assess the expression of CSCs markers, specifically CD133, ALDH1, and CD44. The comparison of the results on TMA with single/whole sections of the same samples demonstrated that TMA is an inadequate technique for the detection of CSCs. A high heterogeneous of CSCs within tumor area could explain the unsuitability of TMA. Finally, the use of whole section is recommended for the detection of CSCs through IHC.

References

1. Clarke MF, Dick JE, Dirks PB et al (2006) Cancer stem cells-perspectives on current status and future directions: AACR workshop on cancer stem cells. Cancer Res 66:9339–9344
2. Krause M, Dubrovska A, Linge A, Baumann M (2016) Cancer stem cells: radioresistance, prediction of radiotherapy out come and specific targets for combined treatments. Adv Drug Deliv Rev 109:63–73
3. Vinogradov S, Wei X (2012) Cancer stem cells and drug resistance: the potential of nanomedicine. Nanomedicine (Lond) 7:597–615. doi:10.2217/nnm.12.22
4. Baumann M, Krause M, Thames H et al (2009) Cancer stem cells and radiotherapy. Int J Radiat Biol 85:391–402
5. Baumann M, Krause M, Hill R (2008) Exploring the role of cancer stem cells in radioresistance. Nat Rev Cancer 8:545–554
6. Cancer Stem Cell Markers. Available: https://www.rndsystems.com/research-area/cancer-stem-cell-markers
7. Ramos-Vara JA, Beissenherz ME (2000) Optimization of immunohistochemical methods using two different antigen retriva methods on formalin-fixed, paraffin-embedded tissues: experience with 63 markers. J Vet Diagn Investig 12:307–311
8. Ramos-Vara JA (2005) Technical aspects of immunohistochemistry. Vet Pathol 42:405–426
9. Van der Loos CM (1999) Immunoenzyme multiple staining methods. Bios Scientific Publishers, Oxford, UK
10. Atkins D, Reiffen KA, Tegtmeier CL et al (2004) Immunohistochemical detection of EGFR in paraffin-embedded tumor tissues: variation in staining intensity due to choice of fixative and storage time of tissue sections. J Histochem Cytochem 52:893–901
11. Fergenbaum JH, Gracia-Closas M, Hewitt SM et al (2004) Loss of antigenicity in stored sections of breast cancer tissue microarrays. Cancer Epidemiol Biomark Prev 13:667–672
12. Mirlacher M, Kasper M, Storz M et al (2004) Influence of slide aging on results of translational research studies using immunohistochemistry. Mod Pathol 17:1414–1420
13. Blind C, Koepenik A, Pacyna-Gengelbach M et al (2008) Antigenicity testing by immunohistochemistry after tissue oxidation. J Clin Pathol 61:79–83
14. Wood GS, Warnke R (1981) Suppression of endogenous avidin-binding activity in tissues and its relevance to biotinavidin detection systems. J Histochem Cytochem 29:1196–1204
15. Henwood AF (2005) Effect of slide drying at 80°C on immunohistochemistry. J Histotechnol 28:45–46
16. Malik NJ, Daymon ME (1982) Improved double immunoenzyme labeling using alkaline phosphatase and horseradish peroxidase. J Clin Pathol 35:1092–1094
17. Cantile M, Collina F, Scognamiglio G et al (2013) Inadequacy of tissue microarrays for the immunohistochemical detection of cncer stem cells in solid tumors: a viewpoint. Expert Rev Anticancer Ther 13:1139–1141

Chapter 18

Circulating Tumor Cells

Sebastián A. García, Jürgen Weitz, and Sebastian Schölch

Abstract

In most solid tumors, it is distant metastases rather than the primary tumor which limit the prognosis. Distant metastases are caused by circulating tumor cells (CTCs) which actively invade the blood stream, attach to the endothelium in the target organ, invade the surrounding parenchyma, and form new tumors. Among many other capabilities such as migration or immune escape, CTCs require tumor-forming capacities and can therefore be considered stem cell-like cells. This chapter describes the enrichment and isolation of live CTCs from clinical blood samples for molecular characterization and other downstream applications.

Key words Circulating tumor cells, Distant metastases, EpCAM

1 Introduction

While many primary tumors (e.g., colorectal cancer) can be controlled locally by surgery and/or irradiation, distant metastases are difficult to treat and lead to the death of the patient in most cases [1–3]. Hematogeneous metastases are the result of tumor cell shedding into the blood stream [4]. The resulting circulating tumor cells (CTCs) are therefore the molecular basis of metastasis and define the fate of the majority of cancer patients [5].

The frequency and number of CTCs vary strongly between tumor entities; while many gastrointestinal tumors such as colorectal cancer (CRC) shed only few CTCs [6–8], other entities such as breast or prostate cancer produce CTCs in large numbers [9, 10]. This variable availability of CTCs for molecular analysis results in a highly heterogeneous body of knowledge about the molecular biology of CTCs across different tumor entities. However, by simple observation, two universal facts about CTCs can be deducted:

Firstly, as distant lesions do occur as a result of hematogeneous tumor cell dissemination, *CTCs must have tumor initiating capacities and hence stem cell characteristics.*

Gianpaolo Papaccio and Vincenzo Desiderio (eds.), *Cancer Stem Cells: Methods and Protocols*, Methods in Molecular Biology, vol. 1692, DOI 10.1007/978-1-4939-7401-6_18, © Springer Science+Business Media LLC 2018

Secondly, not every CTC is tumorigenic. Solid tumors shed thousands to millions of tumor cells into circulation every day [11]. Even in highly disseminated situations, the number of distant lesions rarely exceeds a few hundreds in a single patient; therefore, *not every CTC leads to a metastasis.*

The clinical relevance of CTCs is therefore defined by a stem cell-like subgroup of CTCs which is able to form distant metastases. However, this subgroup of CTCs is ill-defined and its molecular characteristics are largely unknown due to the limited number of CTCs available for molecular analyses in many tumor entities [5]. CTCs are usually found at concentrations of a single CTC among millions of blood cells. As a consequence, the isolation of CTCs is most frequently performed by a combination of enrichment, identification, and isolation techniques. Isolation criteria to differentiate CTCs from normal blood cells can be subsumed under physical (e.g., size, density, deformability) and biological characteristics (surface protein expression, intracellular protein expression, migration capacities) [12].

In order to further study the biology of CTCs from epithelial tumors, we have developed a protocol for the enrichment, isolation, and characterization of CTCs from patients [13] and mouse models [14, 15] of colorectal cancer in order to enable molecular studies of this rare cell population. We use a density gradient centrifugation protocol to enrich the mononuclear cell fraction from human or murine blood samples, followed by an immunofluorescence staining for EpCAM, the most frequently expressed surface protein on epithelial CTCs [9]. The CTCs are then isolated with a micromanipulator and can be used for virtually all downstream analyses including expression profiling or culture.

2 Materials

1. EDTA tubes.
2. Density gradient medium (e.g., Lymphoprep, Stemcell Technologies #07801).
3. 50 mL tubes for density gradient centrifugation (e.g., SepMate tubes, Stemcell Technologies #86450).
4. Fetal bovine serum (FBS).
5. Magnetic beads CD45 (e.g., Dynabeads Invitrogen, Thermo Fisher, Waltham, USA).
6. Magnet rack Dynal MPC®-S (2 mL) and Dynal MPC®-L (15 mL) (Thermo Fisher Scientific, Waltham, USA) or equivalent.
7. EpCAM antibody (e.g., BioLegend #324209).

8. Beads buffer (50 mL PBS + 400 μL EDTA 0.25 M (final EDTA concentration 2 mM) + 50 μL Human AB-Serum). Store it at 4 ° C.
9. Picking buffer (45 mL PBS + 400 μL EDTA 0.25 M (final EDTA concentration 2 mM) + 5 mL FBS + 500 μL 1% Penicillin/Streptomycin. Store it at 4 ° C.
10. Petri dish ø 60 × 15 mm, 21 cm^2 or μ-Dish 35 mm dish, high Glass Bottom (ibidi, München, Germany).
11. Microelectrode Puller (e.g., DMZ Universal, Zeitz-Instruments, Martinsried, Germany).
12. Borosilicate glass capillaries, ends cut.
13. Fluorescence Microscope (e.g., Leica DMI3000B, Leica Microsystems, Wetzlar, Germany).
14. Micromanipulator (e.g., TransferMan NK 2, Eppendorf, Hamburg, Germany).
15. Microinjectors (e.g., CellTram Air, Eppendorf, Hamburg, Germany).

3 Methods

3.1 Circulating Tumor Cell (CTC) Enrichment (See Note 1)

1. Collect blood samples into EDTA tubes (8–10 mL).
2. Pour blood samples (max. 25 mL blood) into a 50 mL tube, add PBS in equal parts.
3. Mix gently by inverting the tube several times (*see* **Note 2**).
4. Pre-fill SepMate tubes with 15 mL Lymphoprep.
5. Carefully pipette the diluted blood sample onto the wall of a 50 mL SepMate tube, holding the tube with an inclination of ~45° degrees, avoiding to mix both solutions (max. 25 mL blood-PBS mix per 50 mL SepMate tube) (*see* **Note 3**).
6. Centrifuge at room temperature for 30 min at 300 × *g* without brake (*see* **Note 4**).
7. Carefully discard the upper 10 mL supernatant with a pipette.
8. Pour the rest into a new 50 mL tube (Lymphoprep medium and erythrocytes must remain under the insert of the SepMate tube).
9. Fill the new 50 mL tube with PBS to a final volume of 40–50 mL.
10. Centrifuge at room temperature for 15 min at 300 × *g* with brake.
11. Discard the supernatant and resuspend the cell pellet with 500 μL beads buffer and leave the tube on ice (*see* **Note 3**).

3.2 CD45 Depletion

12. Resuspend Dynabeads CD45 by pipetting up and down.
13. Pipette 200 μL Dynabeads per 10 mL blood (pre-enrichment volume) into a 2 mL microcentrifuge tube (i.e., use 300 mL Dynabeads for 15 mL whole blood).
14. Insert the tube into the magnet rack, wait for 1 min, and discard the supernatant.
15. Remove the 2 mL tube from the rack and resuspend the beads with 1 mL beads buffer.
16. Reinsert the 2 mL tube into the magnet rack, wait for 1 min, and discard the supernatant.
17. Resuspend the beads with 500 μL bead's buffer and leave the tube on ice.
18. Mix the cell suspension from Subheading 3.1, **step 11** with the beads suspension in a 2 mL microcentrifuge tube. Use another 500 μL beads buffer to wash the 50 mL tube and add them to the beads.
19. Incubate the 2 mL microcentrifuge tube at 4 °C on a roller-mixer (rotator) for 20 min.
20. Fill a 15 mL tube with 6 mL beads buffer and insert it into the magnetic rack.
21. Add the solution of cells and beads into the 15 mL tube. Wash the 2 mL tube and the cap with 1 mL beads buffer and add it into the 15 mL Falcon tube.
22. Wait for 1 min to let the beads attach to the wall of the tube.
23. Pipette the supernatant into a new 15 mL tube, discard the other tube.
24. Centrifuge at room temperature for 5 min at 300 × *g* with brake.
25. Remove the supernatant without disturbing the cell pellet.
26. Resuspend the cell pellet with 200 μL beads buffer.
27. Pipet the cell suspension into a new 1.5 mL microcentrifuge tube and leave it on ice.

3.3 EpCAM Staining

28. Add 4 μL of EpCAM antibody into the suspension (*see* **Note 5**).
29. Vortex the microcentrifuge tube for a couple of seconds and incubate it on ice for 20 min, protected from light (cover the microcentrifuge tube with aluminum foil).

3.4 Screening for CTC

30. Draw a ~1 cm circle in a 6 cm sterile petri dish using a PAP pen to keep the cell suspension from dispersing or use a μ-Dish 35 mm, high Glass Bottom. Add 20–40 μL cell suspension onto one of them.

31. Add 400 μL picking buffer onto the petri dish, mix both solutions by pipetting.
32. Put the petri dish under the microscope (*see* **Note 6**) and leave it for 5 min to allow the cells to settle down.
33. Start the screening using a 10× magnification objective and the appropriate fluorescence filter.
34. Systematically go over the whole petri dish leaving no parts without screening.
35. EpCAM-positive cells (CTCs) should exhibit membrane-bound green fluorescence (*see* **Note 7**).

3.5 Cell Picking

36. Use a puller to manufacture capillaries appropriate for picking according to the manufacturer's instructions.
37. Insert a new capillary into the micromanipulator.
38. Using the joystick, move the tip of the capillary over the surface of the petri dish.
39. Use the Air pump to expel cells and buffer from the capillary, leaving a small volume of buffer in the tip of the capillary.
40. Move the capillary tip close to the cell of interest.
41. Carefully use the air pump to aspirate buffer and let the cell smoothly move into the capillary, then immediately stop the aspiration process.
42. Observe the cell for a couple of seconds to verify that it does not move anymore. This indicates that the system is well sealed. Capillaries are sometime not well adjusted and cells can be lost due to an air leakage.
43. Remove the capillary from the petri dish.
44. Turn the micromanipulator to the right and insert the tip of the capillary into the desired solution (min recommendable 10 μL).
45. Expel the contents of the capillary using the air pump; the appearance of air bubbles in the solution indicates complete evacuation of the capillary.
46. Remove the tip from the solution and put the microcentrifuge tube on ice.
47. Perform the intended downstream analysis with the isolated CTC.

4 Notes

1. Verify if all reagents and materials are available. Try to work quickly. If a break is needed, samples should be left on ice.

2. When blood samples are mixed with clots inside, it is recommended to filter the blood samples through cell strainers (100 μm). Clots can block the small holes of the SepMate tubes' inserts and interfere with the density separation.
3. When the mixture of whole blood and PBS exceed 25 mL, samples should be split in separate SepMate tubes. Cell pellets from Subheading 3.1, **step 11** can be pooled in one 2 mL tube.
4. If after a centrifugation step no clear pellet is seen, the tube can be centrifuged for another 5–10 min at 300 × *g* with brake.
5. After staining, samples should be kept on ice and protected from the light at all times.
6. Once an aliquot of the cell suspension is pipetted onto the petri dish and mixed with picking buffer, the cell density must be adjusted for an optimal CTC screening. To do this, visually check the sample under the microscope and verify if the density is not too high to identify single cells. If the sample is too concentrated, dilute it with another 400 μL picking buffer and split it into two different petri dishes. Repeat this step until the density is appropriate for single cell picking.
7. During the screening process, you may encounter cells that are false positive. EpCAM-positive cells display normally a brighter border and a lesser intense center (membrane-bound staining, cf. Fig. 1). In addition, fluorescence should be observed only through the appropriate filter (e.g., green if using Alexa-fluor488). If the cell is fluorescent in other channels (i.e., TRITC) as well, the signal should be considered unspecific due to autofluorescence.

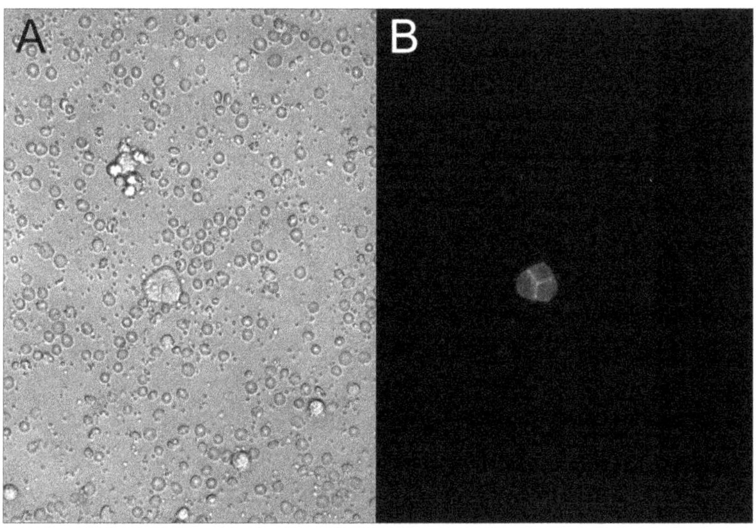

Fig. 1 A triplet of colorectal cancer-derived CTCs in a patient with metatatic disease. (**a**) bright field. (**b**) Anti-EpCAM-Alexa488. Note the membrane-bound EpCAM expression

References

1. Siegel RL, Miller KD, Jemal A (2016) Cancer statistics, 2016. CA Cancer J Clin 66:7–30
2. Steinert G, Schölch S, Koch M et al (2012) Biology and significance of circulating and disseminated tumour cells in colorectal cancer. Langenbecks Arch Surg 397:535–542
3. Weitz J, Koch M, Debus J et al (2005) Colorectal cancer. Lancet 365:153–165
4. Pantel K, Alix-Panabières C, Riethdorf S (2009) Cancer micrometastases. Nat Rev Clin Oncol 6:339–351
5. Schölch S, Bork U, Rahbari NN et al (2014) Circulating tumor cells of colorectal cancer. Cancer Cell Microenviron 1:10–14800
6. Rahbari NN, Bork U, Kircher A et al (2012) Compartmental differences of circulating tumor cells in colorectal cancer. Ann Surg Oncol 19:2195–2202
7. Rahbari NN, Aigner M, Thorlund K et al (2010) Meta-analysis shows that detection of circulating tumor cells indicates poor prognosis in patients with colorectal cancer. Gastroenterology 138:1714–1726
8. Bork U, Rahbari NN, Schölch S et al (2015) Circulating tumour cells and outcome in non-metastatic colorectal cancer: a prospective study. Br J Cancer 112:1306–1313
9. Allard WJ, Matera J, Miller MC et al (2004) Tumor cells circulate in the peripheral blood of all major carcinomas but not in healthy subjects or patients with nonmalignant diseases. Clin Cancer Res 10:6897–6904
10. Miller MC, Doyle GV, Terstappen LWMM (2010) Significance of circulating tumor cells detected by the CellSearch system in patients with metastatic breast colorectal and prostate cancer. J Oncol 2010:617421
11. Chang YS, di Tomaso E, McDonald DM et al (2000) Mosaic blood vessels in tumors: frequency of cancer cells in contact with flowing blood. Proc Natl Acad Sci U S A 97:14608–14613
12. Alix-Panabières C, Pantel K (2014) Technologies for detection of circulating tumor cells: facts and vision. Lab Chip 14:57–62
13. Steinert G, Schölch S, Niemietz T et al (2014) Immune escape and survival mechanisms in circulating tumor cells of colorectal cancer. Cancer Res 74:1694–1704
14. Schölch S, García SA, Iwata N et al (2016) Circulating tumor cells exhibit stem cell characteristics in an orthotopic mouse model of colorectal cancer. Oncotarget 7:27232–27242
15. van Noort V, Schölch S, Iskar M et al (2014) Novel drug candidates for the treatment of metastatic colorectal cancer through global inverse gene-expression profiling. Cancer Res 74:5690–5699

Erratum to: Introduction to Cancer Stem Cells: Past, Present, and Future

David Bakhshinyan, Ashley A. Adile, Maleeha A. Qazi, Mohini Singh, Michelle M. Kameda-Smith, Nick Yelle, Chirayu Chokshi, Chitra Venugopal, and Sheila K. Singh

Erratum to:
Chapter 1 in: Gianpaolo Papaccio and Vincenzo Desiderio (eds.),
Cancer Stem Cells: Methods and Protocols,
Methods in Molecular Biology, vol. 1692,
DOI 10.1007/978-1-4939-7401-6

Sheila K. Singh, one of the authors of Chapter 1, had the letters of her name transposed in the original published version of the chapter. Her name has been corrected in the current version of the volume.

The online version of the updated original book can be found at
https://dx.doi.org/10.1007/978-1-4939-7401-6_1

Gianpaolo Papaccio and Vincenzo Desiderio (eds.), *Cancer Stem Cells: Methods and Protocols*, Methods in Molecular Biology, vol. 1692, DOI 10.1007/978-1-4939-7401-6_19, © Springer Science+Business Media LLC 2018

Index

A

B

C

D

E

Gianpaolo Papaccio and Vincenzo Desiderio (eds.), *Cancer Stem Cells: Methods and Protocols*, Methods in Molecular Biology, vol. 1692, DOI 10.1007/978-1-4939-7401-6, © Springer Science+Business Media LLC 2018

Lightning Source UK Ltd.
Milton Keynes UK
UKHW05n1139200918
329223UK00006B/94/P

9 781493 974009